Drawing the Line

Drawing the Line

*Healthcare Rationing and
the Cutoff Problem*

Philip M. Rosoff

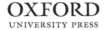
OXFORD
UNIVERSITY PRESS

OXFORD
UNIVERSITY PRESS

Oxford University Press is a department of the University of Oxford. It furthers
the University's objective of excellence in research, scholarship, and education
by publishing worldwide. Oxford is a registered trade mark of Oxford University
Press in the UK and certain other countries.

Published in the United States of America by Oxford University Press
198 Madison Avenue, New York, NY 10016, United States of America.

Library of Congress Cataloging-in-Publication Data
Names: Rosoff, Philip M., author.
Title: Drawing the line: healthcare rationing and the cutoff problem /
Philip M. Rosoff.
Other titles: Healthcare rationing and the cutoff problem
Description: New York, NY: Oxford University Press, [2017] | Includes
bibliographical references and index.
Identifiers: LCCN 2016013207 | ISBN 9780190206567 (hardcover: alk. paper)
Subjects: | MESH: Health Care Rationing | Health Care Costs | Consensus |
United States
Classification: LCC RA410.5 | NLM WA 540 AA1 | DDC 362.1068/1—dc23 LC record
available at http://lccn.loc.gov/2016013207

1 3 5 7 9 8 6 4 2

Printed by Sheridan Books, Inc., United States of America

TO DONA

CONTENTS

PREFACE

On March 23, 2010, President Barack Obama signed the Affordable Care Act (ACA) into law after the US Congress passed it by the slimmest of margins. It has been hailed as the central domestic accomplishment of his presidency. Its many provisions to expand access to health insurance, both public and private, increase benefits available to those with policies and eliminate discrimination against those individuals with "pre-existing" conditions have undoubtedly led to decreased misery and suffering due to both disease and poverty. At the same time it has come under constant legal and political attack, including two challenges that resulted in Supreme Court decisions (upholding most of the law). The first, in 2012, *National Federation of Independent Business v. Sibelius*, eliminated the national statewide requirement for the increase of the Medicaid program by expanding eligibility.[1] The second, *King v. Burwell,* in 2015, upheld the remaining parts of the law.[2] Unlike the doomed attempt at comprehensive healthcare reform from the early 1990s during the early years of the Clinton Administration,[3] it appears as if the ACA is here to stay, the only caveat being that it is conceivable that a future Congress could vote to repeal the law.

The United States remains the only advanced, industrialized nation on earth without comprehensive, universal healthcare coverage for its population when it can readily afford to do so. The story of the repeated efforts to bring comprehensive healthcare coverage to most, if not all, Americans through either public or private funding (or, more commonly, a hybrid of the two) is both complex and, in many ways, quite sad.[4] The saga of the numerous failed attempts to bring the fruits of the truly impressive gains in medical knowledge and their consequent improvements in diagnosis and treatment is one of constant hope met with regular defeat. Unlike other wealthy, industrialized nations, the United States stands alone in not guaranteeing access to high-quality, affordable healthcare to all of its people. The reasons are many and tortuous, but clearly represent a mix of the cultural, historical, and political. It would be simplistic to lay blame at the doorstep of any one group or individual as this is a case of collective responsibility. It is probably not too much of a stretch to say that we have evolved to the current state of affairs. Retrospective analysis demonstrates many missed and failed opportunities to change the course of events and create a system more in step with other wealthy democracies.[5] Even the existence of employer-funded insurance that formed the basis for most private insurance after World War II was due to the exigencies of wartime labor shortages and wage and price controls.[6] And the creation of Medicare and Medicaid as government-funded programs to bring healthcare to the elderly and the (very) poor was an extraordinarily difficult birth.[7] While the ACA undoubtedly represents a major improvement on the existing patchwork and porous "system" (I use this term cautiously) and promises to reduce the unconscionable numbers of completely uninsured people, it is merely another program to plug some holes in an amalgam of programs that promise neither universal access nor universal care to anyone. Perhaps not surprisingly, the lack of any sort of guarantee to economical, readily accessible, and reliable healthcare to all who live in this country has consistently produced data demonstrating that the United States has dismally poor health statistics for a nation of such wealth and prosperity.[8] And many of those fortunate enough to be able to purchase subsidized insurance policies have only been able to afford to do so because the least expensive ones come with very high co-insurance costs, such a high deductibles and co-payments; this has led to a significant hardship of medical debt.[9]

At the same time, the healthcare enterprise in the United States is one of the largest "industries" in the country, annually consuming trillions of dollars.[10] While the healthcare-related inflation rate has slowed considerably over the past few years, at least partially due to the recession in 2007–09, there are some indications that the ACA may also be contributing to this phenomenon (at least in part).[11] Nevertheless, there are also worrisome signs that the growth in health costs may be starting to rise again, and the looming aging of the baby boomers has the potential to lead to explosive and long-term escalation. Numerous economic analyses have warned of the fiscal calamity that waits the country if something is not done (and soon) to halt the apparently inexorable trajectory. To buy so little at such cost seems foolish at best and ethically irresponsible at worst. The lack of comprehensive, universal, and affordable healthcare for all represents a moral hole in the social fabric of life in the United States for which various smaller programs—Medicaid, Medicare, the Veterans Administration system, assorted charities—offer only partial and insecure patches. It seems inconceivable that a modern, technologically advanced country that prides itself on its material abundance and constantly touts the opportunities available to all permits so large a breach in the social contract that leads to such avoidable suffering. It is shameful.

In my first book, I presented an argument for the rationing of healthcare that was predicated upon the creation of a universal, comprehensive, and generous healthcare system in the United States. I based my discussion on the necessity for healthcare reform on both financial and moral grounds. The first was simply an analysis of the math of how expensive our disjointed and poorly functioning healthcare system actually is and the fact that it is almost certainly going to be much more costly in the future unless major changes are made. If we keep things as they are, we would have to drastically increase what is euphemistically known as "cost-sharing," whereby the financial burden borne by patients continues to rise before the bills begin to be paid by whatever insurance plan one has. We already see this as an almost annual event with increases in co-pays, deductibles, and the like, as well as decreases in what might be covered. This phenomenon is most acutely observed with those patients new to the private insurance markets because the ACA has enabled them to buy "affordable" insurance plans. However, the Catch 22—the "small print," if you will—for the newly insured, especially those with the least expensive policies, is the enormously high annual deductible payments. Thus, while it is true that the ranks of the uninsured have shrunk, many of these people cannot afford to go to the doctor unless they judge themselves to be seriously ill due to the up-front, uninsured costs they will incur.[12] In addition, even if the ACA is successful within the legal and political boundaries that have defined its scope, there will continue to be many millions of people who will lack health insurance of any kind. They will endure as an abiding challenge as well as a constant reminder of how we fail to care for our fellow Americans who are less fortunate.

I also argued that there was a substantive moral argument to be made for comprehensive healthcare reform in the United States. Why don't we subscribe to the simple notion that modern, effective healthcare is a public good that should be available to all simply because it has the power to save lives, relieve the suffering of the sick and injured, and offer almost everyone the possibility to take advantage of the opportunities to improve their circumstances? What is so peculiar about America that distinguishes us from Great Britain, the Netherlands, France, and Germany? All of these countries have universal healthcare systems that differ greatly in how they are constructed, financed, and implemented but are united in their dedication to the proposition that healthcare is important enough to be treated as if it were a human right and one that is necessary to provide to their citizenry (and in some cases, to *all* who reside within their borders)?

I will not presume (nor is that my aim in this book) to dissect all of the various sociological, psychological, and political-historical reasons that have been offered to account for this unique position. Suffice it to say that, except for private charitable impulses, we have never been particularly disposed to systematically care for the needs of the poor and otherwise disadvantaged. We Americans have a long history of aversion to government-funded aid, except in disaster, emergency situations (and sometimes not even then, perhaps depending upon who the victims are, such as the initial response to Hurricane Katrina). We also uphold the ideal of individual effort and merit for the fruits of one's labors and the attendant notion that what we earn is due to our own unfettered achievements accomplished without the aid of "handouts." The idea of "just deserts" is one that is seemingly ingrained into the American psyche and culture, leading to the corollary view that those who haven't been successful also deserve their fate. Those less fortunate in one sphere (say, in the realm of income) also tend to have more than their "fair share" of other difficulties, including illness. But the propensity to hold people accountable for their failures also seemingly transfers to a neglect of the consequences of misfortune and disadvantage resulting in benign neglect (at best) to a form of mild to even overt contempt.[13] And, of course, the social, economic, and biological divisions of society often are reflected in similarly uneven divisions of power, which is the mechanism to effect their will on the distribution of benefits.

I suggested that to restrict access to modern, scientific, and effective medicine in the 21st century, especially on the basis of the commercialization of interventions and what they can offer to improve people's lives and opportunities to pursue their goals and aims, is to debase the very meaning of medicine and healthcare.[14] It also demeans us a nation and a people that we would deny or limit the amount of such an essential good to those who cannot afford to buy as much as they need (or want). That being said, we also cannot look at the expenses of technologically advanced healthcare as something that we must absorb unquestioningly and without scrutiny as to value and efficacy. To do so would be both short-sighted and imprudent. One thing is clear from even a cursory analysis of the post-World War II finances of American healthcare: there has been a steadily increasing amount of it available at an ever-escalating price tag. To argue that we should expand access to all without curbing what is available (and its associated costs) would be fiscal suicide and most certainly could be both unsustainable in the long term and drain needed resources from other vitally important social needs.

There are good reasons to believe that there is enormous waste and inefficiencies in the current system, and altering the ways in which business is done to rein in these excesses would undoubtedly save money. But that would do nothing to address the fundamental moral issue that we have millions of people in this country who lack access to decent, affordable, and comprehensive healthcare despite the benefits promised as part of the ACA. Even if the ACA were wildly successful (and it can't be), there will still be enormous numbers of people either without health insurance or underinsured. It can only be a poultice on the suppurating wound that is American healthcare. It is not even close to a cure. But suppose we wanted to rectify the patchwork system that has been permitted to grow, put together slowly and in fits and starts over the past 70 years?

In *Rationing Is Not a Four-Letter Word: Setting Limits on Healthcare* I argued that limiting what interventions were available in a sensible and fair way, combined with a generous and comprehensive universal single-payer healthcare system could help restrain costs and extend the benefits of decent and good medicine to everyone in this country.[15] I suggested that we should also control some of the excesses of commercialism that have led to such gross abuses of the system and that this could lead to a further lowering of costs. I also presented an outline of how limits might be drawn and discussed that the best approach might be to restrict what was available to those interventions that could be shown to be effective, thus eliminating access to unproven therapies (except within the confines of a revitalized and well-supported clinical trials enterprise) and marginally effective treatments. But I did not delve into great detail on how this could be done or offer a deeper rationale and justification for how to make these kinds of important clinical and moral judgments. The devil is most certainly in the details, and that aphorism is no more aptly applied when proposing how to rationally and fairly create cutoffs. That is what I will do in the chapters that follow.

The extended and progressive argument I will present will first focus on establishing the basis by which people may have justifiable claims to healthcare interventions if there were the financial and infrastructure means to deliver them. I will address fundamental questions such as what kinds of patients *qua* patients should be eligible for healthcare? Should some people be excluded because of who they are? Should some sorts of interventions (medicines, diagnostic tests, treatments, operations, etc.)

be off-limits no matter what? And, how can we cope with the inherent uncertainty that is pervasive in the practice of medicine and that makes determinations of outcome (and hence efficacy) probabilistic? I will begin with an introduction to the problem, both the challenges of healthcare reform and then more specifically the issues surrounding cutoff points or where to draw lines between what is and is not reasonable to offer and to whom. I will then follow with a detailed discussion of different kinds of cutoffs that have been proposed by other authors and their benefits and advantages. I will then argue that the most reasonable approach would be to focus on an expansive but justifiable definition and application of patient need for medical care, one predicated on there being beneficial and effective interventions that match the need. Finally, I will devote the latter half of the book to various objections and potential complications of my proposal. In this way, I hope to construct an argument that lays out a detailed strategy for developing and implementing a mechanism for creating cutoffs that could be tolerable, if not acceptable to most people.

ACKNOWLEDGMENTS

I would not have been able to write this book without the help and assistance of a number of people who have generously given me their counsel and criticism. My colleagues at the Trent Center for Bioethics, Humanities and History of Medicine at Duke University's School of Medicine—Jeffrey Baker, Gopal Sreenivasan, Ross McKinney, and Nikki Vangsnes—have been incredibly helpful and I am grateful for their assistance. I would also like to extend my thanks to Kevin Sowers and Lisa Pickett, respectively, President and Chief Medical Officer of Duke University Hospital who have supported me throughout this project. Professors Elizabeth DeLong and Maragatha Kuchibhatla of Duke's Department of Biostatistics and Bioinformatics offered invaluable advice and assistance in my initial research into the details of drawing cutoff points in populations that distribute their numerical descriptive characteristics continuously. I found these discussions both illuminating and somewhat disheartening as the solution remained unsatisfactory (at least mathematically!). Finally, there is little question that without the constant support and counsel of my wife, Dona Chikaraishi, I would have been unable to complete this book.

1

THE PROBLEM

Most wealthy industrialized nations accept that good health and the means to secure it are of fundamental, intrinsic importance to human welfare. They also subscribe to the idea that a central function of government is to provide the resources and services to guarantee that all who live in their countries receive some basic, decent level of healthcare (and often a great deal more). Of course, some are more generous than others, and the methods employed to finance and deliver healthcare services differ. But a common denominator is the view that good healthcare and the good health of their people is a human right and that it is a moral duty of government to ensure that this occurs. They view the provision or warrant of healthcare as a vital component of the social contract, in the same way as education, safe roads and bridges, and other measures underwritten by government on behalf of the people.

The United States is different. While we have slowly and haltingly increased the breadth of a guaranteed social safety net, we have yet to embrace the notion of universal healthcare as something that Americans deserve simply for being here and, like all people, need. Moreover, the United States commoditizes healthcare to a far greater extent than any other country from the group of advanced industrialized nations. While regulated in many ways, the American market for healthcare goods and services still belies the fact that health and the mechanisms to obtain the best state of health one can are available for purchase. These peculiar features of the American healthcare system can in part explain the extraordinary differences in health disparities that are found between those who can afford healthcare and those who cannot. Indeed, whether one is healthy or not, whether one lives longer or not is in large part related to the ability to access and take advantage of the incredible advances in modern healthcare. The fact that healthcare is for sale in the United States also explains why we all fare so poorly in comparison to other similar nations in standard measures of population health. Many in the United States subscribe to a philosophy of American exceptionalism, by which they mean that this nation is different from all others, and, as such, we do not need to play by the same rules as others.[1] By this reckoning, many scoff at the demands of an internationalist and common morality that would require that we hew to common standards of human welfare with respect to healthcare. However, what is most exceptional about American healthcare are the appalling and indefensible disparities in outcomes that are largely stratified by socioeconomic class, race, ethnicity, and where one lives (rural or urban).

The healthcare system in the United States is at a critical point in its history. Even as the enactment and implementation of the Affordable Care Act (ACA), which President Barack Obama signed into law on March 23, 2010, leads to a greater degree of equity and some cost savings in the healthcare budget outlay, it will do relatively little to stem the seemingly inexorable increase in the total costs of healthcare in this country. After a short period during the Great Recession of 2008 (and a few years following) during which medical costs slowed their rise, they have now resumed their previous move upward, still following their prior seemingly inexorable course.[2] The financial incentives that exist for doctors, hospitals, medical device and products companies, and pharmaceutical manufacturers continue to foster the development of bigger, faster, and ever more expensive devices, implants, machines, drugs, palatial buildings, and executive salaries. Drug companies are constantly bringing to market the fruits of the biotech revolution, the majority of which add enormous costs to patients' bills but only rarely pay off with comparable improvements in meaningful outcomes.[3] Physicians also persist in doing more and more "stuff"—surgeries, procedures, diagnostic tests—because reimbursement models frequently reward quantity over quality (although there may be some changes coming to this approach).[4] And, of course, we somehow continue to pay for it all (or at least most of it), the consequences of which are a greater and greater plundering of the national treasury, an increasing debt burden, and growing competition for both government and private dollars. Meanwhile, even with the ACA, we remain a nation with millions of Americans without any health insurance or who have policies with very high annual deductibles that can discourage early consultations for possibly serious medical problems.[5] By any reasonable measure of social justice, the situation has only marginally improved for some and remains significantly vulnerable to both political whimsy and financial ruin, with millions of people susceptible to insolvency or untreated illness.

Technological medicine has an insatiable maw that must be fed (as it has been), and there is no question that if we maintain the current funding model whereby healthcare and the paraphernalia and materiel required to support it are commodities (and very profitable ones at that), increasingly more expensive machines, devices, and medicines will be developed for an available and ready market.[6] It is commonly understood and accepted that something must be done to control costs, if not reduce them, or the economic consequences for the country could prove catastrophic.[7] Budgets must be trimmed somewhere, whether it is by limiting the generosity of Medicare for the nation's senior citizens, reducing access to Medicaid, or perhaps aiming at some other juicy target. But it is generally agreed that some group or groups of people will have to do without services they have previously had or would like to have. The alternative is to continue on our current course, with healthcare sucking increasingly more resources from other important projects. Rationing in one form or another must be imposed. Therefore, the vital questions will be what kind, in what context, and how will it be done?

To my knowledge, no modern society has unlimited money that it either wishes to or does spend on healthcare for its residents. This is true even in wealthy, industrialized nations, including those that have so-called socialized medical systems that offer a defined package of benefits to all their people (like France or England) from general or designated tax revenues. In the United States, it may often appear as if we have no cap on how much we are willing to devote to funding healthcare in our mixture of public and private disorganized delivery systems, but even here there is some theoretical maximum or ceiling that would prove intolerable. Rising healthcare costs and generous benefit plans (at least for some) compete with other important social programs for a share of the economy (including that funded by the government) such as national defense, education, the creation and upkeep of physical infrastructure, pension plans for the elderly and disabled, and so on. Rivers of ink (and now pixels) have been expended decrying the escalation in American healthcare costs and the fact that the current system is not sustainable in the long term. Most reasonable analysts have concluded that some form of restraint or rationing—meaning a limitation on what is available—must be imposed so as to establish some order and control. This cap could be imposed on total funding, on specific interventions (thus saving money), or on some combination. How to accomplish this effectively and fairly are the big questions. Whereas some commentators mold their discussions of controlling costs within a framework that incorporates healthcare for all, most seem to ignore the subject and concentrate on reining in the costs within a template of the existing system rather than questioning the fiscal stability and moral failure of a system that has been permitted to evolve over the past 80 years.

However, the fact remains that the United States is the sole country among the group of technologically advanced nations that has not—as a society—created a universal healthcare system that guarantees a comprehensive set of medical benefits to those who live here. The other wealthy industrialized democracies have viewed healthcare as a fundamental right and the government as a guarantor of that right and as the mechanism to fulfill it. The United States is different.

Even so, there are few people who are able to offer a comprehensive and coherent defense of the American healthcare system. This is not to say that many individuals are not satisfied with their own healthcare; indeed, many people who have good, employer-provided health insurance are in general quite pleased with the range of their benefits, even if they do sometimes grumble and complain about the increasing co-insurance costs such as co-pays, deductibles, limited preferred-provider networks, and the like. It is likely that the prevailing level of satisfaction—among those who have insurance—contributes to the prevalent antipathy to major overhauls of the system as it currently stands.[8] Not surprisingly, a significant effort in both the crafting and selling of the ACA was devoted to assuring the American public with health insurance that the only changes they might notice would be for the better, such as the ability to keep their children on their policies until the latter reached age 26, the elimination of pre-existing condition exclusions, and the like.

Nevertheless, almost everyone recognizes that something must be done to rein in the seemingly inexorable upswing in the healthcare cost curve. But how to reform healthcare is integrally related to one's political and social philosophy. The more libertarian-minded might suggest that individuals are responsible for their own welfare, and whatever benefits we offer to others less fortunate than ourselves should be done as an act of personal beneficence and charity rather than a duty compelled by government enacting a social policy.[9] Other, more communitarian types (such as myself) would argue that healthcare reform is required as a matter of social justice, not in a pure redistributive sense, but rather as a societal moral duty to provide certain necessary and vital goods to all those who cannot provide them for themselves. These goods are varied and compete for societal resources. They include public safety and national defense, roads and bridges, education for the general public, and some forms of social welfare security to avoid the most grievous harms resulting from impoverishment and penury. Due to the phenomenal success of scientific medicine over the past century, with the proven ability of both public health measures (good sanitation, clean water, etc.) and what we might call "private" or individual health interventions (antibiotics, vaccinations, advanced surgical techniques, life support technologies, organ transplantation, etc.) to directly improve (and lengthen) peoples' lives, it would be absurd to argue that 21st-century healthcare is not a social good analogous to education in the benefits that it can offer.

Why is good healthcare so important to individuals and society? This may seem a rhetorical question with an answer that is obvious, but it is worth pointing out that not everyone subscribes to the same rationale. While there are few in modern societies who shun the input of physicians when they are sick or injured, there are a disturbing number who appear to view the subject differently for others less fortunate. One compelling explanation for the singular significance to people of good healthcare is offered by Norman Daniels. He explains that decent and adequate healthcare (how much is adequate is arguable, and I will discuss this in detail in Chapter 3) can perform a crucial role in enhancing personal welfare by maximizing the ability of individuals to take advantage of the opportunities available to them to pursue and accomplish various goals in life (subject, of course, to inherent capabilities, more or less).[10] But society also benefits from the better health of its citizens because of improved productivity, less social unrest, fewer disparities in the outcomes of life associated with a healthier populace (such as less poverty), and the like. It also marks a society as caring about its citizens as opposed to indifferent to suffering due to disease and its consequences. And, unlike what some may declaim, systematic, public caring about suffering is not demeaning or debasing of personal initiative; but poor health, inadequate nutrition and deep-seated, inescapable poverty and destitution is. From good (or better) health may flow numerous secondary benefits.

Interestingly, the United States has approached the acceptance of the social and individual importance of healthcare in fits and starts and sometimes grudgingly. Despite the vociferous (and at times, vicious) objections of organized medicine (personified as the American Medical Association), we have Medicare, which warrants that people over the age of 65 years (as well as smaller populations such as the permanently disabled, those with end-stage renal disease, etc.) will be able to obtain healthcare that is either completely or mostly paid for out of tax and general government revenues. We also have established Medicaid for many indigent people (especially children), even though the benefits can vary widely between states. Thus, we have haltingly accepted the general notion that it is not unpatriotic or undemocratic or un-American to have established general welfare programs for the most vulnerable among us. Even incarcerated prisoners are guaranteed general healthcare (and sometimes considerably more) as a result of Supreme Court rulings dating back to 1976.[11] The Veterans Administration (VA) healthcare system is extensively "socialized" and, despite its flaws, is frequently admired as both comprehensive and effective, as well as accepted by patients, so there seems to be little deep-seated objection to the general idea of subsidized healthcare for all (in defined populations). But there still remain huge numbers of people who continue to be vulnerable to the fickleness of the marketplace, the caprice of employers and politicians, and the ups and downs of the economy.

But if one could be persuaded to accept that it is both in the national interest and a cardinal virtue of social justice that all should have the means to achieve the best state of health that can be reasonably attained—for both instrumental and substantive moral reasons—then there are a number of hurdles to overcome. First and foremost is the formidable political obstacles that would be arrayed against any kind of major change to the status quo. While I will mention these frequently and throughout the course of this book with suggestions on how to possibly meet some objections, my focus will be more on the methodologies used to balance the inevitable competition between fiscal responsibility and offering an array and range of benefits that would be both politically palatable and reasonable. One cannot simply write a blank check; the treasury is not limitless. Negotiating the friction between these two parts of the healthcare equation—recognizing that there are limits to what we can spend, what we want to spend, and what we should spend and the desire to provide a decent package of healthcare insurance to all—defines a large space that must be delineated. Since we cannot buy all the healthcare we can conceivably want to satisfy the needs and desires of everyone, we must draw boundaries or cutoffs. How we go about accomplishing this task is a matter of economics, medicine, and justice, all of which may make competing claims of primacy. Limiting what is available and to whom is not really the issue; indeed, we ration on a massive scale already, albeit irrationally, unfairly, and inequitably. Rather, it is how we ration that remains a puzzle, that has both fundamental moral and practical dimensions.

RATIONING

Scarcity—in this case of the amount of money that we think sensible and practicable to devote to healthcare in this country—will require an acceptance of the fact that we must say no to some people sometimes, that not everyone can get everything he or she wants, and that denying some patients some kinds or types of interventions under certain circumstances must occur. This is by no means easy medicine to swallow, especially for those who stand to lose financially and/or politically due to modifications or restrictions on whatever it is they sell or buy. Of course, there are many different ways this could be accomplished, all of which have their merits and downsides, especially when one factors in features of inclusiveness and fairness (social justice).

For instance, we could probably extract significant savings from our healthcare budget if we simply restricted who had access in a systematic way.[12] In an extreme example, we could offer (and pay for) full access to anything people could convince their doctors to prescribe or do but only to a relatively small segment of the population (say, by eliminating even emergency services to all non-citizens or permanent residents, convicted felons, etc.). Alternatively, for the same amount of money, we could be broadly inclusive in providing healthcare benefits but at the price of placing (for instance) constraints on what could be "purchased." Both approaches require tradeoffs, and which one would be more or less palatable to the people who would be funding the system (the American taxpayer) and to those affected by the decisions would be an empirical question that would need to be studied. I have previously argued that in a wealthy country like the United States with at least a recent history of moderate public fairness and inclusiveness, it would be both more politically acceptable and just to create a system closer to the latter than the former. However, I have also noted that the level of public tolerance for inclusiveness in a health insurance scheme involving rationing (or anything for that manner) may be more questionable for some marginalized social groups, even to the point that mandating their inclusion could threaten the viability of any system.[13]

Thinking idealistically for the moment, an ethically justifiable, affordable, and rational healthcare system that strove to be expansive, comprehensive, effective, and manageable would probably have the hallmarks of a centrally administered national health insurance plan. It would minimize administrative overhead, maximize availability and accessibility, and aim to provide the most effective treatments possible. Doctors would be paid generously, not based on piecework, but rather for the quality of the care they provided. Investigation into both the causes and cures for diseases would be a high priority, along with comparative effectiveness research so that the public could take advantage of what works best and not what advertises best. Would such a Panglossian model require rationing? Of course. If not, then there would be little reason to restrict access to almost anything a patient might want, irrespective of what it costs or how remote the chances of it being effective.[14]

Therefore, rationing necessarily means that some people might not receive what they might want or think they need. Depending on the level of generosity in the funding mechanism, the number of people who would be unsatisfied would vary; one might think that, for a variety of reasons both moral and politically practical, a wealthy and extremely diverse and politically polarized country like the United States would go out of its way to be munificent in funding this kind of healthcare reorganization.[15] This does not mean that controlling the healthcare budget using this approach is a Sisyphean task. On the contrary, as I will analyze and argue in detail throughout this book, there may be methods that could be employed that would meet the multiple coextensive goals of equity, affordability, excellent health outcomes, and a (mostly) satisfied public.

A further point is that the amount of funding devoted to healthcare would be a complex function of competing interests, the willingness of the people to support this sector, and what could be "bought" for the amount of money that was believed to be reasonable to spend. It could certainly be true that the initial estimates would be found to purchase not nearly as much as might be desired, so revisions upward might be necessary. One could label these as *money-primary* and *benefit-primary* approaches. The former would allocate a fixed budget, and the benefit level would be dependent on how much was authorized (the Oregon Health Plan [OHP] was a good example of this method);[16] the latter would first define what would comprise a reasonable benefit package, and the budget would be dependent on the costs, which would presumably vary. Clearly, there is more budgetary control in the first, but the latter might be better able to withstand charges of unfairness and one of the central challenges of the cutoff problem (see later discussion).

Either general method would entail drawing lines and creating cutoff points where those who are classified or defined in a manner that puts them on one side of the line establishes them as fortunate enough to be recipients or not. For example, I referred to the OHP. Created in the late 1980s as a mechanism for improving the delivery of healthcare to the Medicaid population in the state and expanding the population of those who could be covered, a fixed budget was set by the legislature that was felt to be reasonable and affordable. In a series of somewhat controversial approaches (sometimes tragicomically so), a list of covered interventions was created utilizing a hybrid form of cost-effectiveness analysis.[17] The funding level set by the legislature determined how far down on the list one's coverage would go for a given budget period. If one had a condition that was on the part of the list that was within the coverage umbrella, one would be in luck. If one were sick with something further down on the list, this would not be covered. Indeed, presumably, one could be afflicted with conditions on both sides of the line and have one covered but not the other. The important point is that the cutoff point was created by somewhat arbitrary budgetary considerations. Whether the legislature voted to spend rather more or less (resulting in perhaps one or a few more or less condition–treatment pairs to make or be deleted from the list) was a matter of political bargaining and horse-trading. They decided the amount of the finite resource they would make available, thus creating the cutoff. There was no analysis that would say that patients with a disorder that was at the bottom of the list experienced significantly more suffering or that the treatment for that illness was notably more successful than the condition–intervention pair that was just above it. Nevertheless, one kind of patient was fortunate while the other was not. Nor was there any attempt to substantively explain to the people who had just-below-the-funding-line disorders why they would be unable to receive state-funded treatment for their condition(s), only that there was insufficient money available. Even if there were an effective therapy for that illness, funding restrictions would not permit payment. This is an example of a money-centered (or primary) approach to creating cutoffs in which the amount of the budget allocated up front determines what (and how much) healthcare could be purchased. A central flaw in this form of rationing is that it neglects to consider equity and fairness as primary foci of distributing healthcare resources. To be sure, the aims of the OHP were noble: to expand the population of poor people with access to at least some reasonable amount of healthcare within the constraints of budgetary largess (and certainly an amount that exceeded what they would have had without the OHP). But this reveals a problem in employing this approach: how much is available has little to do with how much may be needed and would help the most people.[18]

The case of the OHP is a prime example of what I will refer to throughout this book as the "cutoff" problem: the drawing of boundaries that determine who (or what) is eligible for certain healthcare services (and for what) and who is not. At first glance, it may appear as if this is a simple and straightforward issue. But it is anything but simple. If the goals are fairness and justice, the absence of arbitrary and frequently callous decision-making and rules, and the equitable distribution of resources, then considerable careful thought must be devoted to the enterprise. I will first describe some other, perhaps more well-known examples of healthcare boundary problems that have utilized different quantifiers than money to decide who should get what during a resource scarcity. These cases demonstrate the challenges posed by the cutoff problem and will serve as an introduction to the complexity of the issue (I will examine this further in Chapter 2).

INFLUENZA AND OLD PEOPLE

No one seems to like old people, although perhaps a more charitable way to describe this sentiment is that we appear to like—or prefer—young people more than old people. In multiple studies over many years, psychological tests that assess so-called unconscious biases have demonstrated time and again that both the young and even the elderly have a hidden—but deeply felt—prejudice against seniors.[19] One might think that this is a feature or possibly an anomaly of our youth-obsessed society, but it is also discernible in countries that are known for venerating their senior citizens.[20] This common and seemingly ingrained partiality or proclivity might help explain why numerous surveys have suggested that most people favor allocating scarce resources to the young (vs. the old) when a choice between the two must be made. Even when the outcome of such a choice and decision would mean the death of one of the two individuals, the elder invariably gets the thumbs down. For example, when asked in a variety of ways to whom they would give a liver if there was only one organ and two people in liver failure, both of whose lives could be saved by a transplant, large majorities of respondents state that they would prioritize the 10- or 15-year-old over the 65-year-old.[21]

In the mid- to late 1960s, during the growth and early heyday of youth culture, a saying was coined that encapsulated the severe skepticism that many young people had for their elders, those whom they held responsible for all that was wrong with society, such as a Victorian view toward sexuality, alcohol-fueled hypocrisy with respect to hallucinatory drugs, and, of course, the Vietnam War. This maxim was "Never trust anyone over 30," the thought being (if I can go so far as to imply that there was much thought behind this) that this was the age cutoff beyond which only awaited wretched despair. In response to this popular folk belief, a number of movies and books incorporated it as a theme, one of the more popular (and insipid) being the 1968 film *Wild in the Streets*.[22] In this movie, the hero is Max Frost, a somewhat reformed juvenile delinquent who has become a mega-rock star. An ambitious congressmen decides that the youth vote will be his ticket to perpetual political employment and so teams up with Frost to garner the support of the latter's perfervid fans to endorse his electoral move into the Senate. After this taste of power, Frost apparently proves so integral to the now-Senator's success that he (Frost) decides on a run for the presidency himself. Low and behold, he wins and immediately starts issuing decrees to the delight of his "base." One of the first is to state that anyone over the age of 30 (including his former patron, the lamentable and now forlorn Senator) should be confined to "rest homes." There are vivid scenes of the newly turned 4th-decade "seniors" being packed off to their retirement after first being impounded in wire fence enclosures pleading with their former confreres to have mercy. Although a ridiculous and vapid movie, it nonetheless is not subtle about the imposition of arbitrary cutoff points using continuous variables such as age and the catastrophic effects that result.[23]

This is not to say that we do show great affection and love for our own grandparents or perhaps even those of our spouse, but when hidden feelings are investigated using tools such as Implicit Association Tests,[24] we consistently reveal that we believe that generic older people are less likeable than their more youthful counterparts. It is possible that this bias may be an artifact of the way the questions are asked, sacrificing the particular and individual for the population (although the social psychologists who study these phenomena do not believe this to be true). It is also plausible that some erosion of these beliefs can be found when identifiable persons form the choice pair, revealing some influence of what has been called the Rule of Rescue phenomenon.[25] While there are variations in the ways in which these tests are constructed and administered, for the most part they attempt to detect attitudes to gross differences in age (or at least the appearance of age) as opposed to subtle or minor distinctions. For instance, when photographs of young and old people are presented to test subjects, they are manipulated so that their differences in age are easily manifest. These are unconscious, intuitive, often emotional or visceral, automatic nonrational responses to stimuli, what Kahneman has called "system one" thinking, without rational or reflective thought.[26] This kind of cognition dominates much of our daily life and our reactions to many kinds of prompts. Thus, if we as citizens were to participate in an exercise in which our opinions about dispensing scarce resources or supplies were solicited to determine the acceptability of various distribution plans for rationing, discriminatory beliefs of this kind could have a major influence on the sorts of methods used.

These observations strongly suggest that many—perhaps most—people may place a higher value on continued life for younger than older people, especially when the amount of age difference between the two in a comparison (either-or) test is wide. Hence, saving the life of a child or adolescent could count more and should demand greater effort than saving the life of an elderly person when resources are constrained, all other things being equal. Therefore, there are presumably features about the younger individual that are lacking in the older individual and that contribute to this allowance for disproportionate expenditure of supplies and energy. This is not to say that the old are worth less than the young under ordinary circumstances, but simply that when a tragic choice must be made between them, most favor trying to save the life of the latter.[27] It is obvious that this attitude does not play out in real life in the United States, where we generally act as if resources are not constrained and the amounts of money devoted to those over 65 years (such as Medicare and Social Security) vastly exceeds that which is dedicated to youth. Thus, budget cuts to the entitlement programs for seniors are routinely referred to as the "third rail of politics," warning nervous senators and representatives that they would decrease funding at their electoral peril. It's a different matter for budgets for education, Medicaid, Head Start, and other programs that primarily benefit the young and/or poor and that always seem vulnerable to the budget knife.[28] So, this view appears to be brought out mostly when circumstances of scarcity force a choice. How might this play out for healthcare in the real world, and how could this illustrate the cutoff problem in a real-life situation?

In the early part of the past decade, public health experts began to receive worrisome reports from Southeast Asia about the appearance of a new strain of avian influenza that was beginning to emerge in flocks of domesticated birds, especially chickens. Even more concerning was the fact that, on rare occasions, people who routinely came in close contact with these infected animals (often actually living with them) were themselves infected by the virus, got very ill, and an alarmingly high percentage died. Of greatest interest—and unease—was the question of whether this virus, which seemed to be extremely virulent, had already acquired the appropriate mutations that would enable it to be easily transmitted from person to person (or would soon do so), similar to the usual seasonal influenza viruses with which most of us are familiar.[29] Would the identified H5N1 "bird flu" strain jump to humans and cause a worldwide public health catastrophe like the great pandemic in 1918–19 that started in Europe toward the end of World War I and then quickly spread to the rest of the globe by soldiers returning home from the battlefield? This seemed quite possible because modern molecular biological techniques had demonstrated the genetic similarities between the historical virus (isolated from tissue obtained from the bodies of individuals who had died during the pandemic) and the current avian strain.[30] The danger was real, and it was terrifying.

In a period of less than two years, the so-called 1918 Spanish flu caused upward of 50 million to even as many as 100 million deaths, dwarfing the carnage just experienced by the warring parties on the battlefields of France and Belgium.[31] Most frightening of all about this disease was that, unlike the usual seasonal flu that came and went each winter and which mostly killed the old, babies, and the infirm, this struck people in the prime of life who were seemingly brimming with good health. And it killed them quickly—perhaps not as rapidly as the medieval Black Death (bubonic plague)—but within just a few days. Even the then just emerging scientific medicine, fresh from demonstrating its ability to save the previously unsalvageable from their war wounds but without what we now think of as the essential tools of antibiotics, vaccines, and intensive care high technology, could do virtually nothing to halt the inexorable waves of mortality from the virus. This is what public health authorities and infectious disease specialists now feared: that we would have a repeat of 1918 and be virtually powerless to stop it once it really started.

Of course, there were significant differences between the social and medical state of affairs in 2006 and the second decade of the 20th century, at least in industrialized and technologically sophisticated wealthy countries like those in Western Europe and the United States. In the 1918 pandemic, doctors and nurses could care for but only infrequently cure, especially when confronted by the "cytokine storm" that often developed in the previously healthy teenagers and young adults who appeared to be the primary targets of the flu's propensity to elicit major immune system reactions, which was the probable cause of both morbidity and mortality.[32] There were no antibiotics, no vaccines, no intensive care units (ICUs) and mechanical ventilators; none of what we customarily associate with our expectations of medical "miracles" and recovery from even the most severe and complex illnesses. Quarantine and "social isolation" had a limited effect.[33] And people died in droves in the United States and Europe and presumably in even larger numbers in the undeveloped countries that we now call the Third World.

But, rather than the H5N1 virus that originated in birds, the H1N1 strain that eventually appeared in 2009 traced its lineage to pigs, thus earning it the sobriquet "swine flu" (and its genetic sequence demonstrated that it bore a close relationship to the 1918 strain).[34] Even so, public health and infectious disease experts were still worried and for very similar reasons. The standard approach to containing seasonal flu (and hopefully a pandemic) could have comparable obstacles to overcome:

> Vaccine[s] would have no impact on the course of the virus in the first months and would likely play an extremely limited role worldwide during the following 12 to 18 months of the pandemic. Despite major innovations in the production of most other vaccines, international production of influenza vaccine is based on a fragile and limited system that utilizes technology from the 1950s.... To counter a new strain of pandemic influenza that has never circulated throughout the population, each person would likely need two doses for adequate protection.... In addition, because the structure of the virus changes so rapidly, vaccine development could only start once the pandemic began, as manufacturers would have to obtain the new pandemic strain. It would then be at least another six months before mass production of the vaccine.[35]

Clearly, there would be insufficient quantities of a (presumably) effective vaccine for at least 6 months after the causative virus was identified and then for some time afterward until production was ramped up to meet the full demand (in the United States and Europe, we generally have a lead time warning of several months because annual influenza usually begins in Asia and spreads from there to the West). Therefore, some form of allocation plan involving prioritization and hence rationing would have to be prepared. Who should receive the vaccine first? Who should be saved when not all could?[36]

A number of plans were proposed and then revised, mostly by public health experts with some input from medical ethicists and occasionally even contributions solicited from members of the public.[37] This was not a simple matter, largely due to the unprecedented nature of what was being attempted and the lack of complete information about who would be most at risk of getting sick and dying. In a normal flu season, young children and the elderly (plus those who are immunocompromised, such as patients receiving chemotherapy for cancer) are most susceptible to becoming severely ill and succumbing. Should allocation be based upon historical data from 90 years ago? Or should primary recipients be those who usually are the ones who get sickest each flu season?

Eventually, it was decided that healthcare providers (doctors, nurses, etc.), those workers who were involved in vaccine production, and first-responders such as police, firefighters, ambulance personnel, and the like should receive the initial batches of vaccine for reasons that were readily understandable by most people.[38] The demarcation lines distinguishing these people and others were also fairly obvious and definitive: one either was or wasn't a doctor or nurse; one either was or wasn't a firefighter or member of the National Guard. The difficult part was figuring out who should come next. What medical and/or social criteria would be reasonable (and acceptable) to employ to offer a select group of individuals the opportunity to live (assuming the vaccine would be effective)? And the distinguishing characteristics that could be utilized to categorize people for eligibility starkly illuminated the cutoff problem.

One of the more potentially controversial and inflammatory suggestions to cope with this challenge was to privilege the young over the old, presumably acknowledging the existing preferences I discussed earlier. While similar proposals have been made before in the context of resource scarcity, such as with solid organ transplantation, when Ezekiel Emanuel and Alan Wertheimer published their recommendation in the prominent American journal *Science* in 2006, it stimulated significant debate.[39] Essentially, they based their plan on an idea originally presented by John Harris in 1985, which has come to be called the "fair innings" argument.[40] The basic concept is that a reasonable composition of a good life is one that enables an individual to experience the various stages of life and the events that are customarily associated with those temporal periods, or having a shot at a fair innings (or that one should have the opportunity to experience them; there is no warrant for mandating that one take advantage of these opportunities, only that one be afforded them). These events might ordinarily include a childhood phase with an appropriate education and physical development; then a young adult period characterized by establishing a partnership with someone one cares for and starting a family and a working life; and, finally, a well-deserved retirement (presumably something akin to Shakespeare's "seven ages of man").[41] Even without the philosophical rationale, this model accords with our intuitive judgments.

In their account, altered from Harris's original and now relabeled as the "investment refinement of the life cycle principle" (which also included appropriate consideration for those people whose jobs including maintaining "public order"), they created four tiers of vaccine recipients whose needs would be met in ordinal order depending on the available supply of vaccine. Like the official plan promulgated by the Centers for Disease Control,[42] the initial lots of vaccine would be first granted to those whose job it was to produce the vaccine as well as primary healthcare providers—presumably doctors and nurses and ancillary supportive staff. Next came a series of younger (and some older) individuals with sharp demarcation lines based on age such as "people 13 to 40 years old with < 2 high risk conditions" or "7 to 12 years old and 41 to 50 years old," and so on.

By this account, we could presumably think of years accumulated as a form of interchangeable currency, a currency of accumulated experiences. That way, it could be quantitatively compared with other years experienced by other people. Of course, one could perhaps argue that not all years are commensurable between different individuals. Those whose lives are particularly grim, harrowing, or destitute, or who were born with or acquired a physical or cognitive disability and hence had fewer opportunities to enjoy the kinds or amounts of experiences, would be lumped in with those of similar age whose lives were perhaps more rich and successful. This form of cutoff is thus a blunt tool, indifferent to these distinctions. By using this measure, people would not necessarily be thought of as unique individuals, but only as parts of a large population and as numbers symbolized by their age. A life filled with great privation (say, by extreme poverty or neglect by one's caregivers) would be considerably less fulfilled than one blessed with the proverbial silver spoon. Alternatively, the "natural lottery" of birthright and genetic circumstances (when coupled with what nurture has made available) can present similar congenial or malefic impediments to achieving "normal" goals in life. Should those unfortunate people who have, for one reason or another, been less fortunate than others in attaining these notable landmarks as they pass through life be given the same priority as similarly aged peers who have been luckier?

The simple answer was "yes" since other considerations were not relevant in this scheme. All that mattered was the easily quantified and interpersonally comparable metric of age. Therefore, if age is the primary determinant of who gets what, then the kind or quality of the life one has led is irrelevant to this calculus; quantity is taken as an adequate surrogate marker for worthiness for access to the vaccine. But, as these last points suggest, unlike money, time and its accumulated life-years are not fungible. Furthermore, age has often been used as a "surrogate marker" for some other less quantifiable variables such as disease or infirmity. For example, we might say that old people are sicker on average than young people, which is no doubt true in an aggregate basis, but much more complex in the particulate. When one begins to delve a bit deeper into this issue, one begins to see that one's age is a very poor indicator of illness except when one uses it as a general term to describe some gross characteristics of a population whose boundaries are often quite fuzzy and most certainly have significant overlap with adjacent groups.[43] Moreover, when these analyses and explanations are performed in this statistical manner, it becomes all too easy to reify these combinations such that the result is old = sick or old = has experienced more qualifying events (or so it is presumed). As I will discuss in greater detail in Chapter 2, using age as an accessible and quantifiable measure for apportioning scarce resources has significant drawbacks for a morally justifiable implementation.

But no matter which way one analyzes their proposal (and many more like it for a variety of other health conditions or kinds of resources), it still relies on distributing a precious and scarce resource on the basis of age, a continuously distributed variable that is an essential feature of us all and which changes on a daily basis (if not second-by-second). And when they impose cutoffs at strict boundaries (as in "7 to 12 years"), this implies that, at the moment of distribution, a child who is just shy of her 7th birthday (say, by one or two days) or who just turned 13 the day before is out of luck, with no discernable or significant difference between them and those fortunate enough to fall within the borders that have been arbitrarily designated. Indeed, for some of these children, misfortune cannot even be ascribed to nature if their mothers happened to have an elective cesarean section on this day or that. In life's celestial roll of the dice, they lost. It is difficult to imagine how one could explain the practical implications of such a plan to those who would lose out for reasons like this. And this reveals an inherent problem, perhaps a fatal flaw, in proposals of this type: relatively simple to generate, extraordinarily *demanding to accomplish in real life*, because they are not really fair.

Age is a continuous variable (see Figure 1.1). When we examine two people, unless their birthdays and times of birth are identical, they can be absolutely differentiated by the fact that one is chronologically older (or younger) than the other. But when we expand the number of members in the group to a large population (as we necessarily must if we are considering how to dole out a vaccine that is in short supply), the distribution of ages begins to assume the shape of a smooth curve.[44] Let us assume we decided that everyone below the age of 35 years would receive the influenza vaccine because they had not really had a chance to experience all of the benefits, opportunities, and experiences of a full life; all those over 65 would not receive the vaccine because they had already experienced most of what life has to offer; and all those in between would have a lottery for any vaccine that may remain after everyone in the youth group was immunized. How might this actually work?

Let us next assume that the vaccine would be administered today. Most importantly, let us also suppose that Sally's 36th birthday is tomorrow and Ted's was today; their ages are separated by a mere 24 hours, but the allocation plan states unequivocally that Ted can get the vaccine and Sally can't. His life will be saved and hers will not simply because of a quirk of birth dates and a vaccination strategy that was designed to draw a line somewhere to distinguish the haves from the have-nots. I think most people would be hard-pressed to say that Ted is substantively different from Sally—in a meaningfully moral or even medical sense—simply because Ted was sufficiently lucky to have his birthday fall one day before Sally's. It would be quite difficult—if not impossible—to justify an assertion that he *deserved* the vaccine because of the fortunate juxtaposition of their birthdays (in their relative order) and the arbitrarily decided distribution date. Indeed, if their birth dates were even further apart than say, 24 hours or 2 or even 3 days, it would still be implausible to argue that they were different enough to justify saving his life and not hers.[45] One could ask

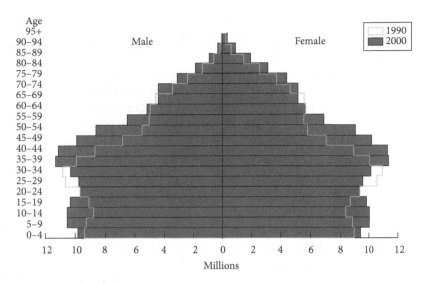

FIG 1.1 This graphic shows the distribution of ages in the United States at 1990 and 2000. It is not exactly a "normal" Gaussian distribution (nor would one necessarily expect it to be), and the data are "chunky" because they are presented in 5-year groups. If presented in smaller increments—for example, in annual increments—the edges would be much smoother. (Graph obtained from http://nationalatlas.gov/articles/people/a_age2000.html, accessed October 11, 2013.)

oneself the question of how separate or far apart their ages would have to be to really make a difference that would and should count?

That is one of the prime challenges of the boundary or cutoff problem. This is an extremely important and complex issue, one that begs an answer that has proved to be elusive. Indeed, I have not been able to find any authors who have truly attempted to solve it, indicative of either its extreme difficulty (I don't disagree with this conclusion) or perhaps even its insolvability (however, I disagree that a practical solution cannot be found). Nevertheless, this problem demands attention and a feasible (and morally defensible) solution. Let me give another related example, also from the pandemic flu scare from a few years ago.

For several years, I have served as a member of the Ethical and Judicial Affairs Committee of the North Carolina Medical Society. In the fall of 2009, we were asked by the State Department of Health to develop a plan to allocate healthcare resources—especially intensive care—for the anticipated pandemic that could possibly overwhelm the available ICU beds and staff relatively quickly, presenting a classic scarce critical resources problem. Simply put, we were expected to create a consensus proposal that would prioritize and distribute ventilators and their associated high-technology paraphernalia to those patients who could perhaps most benefit from having access to them. Importantly, we would also have to provide both medical *and* ethical justifications for the recommendations we would make. This committee was mostly composed of physicians and some legal staff from a wide variety of backgrounds, none of which was critical care medicine. Therefore, we invited several experts in this area to advise us. One of the most potentially contentious and controversial issues we confronted was how to cope with the elderly if there were a competition for ICU resources between them and the generic "young" (perhaps not surprisingly, the definitions of young and old were left somewhat ill-defined).

A fellow member of the committee, a retired physician in his mid-70s and a former academic surgeon who lived in a local retirement "village," offered that he had conducted an uncontrolled but nonetheless interesting experiment with his fellow seniors and neighbors. He asked them to imagine that they or their spouses or significant others contracted the flu and became very ill with impending respiratory failure to the point that they would require a ventilator and ICU care to possibly survive, resources that would unquestionably be available to them under normal circumstances. Then he asked them to picture one of their grandchildren becoming sick at the same time and also needing the same kind of treatment. However, there was only one ICU bed and respirator remaining, and thus there would have to be a choice between them or their grandchild possibly living: which would they choose? Would they grab the ventilator, or would they give it up so their beloved granddaughter could have the opportunity to live a life that they had already experienced? Not surprisingly, the unanimous answer was that they would gladly die so that their relative could live. But he also asked them if they would make the same decision if it were a child unknown to them. Even then, for a stranger, almost everyone he asked (but not all) gave the same answer. This unscientific study was presented to the group and reinforced our endorsement of a variant of the life cycle opportunity views expressed by Emanuel and Wertheimer (and many others). However, it is significant that my colleague did not ask his friends if they would voluntarily give up an ICU bed for a middle-aged stranger or at what age their overriding concern for younger people would stop.

While this story again reinforces our common intuition that unspecified "children" should receive priority over unspecified "old people," it does not address at all how such a belief should be implemented.[46] Furthermore, once these nameless or anonymized youngsters or seniors become identified and, most significantly, become recognized as our friends or relatives, our selfless devotion to these moral intuitions may vanish or, at a minimum, be seriously eroded. This belief raises significant questions and problems about how to actually create meaningful, practical, and socially and morally justifiable (and thus publicly legitimate) cutoffs.

I am not asking whether we should ration healthcare resources. I will take it as a given that we must, either because indivisible things like organs (e.g., hearts) cannot meet demand or fungible assets like money must be limited because of other pressing demands.[47] How should we go about distributing resources—stuff—to some people rather than others? How should we determine where the cutoff should be between those who receive what may be a life-saving vaccine and those who don't and thus must trust to luck not to get sick and die? And what kind of cutoff should be used? One or more different categories of boundaries might be better for a variety of reasons. This means we can compare and contrast them and that we can thus make a choice. It's all well and good to say that children should be given the vaccine and seniors should not, but how exactly do we draw the line that distinguishes these two groups from one another? The legitimacy of any plan to be actualized in the real world must achieve minimal tolerability and acceptance by those to whom it would apply, and that is a challenge that has never been successfully met in all the proposals that have been advanced. I will present a workable solution in this book.

CUTOFFS, PROBABILITIES, AND RATIONING

Why discuss these nightmarish scenarios, which thankfully never really had to be implemented (although, to be sure, it is only a matter of time before we experience a major influenza pandemic)? I think they reveal the kind of analysis and thought that large numbers of people—ethicists, physicians, public health experts, and government officials, to name but a few—participated in in an attempt to devise strategies to cope with what were forecast to be both temporary and durational shortages of many different healthcare resources. In essence, the people who worked on these plans were tasked with formulating rationing schemes, creating algorithms of allocation priorities that decided who should get what and when, and necessarily, who should not. While concerned with what was hoped to be an episodic one-time event, pandemic rationing was related to other forms of systematic healthcare rationing in which we are already engaged, such as the distribution of solid organs for people with liver, heart, and kidney failure. In both general situations there exists a mismatch between the availability of a needed resource (vaccines, ventilators, and organs) and the numbers of people who could possibly benefit from receiving them. Creating a plausible approach that would be deemed acceptable and reasonable by the people to be affected by it was and remains a major challenge but, in the case of organ transplant, one that has been largely successful in the United States.[48]

Virtually all of the characteristics or measures that might be used (and those that have been discussed) to determine how healthcare resources should be rationed, either electively or because we must, share some features: they all involve some form of what has been called a continuous variable. Many have what I shall frequently refer to as "fuzzy" borders. Age is a perfect example, and I have already illustrated some of the problems that this and similar metrics have in attempting to create cutoff points. Being a continuous variable does not mean that the distribution of the measurements at any given time resemble the so-called normal curve or Gaussian distribution, such as IQ (see Figure 1.2).

But it does signify that, given a sufficiently large population of data points, they will vary continuously from small to large, with greater or lesser density of quantities (represented on the ordinate or "y" axis). So, looking at the scatter of IQ, which by definition is designed for the Wechsler testing scale to be normally distributed, is a perfect example of such a continuous variable.[49] One noteworthy feature of this figure is how smooth the curve is (of course, it is describing data collected from large numbers of individuals in a population). How is it possible to decide the cutoff

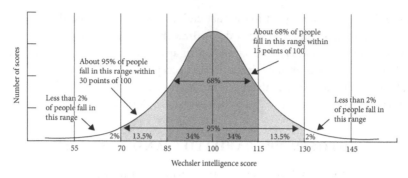

FIG 1.2 Distribution of IQ in US adults. (From https://new.edu/resources/the-social-cultural-and-political-aspects-of-intelligence#stangor-ch09_s02_s01_f01, accessed October 11, 2013.)

points that distinguish between say, people of extremely high intelligence and those who are smart, just not that smart (although this analysis may be more socially relevant to those people who find themselves on the other end of the curve distribution)? The mean (or average) IQ score is arbitrarily set to be 100, indicating that half of people taking the test are higher than this and half are lower.[50] Then, using the common statistical calculation known as the standard deviation, lines are drawn on either side of the mean to indicate one or more standard deviations. The further one gets from the mean, the fewer individuals (or data points) there are. Thus, if you happen to have an IQ of 130, you are "smarter" than 98% of all the people taking the test and only 2% of the population are smarter than you. Conversely, if your score is 70, 98% of test-takers are smarter than you, and you are only smarter than the remaining 2%. Of course it is extremely controversial if what these IQ tests measure actually represents what we commonly envision or conceptualize as "intelligence" (somewhat tautologically, it is IQ), but the point for my purposes is a different problem. The challenge arises because of our need to classify people using subjective descriptors applied to objective measurements. In the case of IQ, the former may be smarter or "cognitively" or "intellectually" disabled (these are the more modern terms describing what in the past were called "mental retardation," "feeblemindedness," and the like).

Let us assume that John's IQ is measured at 71, and the cutoff for being classified as having an intellectual disability is 70. Being labeled as having such a disability would entitle John to many state-supported services, such as life-long Social Security Income payments each month, perhaps subsidized housing, and more. However, because John is on the higher side of the cutoff line, even though he occupies a boundary position right next to it, he fails to meet the criteria that have been set (based on fairly routine statistical analysis and agreed to by committees sitting in a room and discussing what sounds reasonable for classification purposes) and is out of luck. His doctors and family argue that there is no reasonable substantive difference between him and any similar people whose IQ measures at 69 or 70, but because his test score falls on the wrong side of the line, he is not intellectually disabled enough to obtain the sorts of services that are reserved for those who have profound cognitive disabilities that have been arbitrarily (but perhaps reasonably) set at 70.[51] Is this fair? Of course, this is no different from the examples I gave earlier about age cutoffs for vaccines or any other form of line-drawing cutoff that attempts to apply firm, distinct boundaries to characteristics that are inherently blurred or fuzzy.[52]

Another current and extremely controversial cutoff example is the legal gestational age limits on abortion. If one believes that a person is created at the moment of conception, then the issue is relatively straightforward and simple; indeed, there is no cutoff problem because it is reasonably distinct, without blurred edges. Jonathan Glover alludes to this quandary when he discusses where to draw a line for when abortion may be permissible (or not) with respect to when a fetus becomes a "person" (in the morally relevant sense): the transition from fertilized egg to adult, like many biological developments, can better be represented by a fairly steady upward curve than by a series of obviously discrete stages with abrupt transitions. To ask "when does one start to become a person?" is like asking "when does middle age begin?".[53] However, if one will admit that some elective pregnancy terminations are morally permissible, one then has to decide which ones would qualify. If one then utilizes the most common qualifier—that of *ex utero* viability—then one is of course faced with a boundary issue. When the Supreme Court ruled in *Roe v. Wade*, in 1973 that this was the standard that should be used, it was not a major stretch to say that 24 weeks' gestation was the absolute lower limit of viability because the data for premature infant survival at this stage of development was (and remains) extraordinarily poor.[54] However, in the succeeding 40 years, a number of technical and medical advances have been made in neonatology such that the same babies we would have written off as not salvageable in the late 1970s, when I was a pediatric resident, are now considered to be "big babies" with an excellent chance of both survival and disability-free outcome.[55] Nowadays, the big debate in the field of neonatal intensive care is if infants of 22 or 23 weeks' gestation should be resuscitated and offered intensive care. Due to their often poor prognosis, whether it be the dismal survival statistics or even worse quality of life estimates, this is a hotly contested question.[56] How little a chance (or conversely, how big a chance) of viability (i.e., the possibility of survival outside the womb) is so little that one can say that it is equivalent to no chance? This is clearly a cutoff problem and, as I will be describing in this book, one with inherently fuzzy borders.

Cutoff problems are widespread and common in our everyday lives, even if our attempts to confront them and solve them are somewhat feeble. For example, college admissions officers are confronted with cutoff problems all the time. They are constantly forced to choose between hundreds, if not thousands, of applicants all of whom have minimally differentiated SAT and GPA scores, and they must somewhat arbitrarily pick who will be admitted and who will not. Not surprisingly, they readily confess that they could easily have chosen a number of mostly indistinguishable first-year freshman classes without a noticeable change in the qualifications or performance of their entering class. But, of course, they do have to make a decision, and, much to the dismay and chagrin of those who are not admitted and much to the everlasting joy of the others, it is actually somewhat arbitrary who gets in at the cutoff boundary. Admission to college is not the same thing as admission to an ICU or access to medicines or other types of therapies or medical interventions that have the opportunity to make a significant change in one's quality of life and health. But those charged with deciding who gets what (and of course who doesn't) face the same problems and same issues as the college admissions officers.[57]

Some variables that are used in healthcare allocation are less obviously continuous than others. One of the more notable is money. This is a manifestly important one because money is one of the central issues that is driving the discussion (or argument) about rationing. We are spending too much, and we are certainly not receiving the sorts of benefits in terms of health outcomes that one might expect considering the total amount of dollars we spend each year. For example, a recent report has noted that the United States continues to have a higher infant mortality rate and rate of premature births (the two are related) than most other industrialized developed nations. We also have a lower life expectancy, both overall and even more blatantly in some populations such as African-American men. Indeed, those who aren't appalled and ashamed of these statistics are at least embarrassed when they consider which countries do better than us on these metrics, including some of our most nettlesome neighbors (like Cuba).[58] It surely isn't because we can't afford to spend the money to obtain good health outcomes because we spend more per capita per year on healthcare than any other country in the world.[59] Clearly, it must be *how* we spend the money. Presumably, if we could reorganize the way we spend our healthcare funds, we could be healthier and save significant sums to devote to other projects we think important.

Money may not be able to buy you love, but it can (and does) buy you stuff, and it is almost unconditionally fungible, meaning that one can buy and spend it in a virtually infinite number of ways. That is most certainly true for healthcare funding. Much of the debate on the complex American healthcare system is centered on how the money is allocated and on whom it is spent. Nearly everyone agrees that we are spending more than we need to and that the continuing escalation in annual costs is fiscally unsustainable. A multitude of suggestions and plans have been proposed to control (or even reduce) costs, including a single-payer national insurance plan perhaps modeled on Medicare and some more expansive form of the ACA (including a "public" option) that continues to rely on the private marketplace and all of its associated administrative costs.[60] Others have noted that a privatized system that continues to employ the financial incentives that currently exist (such as fee-for-service reimbursement schemes for doctors, an inability to factor in costs and efficacy when approving items for Medicare reimbursement, and the like) cannot realistically be expected to drive down costs or enhance quality.[61] I have previously proposed a general outline of a national insurance program that could be generous and cost-effective if it incorporated a form of rationing, minimized administrative costs, and substantially altered how physicians are paid.[62] But all of these ideas lack the specifics of how it might work and do so in a manner that made fairness and equity a central hallmark to engender legitimacy and acceptance. An essential requirement of implementation of any rationing plan would be how to draw the line—how to establish cutoffs—that people could accept as reasonable, understandable, and acceptable.

My goal in this book is not to argue whether the young should be preferred over the old or that those with so-called self-induced conditions should receive less consideration than those who have purportedly led a pristine life, always eating their vegetables, exercising daily, and essentially living the Aristotelian ideal of moderation in all things. Rather, it is to discuss a practical approach to solving what may appear to be the intractable problem of not only where to draw a line, but how to do so. While I have previously argued that healthcare rationing is not only necessary as a central component of overall healthcare reform but could be acceptable if implemented and accomplished in a certain way,[63] a crucial and critically missing component of my (and virtually all other) proposals on rationing is how to accomplish it in the real world. For to do so means that one must devise a method to both appreciate and find the key to the cutoff problem. This is both a practical and a moral issue, for the approach that is taken has enormous implications for the acceptability or tolerability of any kind of rationing plan in general and the ease with which one can actually execute the scheme that is formulated. These two aspects are inextricably related. Some strategies will be more reasonable and plausible than others by virtue of the fact that they have less complex boundary issues, and I will argue that those they do possess are more amenable to overcoming objections raised by fewer people than others.

What has been totally lacking in both the academic literature and in the discussions of policy-makers is what Williams has referred to as the "quantification" of the application of the various theoretical approaches.[64] While some may argue that the proposal put forth by Emanuel and Wertheimer and discussed earlier was both specific and quantitative, I would suggest that it was neither because it completely avoided the practical aspects of policy implementation: how would it actually work in real life? Ethical arguments of this type often take the form of philosophical discussions that, while they have their merits and place, tend to lose focus—and thus force—when it comes time to make decisions on what is to be done. Stating that young people or even "people 7–12 years old and 41–50 years old with < 2 high-risk conditions" would be first in line for a life-saving vaccine is all well and good except when one must translate these suggestions into a workable, tolerable, and thus acceptable policy and method for delivering vaccine in the midst of a crisis of unknown proportions.[65] One would obviously wish to minimize both any controversy and the number of people who would think themselves ill-served or rejected (for whatever reason). But when the strategy for allocating and administering a potentially life-saving preventative treatment eliminates large swaths of the population who would undoubtedly have difficulty understanding the justification for their exclusion on the basis of substantive differences (which they may not see or comprehend or certainly contend are not substantive) with others who are lucky recipients, the ability to garner legitimacy is undermined. Trying to convince the parents of just-turned-13-year-old children that they cannot get the vaccine solely because of a quirk of birthdate while their neighbor's child whose birthday is a week (or even a day) later qualifies, presents an insurmountable difficulty, and one that exemplifies that task of where (and how) to draw the line such that one can meet these dual challenges.

Hence, some form of exactitude that can inform the formulation of reasonable rules that would be open to debate and justifiable democratic acceptance would be mandatory. How much arbitrariness could be allowable would undoubtedly constitute a significant component of the possibly acrimonious debate that would follow. And it is likely that some quantifiable measures of differences between people would be more amenable to line drawing than others for either computational or statistical reasons, or perhaps because the conclusions that would be drawn (i.e., where the cutoff would be placed) would affect the smallest number of people. I will discuss some of these various possibilities in detail, along with their merits and drawbacks.

An associated problem that needs to be addressed is that of coping with translating population information or data in which individuals are both anonymized and homogenized to extract specifics or particulars that can be applied and useful for single, unique people. After all, we do not think of ourselves as indistinct members of a population, even though we most certainly are when viewed from afar. We prefer to regard ourselves as separable, distinct persons, and this is most certainly true when we are dealing with our physicians. We don't want to be treated as units or numbers, faceless and indistinguishable from others with whom we are grouped. If, for some reason—which may or may not be known or understood by me—I am refused some resource because of the class or category to which I am assigned (say, those over 50 years of age)—I may find solace knowing that others of my "kind" are in the same boat as I, but I take little comfort in knowing that I am no more than a statistic rather than the one-of-a-kind individual I know myself to be. When my doctor explains to me that I have a 75% chance of cure I, like most people, really have no idea what that means. But when she says that this can translate *for me* as a 100% or a 0% chance, that makes sense. Indeed, one the main fears stoked by those opposed to healthcare rationing or reform (irrespective of whether this is true or not) is that patients will lose the individuality of *their* doctor–patient relationship, which will be sacrificed on the altar of the government deciding what is good (for me).[66] Heretofore, all attempts to discuss cutoffs and drawing lines limiting access to one or more healthcare resources—like vaccines—do so, like Emanuel and Wertheimer, by creating inflection points using population data that fall apart when applied to individuals. Thus, the problem with any policy that is based on averages drawn from data derived from populations of people—thousands or millions of individuals who are merged together (like those of different ages, weights, heights, etc.) to make a smooth variable curve—is that it necessarily loses the specificity and particularity we want. We are not accustomed to thinking of ourselves as members of populations, with the associated anonymity, unless we do so abstractly. The more cerebral and statistically sophisticated among us might readily agree and intuitively understand that we are of course just one bit in a large bunch, but that ordinarily doesn't matter when we are working with our physician to determine what is the correct course of action or therapy for our body with our disease. I will discuss this problem in detail in Chapters 4 and 5 because the challenge of applying the theoretical concerns and constraints offered by population analysis to the practical needs of unique persons presents some major conceptual and feasibility implementation obstacles.

It may be thought that the classic or prototypical case of how and where to draw a line defining a cutoff would be organ transplantation. In this situation, there is a finite and ineradicable difference between the number of organs available (e.g., lungs, livers, or hearts) and the number of people who could potentially and reasonably benefit from receiving them; there are always many more of the latter than there are of the former. This permits transplant doctors to set up an allocation system that is quite "choosy," in that they can afford to pick candidates who may derive more benefit (such as both quality and length of life) than others. Furthermore, they give a great deal of deference to the fact that cadaveric organs are a public resource, donated in a spirit of altruism for which there is no material compensation, and thus transplanters view themselves as "stewards" of this precious and scarce life-saving resource. Over time, the prioritization system has evolved to consider a balance between both sickest first and those best able to utilize the organ. Once the rules are created and the waiting list is populated (and continuously renewed), the cutoff is then simply determined by the number of organs available at any point in time. In principle, other forms of scarce resource allocation could be approached similarly, although it turns out it is not that simple.

Drawing lines, establishing boundaries, and creating cutoffs are always problematic when one must do so when developing public policy because one must necessarily be fairly immune to subtleties and nuance. Each case is of course somewhat or slightly different from every other one, so in an ideal world one would like to be able to treat each case on its own merits. In the rare event that there is another case that is identical or exactly like one that preceded it, one would then expect (hope?) that they would accordingly be treated identically. However, we do not live in such an ideal world, so we must establish rules that treat *similar* cases similarly. This raises the question of how similar do similar cases have to be to be treated or considered to be *as if* they were identical? Not surprisingly, this points to another aspect of the boundary or cutoff problem because we are again creating artificial categories for the sake of convenience. We have to decide how many categories it is reasonable to have: too many and one might as well not have any; too few and one might ask what the point actually is. What one is aiming for is "just enough" (whatever that may turn out to be). We would like to have rules that are relatively straightforward to understand and that make sense to a broad range of the people to whom they would apply to ensure legitimacy and buy-in. But they can't be so crude that they do not permit some form of (justifiable) exceptions. For example, it is simple to say that killing people is forbidden, but both morality and societies have generally permitted certain kinds of killing under certain circumstances, as in (just) wars, self-defense, and the like. However, if the exceptions start becoming so numerous that they threaten the rules themselves, then one has a further set of problems. So, once again, what one is aiming for is *just the right number, not too many and not too few.*

WHAT I WILL DO IN THIS BOOK

The identification of what I have labeled the cutoff problem is not new. The famous ancient Greek Skeptic philosopher Eubulides of Miletus characterized it with his "heaping" argument (actually utilized as an atheistic reasoning against the actual existence of the gods). This is a version of a "sorites paradox" argument: "The *sorites paradox* is the name given to a class of paradoxical arguments, also known as *little-by-little arguments*, that arise as a result of the indeterminacy surrounding limits of application of the predicates involved. For example, the concept of a heap appears to lack sharp boundaries, and, as a consequence of the subsequent indeterminacy surrounding the extension of the predicate 'is a heap,' no one grain of wheat can be identified as making the difference between being a heap and not being a heap. Given, then, that one grain of wheat does not make a heap, it would seem to follow that two do not, thus three do not, and so on. In the end, it would appear that no amount of wheat could make a heap. We are faced with a paradox since, from apparently true premises by seemingly uncontroversial reasoning, we arrive at an apparently false conclusion. This phenomenon at the heart of the paradox is now recognized [*sic*] as the phenomenon of vagueness."[67] Put simply, it asks when a pile of something (say, grains of sand or seeds) becomes a "heap." Virtually no one would say that one piece of "x" would be a heap, or even two or three. Is there a magic transformation when the cutoff is reached to become a heap, analogous to a phase transition in chemistry? Or is it a gradual transition to a point where one's evaluation of some physical and subjective qualities of the pile of "x" that permits one to pronounce that it is now a heap? It is likely that different people will draw different conclusions about how many pieces of "x" are needed, how they are stacked, and how high or wide the pile is meet the criteria of what they have decided (presumably beforehand) constitutes a "heap." Cutoffs in other domains are remarkably similar: the distinction between a 69.99-year-old woman and a 70.00-year-old is analogous to the variation between 300 and 301 grains of sand. If we use a characteristic like age as a cutoff point, we state that one qualifies to receive some therapy (for example) while the other doesn't, analogous to saying that the pile of seeds with 1,000 is not a heap, but the one with 1,001 is. Importantly, as Hyde also notes, "Predicates such as 'is a heap' or 'is bald' appear tolerant of sufficiently small changes in the relevant aspects—namely number of grains or number of hairs....Yet large changes in relevant respects will make a difference, even though large changes are the accumulation of small ones which don't seem to make a difference. This is the very heart of the conundrum which has delighted and perplexed so many for so long" (p. 6). While the paradox appears to be logically unsolvable, condemned to be forever a puzzle, a resolution must be sought, at least for the problem as I see it in the realm of healthcare. There needs to be an acceptable mechanism for setting the cutoff problem (or sorites paradox) that is politically feasible and ethically justifiable.[68]

I have described the challenges that exist to creating a sensible, acceptable, and legitimate healthcare rationing plan; any metric that can be used short of some form of unjustifiable true dichotomous variable (such as gender or citizenship) will necessarily entail confronting the cutoff problem. This obstacle contains two major components, and I will thoroughly discuss both. The first is a decision about what measure or characteristic (or characteristics) about people and/or their situations in life or their clinical conditions is reasonable to use as determinants of cutoffs for the purposes of limiting the amount and kind of healthcare services and interventions that should be available in a plausible rationing scheme in a wealthy country such as the United States (taking into account the indispensable need to embrace the dual objectives of ensuring both quality and economy). To accomplish this, I will discuss in greater detail the main traits or features that have been proposed by others and myself to serve this function. Each has its attractions and flaws, the latter of which doom most to be discarded because of the challenges—both moral and practical—of implementing them. By this analysis, I will be able to draw lessons from the deficiencies (and occasional strengths) of these strategies as I develop my own proposal. I will settle on a reasonably justifiable and feasible rationing method, concentrating on an amalgam of healthcare needs and clinical appropriateness. In the end, I will contend that the only morally justifiable metric that fulfills these requirements is that of the efficacy of specific interventions and placing the cutoff at the level of marginally beneficial care. The second component will concentrate on building on the argument set forth from the first, and I will present an approach to how such a proposal could actually be implemented in practice: what would it look like and what would be the requisite conditions—both political and social—to enable its application and possible success. This argument will thus include both a philosophical and a practical part. It will essentially be an ethical statement based on the accepted inescapable fact that some form of standardized rationing must occur to avoid bankruptcy and the moral calamity of the collapse of the healthcare system for anyone except the well-off. Throughout this discussion, I will also consider objections that could be raised to the moral basis for my claim as well as deal with concerns about its plausible practicality.

Nevertheless, it must be generally understood that good and *effective* medicine or healthcare does not come cheap. The virtues of MRI or CT scans in their ability to detect previously clinically imperceptible but perhaps suspected lesions is unparalleled and would undoubtedly make the physicians of even 40 years ago green with envy at their power. Our forebears only had plain skull or abdominal or chest x-rays for diagnostic imaging. Cheap, yes; better, no. So the development of remarkable imaging technology, amazing and hugely sensitive blood tests that can be performed by machines (and not individually by hand) extremely quickly, remarkable drugs born of the molecular revolution of the latter half of the 20th century, and innumerable other interventions made possible by modern scientific medicine have revolutionized our ability to cure and care. Even though some of the most effective healthcare is still inexpensive for populations (such as childhood vaccinations, clean water, and sanitation), few would deny that technologically sophisticated medicine has also improved the lives of millions. But there is a large cost to developing and using this kind of medicine. This means that if we want good, comprehensive healthcare in the United States we must be prepared to pay for it. But that doesn't mean we should not be prudent with our dollars and demand efficient, beneficial, and equitable care. That is why developing methods for establishing what is reasonable to provide to people—both the "what" and the "how"—is so vitally important. A system could avoid these difficult and challenging issues by simply saying "yes" to everyone for everything. Of course, that is both ridiculous on its face and obviously unsustainable (i.e., unaffordable). Or, it could say "yes" to some things for some people and no to many others; that is the system we have evolved in the United States today, even with the decrease in the uninsured population as a result of the ACA. However, with a generous system that has as its goals the attainment of the best health outcomes for the most people at a cost the country wishes to (and, I believe, can) afford, we would say "yes" to things that work for virtually everyone. Where and how to draw the line between reasonable "yes's" and "no's" is the trick. That is my task in what follows.

In many ways, my argument is based on a hypothetical: if we were to radically transform the healthcare system in the United States, what sorts of reasonable goals should there be to satisfy the demands of the general aims of medicine to relieve human suffering and of social justice to more equitably make available the goods, bounty, and opportunities of society? These goals are not mutually exclusive; indeed, they are complementary. The very fact that modern scientific medicine has been able to lead to improved lives for so many due to its increasing efficacy has demonstrated that it deservedly should be considered one of those goods that social justice requires be both accessible and obtainable for all so that individuals can maximize the possibilities of their lives. This naturally means that there must be a mechanism to offer a basic and comprehensive set of healthcare benefits to all. There are a variety of ways in which this can be accomplished, ranging from a truly nationalized, government-run system as in France, to public–private hybrids similar to those in the Netherlands and Germany. However, in the current era of technological medicine, these lofty aims are very expensive and the "beloved beast" has seemingly an insatiable (cost) appetite.[69] Hence, there must be sensible restraints upon what can be used to enable people to be as healthy as is reasonable in a just and wealthy society.

In the end, though, solving the cutoff problem and the ethical dilemma posed by rationing of any sort—and, by extension, proposing a sensible approach to constraining healthcare costs—is fundamentally a moral problem in the realm of social justice. We could resolve the issue utilizing a methodology that continues to maintain the vast inequities in access and outcomes that is the current state of affairs in the United States. To do so would be to persist in relying on a system that serves only some people well, many adequately, and inordinate numbers of people poorly or not at all. It seems unconscionable to support a system that is inherently unjust, in which so many must do with so little when the consequences can be so grim. In much the same way that few of us would refuse to help a drowning child when to do so would cost us little, it seems we can similarly extend the enormous benefits of modern medicine to all as a matter of both compassion and moral equity.

2

CHARACTERISTICS USED
AS CUTOFF POINTS

In the previous chapter, I introduced some general features of the cutoff problem and briefly illustrated them with a couple of examples. I explained that a central attribute of rationing, or limiting access or distribution of a good or resource that people want and/or need, is the decision of who should get what and how much of it. This entails deciding where the boundaries or cutoffs should be. Because we are discussing healthcare that can play an enormously beneficial role in the individual and collective well-being of a population by relieving suffering, extending life, and so forth, it is inherently a moral enterprise. This means that the strategies that are used to generate cutoffs and the methods employed to impose them are of paramount importance to judging them to be morally justifiable. I now wish to examine the challenge this presents in greater detail and closely examine some of the most frequently discussed characteristics about patients and their conditions that have been proposed as cutoff measures by other scholars. I will offer substantive critiques of these various proposals and argue that they are fundamentally flawed on both moral and practical grounds because they fail to adequately address the cutoff problem.

I have argued that a fair, equitable, and generous system of rationing healthcare in the United States would require restricting the availability of some potentially beneficial (to some people) interventions. This is the essence of rationing: it would be meaningless to limit access to something no one needs or wants or to patently obvious ineffective treatments. Currently, we ration haphazardly and inequitably, almost always on the basis of the financial ability to pay for services. For example, we discourage (i.e., limit) the use of diagnostic and therapeutic interventions by assigning increasingly onerous co-payments and higher annual deductibles. In and of itself, this may not pose a problem, but the amounts are not graded or proportional to income, and hence this leads to less healthcare for those with less money even if they may be clinically similar—and hence with a similar ability to benefit—to those with greater financial resources. If we were to go about designing a more rational—and more fair—rationing plan, this would necessarily have to apply to everyone—and hence be universal—in order for it to work properly and achieve significant constraints on spending. However, if the system were too generous or lenient, other than offering a wide range of healthcare benefits to all, it would not realize one of the other primary goals of reforming our healthcare system: curtailing out-of-control expenditures and avoiding financial catastrophe in the future. There thus must be a metric that is used to demarcate between what is reasonable to offer to people (and pay for) and what is not. Other writers have proposed formalized approaches using features of people (for example age) or of the community (e.g., money) as convenient and justifiable methods to ration care. In this chapter, I will critically assess a number of these views. I will analyze them from at least two points of view: their practical workability, as well as their moral justification, utilizing a scale in which I judge their ability to withstand a test of equity and fairness to all, especially those who suffer not only straightforward medical diseases but the social ills that frequently accompany poverty, disability, and the like. They all suffer, more or less, from the cutoff problem for which an adequate solution is lacking. In the end, I will argue that this obstacle forms a fatal flaw for each.

I think it important that I begin my argument by setting forth a fairly broad definition for what may be reasonable goals for healthcare (and medicine in particular) because it will help frame the discussion that follows throughout the rest of the book. While it is frequently stated (and assumed) that the sole aim of medicine is to cure, although noble, it is nonetheless both hubristic and a relatively modern conception. After all, for the vast majority of the history of humanity, although attempts to interfere with disease or (broadly defined) cure might have been a hopeful intention, they have been little more than that. Indeed, it is only within the past 100–125 years that this has become a more realistic endeavor, at least for some illnesses. But, for the vast majority of the conditions that affect modern technological society, cure is equivalent to management or minimizing and coping with symptoms and forestalling or possibly preventing complications.

In essence, medicine is a moral enterprise because it is directed to the understanding and relief of human suffering caused directly (and indirectly) by illness. We are all susceptible to falling sick and needing the assistance of others to fend off and cope with the effects of disease. It is this shared liability to similar bodily misfortune and the dedication to the creation of a corpus of knowledge of etiologies and remedies that makes healthcare such a singularly moral undertaking. Thus, a necessary and sufficient goal of medicine (healthcare) is the relief of (human) suffering.[1] If this assertion is reasonable and accords well with my initial suggestion, then the main question becomes how do we best use the tools we have to relieve suffering, both efficiently and equitably? And what follows from this is the necessary adjunct of deciding politically and socially what resources are reasonable to devote to this enterprise.

If possible (and I believe it is), one would wish to create a resource allocation strategy that is both simple and easily understood by the people it affects as well as straightforward to implement. It would be vitally important to qualify rationing or allocation prioritization methods with this essential caveat: if one is discussing denying a patient or group of patients access to a potentially beneficial intervention because others could benefit more or there is a finite shortage of that resource (e.g., solid organs for transplantation), then one must have in place a mechanism for reallocating the resource in question that is acceptable to both the people to whom the resource is reallocated *and* those to whom it is denied. If the resource is money, then there must be a distribution plan to use the money saved from denying a costly intervention to old people (for example) for a good that has been agreed upon that can justify the denial (such as offering free or subsidized pre-school for all 4-year-olds, assuming all or most would agree to this). But if one were to use the money that was saved to fund a tax cut for the wealthy (for instance), this could be more problematic and certainly less justifiable.

With solid organs like hearts or livers, if A doesn't receive the organ, B will, all other things being equal. Money—being fungible—is much more troublesome and challenging stuff.[2] So, one of the major justifications that adds legitimacy to any rationing scheme is *how* one (re)allocates the "saved" resource and *why*. To a very great extent, then, the moral reasons for a permissible redistribution of resources—especially those resources that are fungible (like money) from important welfare uses such as effective healthcare interventions—is the beneficial intentions and outcome for the other use(s). To be a worthy and worthwhile competitor for funding that otherwise could be allocated to healthcare, these other areas must promote similar enhancements to public welfare, broadly construed. Of course, societies could make rational decisions under some circumstances that some non–health-related distributions may be more important than healthcare; for example, in times of national defense emergencies, a plausible case could be made to divert significant budgetary allotments away from their ordinary commitment to (some) healthcare to military-related expenditures, and this could be justified due to the (perhaps) existential threat posed. Nevertheless, as Daniels and others have argued, modern healthcare (including standard public and social health measures) is sufficiently effective in improving the well-being of people and affording them enriched opportunities to plan and pursue their goals in life that programs offering at least similar amounts of good would be the only morally credible competitors for communally held monies.[3] Most important, however, is how the cutoff lines are decided and where they are drawn, needs to be sufficiently good reasons supporting them to ensure a modicum of legitimacy required in a democracy.

Since my focus is on setting limits in healthcare, ideally, the properties of people or their conditions that would serve as markers or indicators for cutoffs should be clinically relevant in some meaningful way. What we are looking for is some attribute that people either intrinsically have or acquire that can be used as a reasonable, acceptable, and plausible indicator of value for rationing or limiting healthcare. The goals are praiseworthy: to identify one or more characteristics that are clinically determinable and measureable (to the extent this is possible or feasible) and hence quantifiable. It would have to stand the test of practical implementation but be sufficiently malleable to withstand alteration and amendment as newer and more reliable information becomes available. It must additionally cross dimensions or domains so that it would not be so specific that its utility would be limited to highly particular situations and very small groups of people. This seems a very tall order, and there is no doubt that it is. Throughout this book, I shall develop an argument for one feature of clinical healthcare that fits the bill, although far from perfectly. However, the inherent uncertainty that is unavoidable in medicine makes the search for a faultless ideal characteristic virtually impossible. Nevertheless, compared with the alternatives, what I will suggest is likely to be, if not the best, the least worst, as well as the most reasonable to use. As a prelude to initiating the substance of my argument, however, I will begin with a presentation of various other approaches that have been suggested to use as methods for limiting healthcare. I will offer detailed critiques of each in turn to demonstrate how they fail both practically and morally as a basis for healthcare rationing.

Generally speaking (and subjective and empirical research strongly supports the notion), people value not only the consequences of their choices (or those that follow from decisions made for them), but also the manner in which they are made.[4] Thus, the tenets of procedural justice—both the rules governing allocations and the ways in which the rules are formulated—are as important, if not more so, than the results of applications of the rules to distributions. This means that people are prone to accept the lack of access or their perceived loss of some good that could be valuable to them if (and perhaps only if, unless they are so oppressed by an autarchic or dictatorial system that they are resigned to always receiving little) they view the procedure by which allocations are made as fair.[5] Often neglected in these analyses, except in the abstract as in Rawls' notion of "primary goods" or Sen and Nussbuam's "capabilities,"[6] is the distinct nature of what is to be distributed (especially in cases of relative scarcity) and the basis on which inclusions and exclusions will be judged.

Very few rationing schemes are grounded on allocating significant goods conditioned on first-come, first-served conditions.[7] Rather, they appeal to more significant features about people or their condition(s) that would make them more or less deserving of consideration. It is not just the procedure that must meet the demands of justice, but the subject to which the procedure is applied. In the absence of either wanting or being able to give everything to everyone—an idea that is both fiscally foolish and morally indefensible (although perhaps politically palatable)—decisions must be made on where to draw the line(s) on what should be available and for whom and for what reasons. Over the years, a number of features about people (patients), their conditions, and circumstances have been offered as more or less attractive properties that could be employed or exploited to generate cutoff points. Thus, we might consider the age of a person (as has been suggested by a number of writers), or how much money he or she may possess (rarely suggested overtly, but this actually occurs in real-life quite commonly in the United States), or some other feature about him or her that is both practically and perhaps morally relevant to allocation strategies. In this chapter, I will analyze and discuss various proposals and methods that have been suggested as a strategy to utilize to limit the availability of healthcare interventions (rationing); all suffer in one or more ways from the cutoff problem as well as somewhat more morally disturbing features that make them less desirable to use for this purpose. I will begin by looking at money: it is both the most obvious and tempting target for rationing because it is numerically finite and precise, and it is the final arbiter of which healthcare interventions to purchase; by limiting the amount of money available for healthcare, one necessarily places restrictions on what one can buy.

MONEY

There are generally two substantive complaints about the US healthcare system. First, it spends an enormous (and increasing) amount of money per capita and, compared with other wealthy industrialized nations, has little to show for the expense by such measures as infant mortality, longevity, and other metrics.[8] Second (and related to the former), is that we also have massive inequities in access to care and huge numbers of people without a regular source of care (presumably related to lack of health insurance or underinsurance), and we focus a disproportionate amount of our medical attention on high-technology and intensive interventions draining resources away from primary care. In this section, I wish to discuss the first of these two separate, but closely associated, issues.

Few would argue that we are spending too little on healthcare, and most would agree that we must rein-in annual spending and attempt to control healthcare inflation, especially before the major expansion expected when the mass of the baby boomers retire. At first glance, the solution may seem trivial: we should just stop spending so much, and the problem will fix itself. Of course, if we utilized this strategy on a wholesale, nontargeted basis, it would only exacerbate existing inequalities and disparities in healthcare access and outcomes. Furthermore, it is likely that such an approach would prove politically more unpalatable to the public (and their politicians) than would complete reform of the system with the institution of a single-payer system that eliminates most commercialization of healthcare, such as I have proposed.[9] However, there is a certain appeal to simply saying that the way to save money is spend less. That being said, it would be both short-sighted and perhaps foolhardy to restrain access (by rationing goods or medical interventions) without at the same time limiting their unit costs. Less and cheaper should be the bywords. But how to decide less of what and cheaper how? How could this be accomplished? This dilemma presents a direct cutoff problem.

The most straightforward approach might be to expand what already goes on in the United States but in a much more draconian fashion. There is little debate among scholars in the field of health economics that America rations by one's wherewithal to pay for healthcare. While this has resulted in little in the way of cost savings, it certainly does limit what people can have by their ability to pay for it. Even though the Affordable Care Act has enabled millions of Americans to purchase private insurance on both state and federal exchanges, what can be purchased by the less-than-well-off is generally a very high-deductible plan that pretty much only covers catastrophic care. The upshot is that, once again, one is limited to what one can afford, notwithstanding the subsidies that are provided. Those poor people fortunate enough to live in states that have expanded Medicaid may be somewhat better off, and the deductibles and co-pays are (for the most part) minimal to nonexistent. Everyone else—including (and perhaps especially) Medicare recipients—can only access what they can afford to buy. While this is certainly rationing of a kind, it is irrational. It permits people to buy stuff that can't help them (indeed, encourages it), and it bars others from obtaining what could help them if they only had the money to acquire it. While aficionados of the current somewhat free-market system that we currently have will continue to defend what they believe to be its virtues, no serious student of reform and/or cost savings would do so, knowing full well the inherent flaws that will almost inexorably lead to financial disaster, not to mention unconscionably barring millions from effective healthcare. That being said, there are potentially justifiable ways of rationing using dollars as the primary target.

One could set a certain budget in which it is decided how much money to spend on healthcare, pass a budget, and purchase what healthcare one can until the money runs out. Presumably, the budget would be set to provide some predetermined esti-mate of a reasonable range of services, but no more. One would have to be quite strict on the amount of annual inflation one would permit; otherwise, the enterprise would be doomed from the start. Alternatively, one could make a list of healthcare services that were deemed reasonable to provide to the target population—let's say Medicare, for example—and then the budget would be dependent on the cost of those services. To a certain extent, the Medicare budget is more like the second system, with its list of targeted populations, than the second with no current cap. The Oregon Health Plan (OHP) in its original iteration was more similar to the system using a budgeted list of items.[10]

The main ethical challenge of rationing money as the primary target is that it transfers the details of the cutoff decision-making process downstream. The OHP took this approach. The state legislature passed a healthcare budget before it was determined what it would be reasonable to fund and with specific allocation deter-minations (i.e., cutoff points) to be decided later but entailed by the total amount of money that was made available. By limiting the funding first, even interventions that could be highly beneficial to a number of people would necessarily be inacces-sible. Of course, the legislature might argue that by limiting funding for this form of healthcare (for the poor) they had more money to spend on other important pri-orities. However, they could also have raised taxes on wealthier Oregonians to pay for more healthcare for the less well off; instead, they made a choice that resulted in denying some plausibly significant treatments to those who would be otherwise unable to obtain them. Certainly, elected bodies make these sorts of priority-setting decisions all the time, and it is not only healthcare that can suffer from parsimonious legislators who may be reluctant to impose taxes on higher income people to pay for services for public school children (for example).

Part of the challenge is surely a psychological one, the idea being that the value of (effective) healthcare can be equated with certain amounts of money and that some interventions (or even categories of interventions) are less valuable using this metric than others. Many (perhaps most) people, certainly in the United States, seem to have a gut reaction against the idea of assigning monetary values to their lives and what is done to improve or even save them. It somehow seems repellent that lives are not invaluable or incommensurable with economics, even though that is how we articulate value in almost everything else we do. But the truth of the matter of course is that it costs money to deliver healthcare. One cannot expect physicians and nurses to work for free or the companies that make medical equipment or drugs to do so for free (although the role of profit and how much is reasonable is a somewhat different, yet related, topic). Thus, we cannot avoid thinking about cost. Nevertheless, making a priori assumptions about how much healthcare to purchase without specifying what to buy seems arbitrary, if not capricious. Certainly, the cutoffs that result or are imposed will depend on whatever fiscal whims are current or winds are blowing in the legislature at the moment, without due regard paid to the impact they may have on the recipients who depend on this generosity (or lack thereof). Rather than making financial allocation decisions based on the needs to the people who will be served, this approach can have the effect of leaving many out of luck. On the other hand, this method can be contrasted to that taken by Medicare, for example, in which the annual budget is only estimated from year to year because decisions on what is purchased are made much closer to the patient; this unfortunately then incentivizes overuse.

While it may be abhorrent to consider how much it is costing to keep a loved one alive in a permanent vegetative state indefinitely during the emotional heat of the situation (after, say, a traumatic brain injury or a massive heart attack with prolonged oxygen deprivation), there is little question that the expense of doing so is both enormous and of questionable value, assuming that the dollars saved from not doing so could be put to a more valuable or better application. But another crucial aspect of this issue is how to assign a monetary value to various interventions on scales that could then be used both comparatively (between patients) as well as on a population basis to estimate the worth on a ordinal ranking. This brings us to the most popular approach that, not surprisingly, has been employed for rationing healthcare. It attempts to quantitatively assess how people value various health states and assign a monetary amount to each "unit" of an optimally healthy life. These elements can then be compared with one another across various diseases, domains, and the like.

CEA AND QALYS

Of course, healthcare interventions cost money because of the equipment and disposable supplies required, the infrastructure necessary to carry out the interventions, and the highly trained personnel needed to decide which interventions are appropriate and then administer them. As we well know, modern, technologically sophisticated medicine is a hugely expensive affair, and it is often difficult to gauge what represents a "good deal" analogous to the purchase and acquisition of other goods and services that we routinely judge to be "worth" the money paid. The complication is that we tend to rate some things more than others, both for their intrinsic significance as well as their instrumental value when they permit us to pursue other aims and goals. Health clearly has components of both, and because its valuation can be so subjective it can be extremely difficult and imprecise to attach a monetary amount per unit of worthiness to an individual, much less to her family and society. Moreover, people and their health states and how much they treasure them (or not) often can be incommensurable, making comparisons quite challenging. Nevertheless, attempts have been made to do so and hence create mechanisms by which numerically derivative cutoffs can be used to draw the limits of healthcare access and avail-ability. The critical question, as introduced in the previous section, is how much healthcare is it worthwhile to buy? If we decide to spend x amount on healthcare, what is the best value we can get for our money? As the rest of this chapter unfolds, I will repeatedly stress that I believe this to be the wrong way of looking at things in a wealthy society. It is not that we shouldn't be looking at maximizing efficiency; instead, simply, it is a moral error to do so at the expense of the most vulnerable *when we can afford otherwise.* I will begin by describing an unfortunate but all-too-real clinical scenario.

Imagine that you have been involved in a terrible and freakish accident at the beach shortly after your 25th birthday. As you run into the surf, you are hit by an unexpectedly large wave in the shallows, you are knocked off your feet, and hit the back of your neck on a submerged rock. Instantly, your life changes forever because you have suffered burst fractures of your third and fourth cervical vertebrae. The spinal cord in this region is crushed, and you stop breathing because your diaphragm and all other muscles and sensation below the neck are now paralyzed. Fortunately, the trained lifeguards on duty observe the accident, and they reach you before you drown or die from lack of oxygen. They immediately begin cardiopulmonary resus-citation techniques, stabilize your neck and head with a brace collar, and call 911. You are transported to the nearest hospital, a major academic medical center specializing in spinal cord injuries. You are placed in the ICU and given large doses of dexameth-asone (a corticosteroid) to attempt to minimize the swelling and prevent any further damage. However, the destruction is permanent. At best, you will require a mechani-cal ventilator to breathe and full-time care to see to your basic bodily needs such as bathing, dressing, bowel and bladder functions, and feeding. With new technol-ogy, you will probably be able to communicate by mouthing words and using a blow tube and/or eye movement-activated computerized speech and typing devices. Even under the most optimal of circumstances with the best care available, you may only live another 10–15 years due to the many complications such patients have because of their condition. Given these facts about your current limitations, the severity of your disabilities, and your guarded prognosis, would you want to live under these circumstances, or would you wish to be given some sedatives and have the ventilator turned off so you could die? If the former, how would you rate the quality of your life?

Many people who are well and reasonably physically able-bodied, especially those in the "bloom of youth" would readily endorse the tragedy of this scenario and either say they would rather die, or, if forced to live under these severely reduced circum-stances or opportunities, would assess their quality of life as poor. Of course, this is a hypothetical situation, similar in many ways to the sorts of questions random people are asked in assessments of health-related quality of life. It turns out, however, that people are incredibly resilient, and many are able to adapt to states of affairs that their premorbid selves (or others) could not begin to envisage coming to terms with.[11] And physicians may be the worst offenders in their ability (or lack of it) to accurately assess the quality of life experienced by their ill patients.[12] Of course, there is an important caveat, as the quality of life of many disabled people is directly affected by the support they receive, especially with respect to maximizing their opportunities and residual abilities.[13] Most important, however, is the fact that assessments of hypothetical quality of life after an injury, onset of a chronic illness, or some other conjectured or imagined situation is simply that: anchored in the mind's eye and colored with all of the associated historically based thoughts that can accompany any invented abstraction. One truly has little accurate idea of how one would react when presented with the actual situation and the torrent of fears and emotions that can accompany it.[14] Yet, this is the way that health economists and others assess and gauge the utility of various health states to incorporate into *cost-effectiveness analysis* (CEA).[15]

As Weinstein and Stason defined it almost 40 years ago, CEA can be described thus:

> The underlying premise of cost-effectiveness analysis in health problems is that, for any given level of resources available, society (or the decision-making jurisdiction involved) wishes to maximize the total aggregate health benefits conferred. Alternatively, for a given health-benefit goal, the objective is to minimize the cost of achieving it. . . . Health-resource costs are inevitably measured in dollars. Health benefits, or health effectiveness, may be expressed in a variety of ways, the most common being either lives or life years, or some variant of them. The use of "quality adjusted life years" [QALY] has the advantage of incorporating changes in survival and morbidity in a single measure that reflects trade-offs between them. The ratio of costs, expressed as cost per year of life saved or cost per quality-adjusted year of life saved, becomes the cost-effectiveness measure. Alternative programs or services are then ranked, from the lowest value of this cost-per-effectiveness ratio to the highest, and selected from the top until available resources are exhausted. The point on the priority list at which the available resources are exhausted, or at which society is no longer willing to pay for the benefits achieved, becomes society's cutoff level of permissible cost per unit effectiveness.[16]

Importantly, CEA utilizes the *health utility function*. This is a method of expressing the usefulness of a particular state of (personal) affairs (related to his or her health) to an individual, as well as to the society in which that person lives and the personal as well as communal resources used to bring about desired states of affairs. As Torrance explains, "a simple definition of utility is that it is a cardinal measure of the strength of one's preference."[17] With some modifications to the method in which the list was created, this was indeed the method used by the state of Oregon in the late 1980s to develop the OHP.[18] An ordinal list of various condition–treatment pairings was created with the ranking according to health utility or CEA (incorporating QALYs; see later discussion). For example, acute appendicitis was listed with appendectomy as a treatment and streptococcal pharyngitis was paired with amoxicillin (or some other suitable antibiotic). In Oregon, the legislature decided how much money it wished to spend on indigent healthcare and, depending upon certain demographic and epidemiological estimates and predictions, that would determine what amount and kinds of healthcare could be purchased during a given budget period. This is an unvarnished example of what I have called "budget-priority" or "dollar-priority" healthcare rationing, in which the amount of money available is set first and how far down on the list one could go was determined by how much money was available to spend, exactly as stated by Weinstein and Stason. Of course, the difference in health utility between the last fundable item on the list and the one next down is likely to be quite small, irrespective of how far down the actual budget permits it to go. Hence, while the quantification aspects of CEA make it extremely attractive for setting limits and establishing firm cutoff points, especially when coupled with a finite amount of money, the boundary problem is still a significant issue, as would be apparent to anyone affected by a condition–treatment pairing that just missed the line.

Nevertheless, these criticisms do not mean that CEA has no relevance to cost-conscious decision-making in healthcare resource allocation. I would argue that it most certainly does. The question is whether it should play a controlling role as it did in Oregon and as it so often does in (for example) pharmaceutical formulary decisions today. Its emphasis on analyzing the costs of outcomes that are hypothetically important to people such as symptom reduction or years of life gained can serve as extremely useful arbiters of both financial and clinical value of a given intervention. The decision about whether the *value* of a treatment or a diagnostic test—it's cost per QALY or any other validated metric one might wish to employ—is *valuable* to the population both affected by the illness and those who must pay for it (which should ideally be one and the same, broadly understood) is in essence a political question.[19] This interpretation however, would mandate a financing approach to healthcare that, *contra* Oregon, is "intervention priority," in which it is decided what is reasonable to pay for first (but not completely blinded to the costs). I will discuss this point later.

One of the truly admirable features of CEA (and related approaches) is its emphasis on actual outcomes as opposed to biological or other endpoints that may bear little relation to what matters to most people. There are exceptions, though, such as blood pressure measurements as a determinant of the effectiveness of anti-hypertensive therapy and serum cholesterol and high-density lipoprotein (HDL) levels in response to cholesterol-lowering interventions. Some of the most expensive and least beneficial interventions in terms of actual effects on the lives of patients that have been introduced over the past 25 years have been based on biological or other surrogate markers that have little connection to what most people with advanced cancer (for example) care about, such as meaningful life extension, relief of burdensome symptoms, and the like.[20] But like any population-based analytic system, CEA employs aggregates in its assessments and assigns weights constructed from data obtained from generalized groups; applying these judgments to individual patients can be extremely difficult.

Any given country or society—say, the United States, for example—that is committed to endorsing the proposition that each of its citizens (and his or her life) counts as equally valuable to the state (and presumably to each individual as well) could be potentially extremely disturbed by the application of QALYs (and their base corollary, CEA) in the distribution of scarce resources due to what has been called the "aggregation problem" or the philosophical and moral challenge of applying utilitarian principles to things that matter to people.[21] When this is done, the lives of individuals matter much less than the averaged or aggregated "lives" of the population for whom the technique is used. A morally significant concern with the use of QALYs and one that stems directly from its inherent aggregative method, is that it fails to pay due concern and attention to issues of equity for individuals, especially the worse off due to health (broadly construed). Inasmuch as utilizing QALYs aims to maximize overall health results from interventions (as well as controlling costs), it ignores the greater needs (and poorer health with poorer outcomes) of those who are worse off to begin with. It thus devotes more resources to those whose "bang for the buck" would be greater and hence tends to reject some of the cardinal principles of distributive justice. Since numerous surveys have suggested that many societies believe in both greater health equity and giving priority or preferences to the most gravely ill first,[22] considerations that standard CEA utilizing QALYs essentially disregard, there have been numerous suggestions on how to modify QALYs and/or incorporate these views into CEA.[23]

On the other hand, even though it is an aggregate function, QALYs are predicated upon the assumption that people value not only how long they live (the time integer) but also how those years are lived (the quality integer). The QALY is equivalent to the product of the two and set with a maximum of 1.0 (perfect health and quality for 1 year) and a minimum of 0.0 (death).[24] How one goes about determining how people view the value of life with various health conditions and the functional quality of how life can be lived with those abilities (or lack of them) and for how long is key. Should one survey physicians with knowledge and experience of caring for a range of patients with a particular disease, for example? Or would it be better and more germane to gather the views of patients with the actual disease and the experience of living with it? Or, should one simply examine the opinions of a large number of the general public? Which should count, and how should they be weighted in the final assessment? The techniques that are employed to elicit peoples' views (irrespective of which population is studied) are also important and can influence the results.[25] It is true that most experts in the field who believe that QALYs can contribute a great deal to matters of allocation and prioritization of scarce resources endorse these methodologies as reliable and valid.[26] Even so, there is evidence that people's preferences can be both labile and subject to significant "framing effects" during the interviews and questionnaires that form the very basis for calculating QALYs; this certainly can give one pause in evaluating how justifiable they are.[27] Nonetheless, this is often how QALYs are determined for specific health states and then combined with economic cost data to yield CEA assessments. Since QALYs emphasize summative totals of health gains or losses (per unit cost) in a population of people, they would seem particularly poor to apply to the United States, with its long tradition of extolling personal freedom and the autonomy of the individual. Indeed, believing oneself to be simply another anonymous QALY-cog in a healthcare system seems sure to inspire the animus of huge numbers of Americans who, rightly or wrongly, believe themselves in large part to be in control of many aspects of their lives. The illusion of mastery over one's fate in the healthcare system, as exemplified by the backlash against the managed care reform debacle of the 1990s, is illustrative of this conviction.[28]

Irrespective of how one may criticize the various methods for calculating QALYs, they do possess the virtue of being comparable across different health domains (and the people afflicted with those conditions) and thus useful for evaluating cost variations that produce similar results and "health utility." When two interventions are therapeutically (or diagnostically) equivalent, to the extent this is knowable by the best available scientific information, it is both reasonable and, I would argue, quite correct to choose between them based at least in part (if not wholly) by their cost. All things being equal, one would naturally choose the cheaper.[29] Unfortunately, this situation is encountered all too rarely. More commonly, there are what could be considered substantive clinical variations between competing interventions such as side effect or toxicity profiles, convenience to patients, and accessibility. Nevertheless, in a financially strapped or challenged system, it makes sense to disregard many of these differences in order to highlight efficiency, as determined by cost savings. And, even if by all usual measures, two (or more) interventions are identical in their benefits *for populations*, there is little doubt that one will be significantly better for some *individual people* than the other, irrespective of cost (meaning that the less expensive could be better for some or vice versa). In the United States, we have customarily and historically permitted physicians and their patients to decide on an independent basis which alternatives to choose for their specifically determined needs; indeed, this is one of the fundamental rationales underpinning the continued acceptance of off-label use of Food and Drug Administration (FDA)-approved medications. But cost-saving measures have put a severe crimp in this liberty to choose, even in this country, by the imposition of prior authorization procedures, pharmacy formulary limitations, and the like.

In the United Kingdom, where the National Institute for Clinical Excellence (NICE) explicitly utilizes QALYs to analyze cost effectiveness of new treatments, diagnostics, technology and so on, the challenge is how to judge the worth or value of novel interventions that offer what could be called "incremental benefits" (if they demonstrated major gains, no matter how one defined "major," that would be simpler).[30] Over the past decade or so, NICE has made major efforts to include "social value judgments" in its deliberations so as to balance the strictly utilitarian modus of "a QALY is a QALY is a QALY" with the demands of equity and the needs of the disabled and especially the terminally ill.[31] In some localities in the United States, programs analogous to NICE have been created, one of the more interesting being the New England Comparative Effectiveness Public Advisory Council, which evaluates various medical interventions for efficacy and "value." They have developed a methodology employing what they call a "comparative value evidence table" that incorporates all of the metrics that stakeholders will find useful to consider in their deliberations.[32]

While the attraction of using a quantifiable benchmark like the QALY is simple to understand due to its presumed universalizability, broad applicability, and comparability, there are significant concerns—and not only the ones I have already mentioned. One of the most worrisome is the fact that CEA/QALY definitively has a cutoff problem that is difficult to resolve. As nice as NICE may be in England, it is merely advisory and its recommendations are at the mercy of the budget-makers in Parliament. Unlike Medicare here in the United States, the budget of which is not fixed until after the money is spent, in the United Kingdom they have to decide how much it is reasonable to spend on healthcare *first*, which of course raises the fundamental question of where to impose the cutoff. There is little reason to believe that the threshold for purchasing interventions has a sharp boundary between what Parliament thinks is acceptable and what is not. Similarly, the threshold for what is adequate or acceptable to spend for a QALY is difficult to determine: why should a life be worth spending $100,000/year to save and not worth spending $101,000? Most important, the justifications for these sorts of cutoffs are extremely thin. Rather than stating that a specific intervention is sufficiently effective that the cost (whatever it may be) is hence worthwhile to support, QALY people resort to analyzing the situation from the wrong end. Even though the National Health Service in its founding documents was dedicated to meeting the health needs of British subjects, they are still enslaved to the budgetary master in a way that those needs can only be met if the financial wherewithal is dedicated to that purpose.[33] For a fiscally constrained nation, tight budgets necessarily should be the tail that wags the dog; in wealthy countries devoted to the welfare and well-being of their residents, that view could be reconsidered.

Unfortunately, the clinical differences between quantitatively or numerically close QALY values above or below whatever is decided to be the cutoff, irrespective of whether the boundary is set by fiscal limitations or an arbitrary QALY number for some other reason, is minimal and hence also arbitrary. Even a generous healthcare budget that utilizes QALYs for distributive purposes would guarantee such capricious imposition of cutoffs between two closely positioned QALYs without meaningful differences between them. The inability to distinguish substantive discrepancies between adjacent or closely related QALYs means that the moral and practical clinical predicaments entailed by the cutoff problem are not solved by employing this approach to rationing.

QALYs and CEA have the virtue of being based on determinant value (both monetarily and subjectively evaluative) derived from the beliefs and views of real people, as opposed to being only theoretical. They also describe clinical situations and the value that people place on the quality of life associated with those health states, at least in the hypothetical abstract. Finally, because they are reduced to ordinal units, they can be compared across starkly different diseases, ages, and other characteristics. My concern is with the impersonal and detached mechanism by which they are applied to suffering people. While I do not dispute the fact that money to fund healthcare in the United States is not limitless and hence a cutoff must be made, we are far from the situations present in less wealthy countries where the discretion with which their wealth can be dispensed is much more confined than it is in this country. Our wealth gives us the luxury of choices. In some respects, severely restricted fiscal resources are, in some respects, similar to the situation that we face with solid organ transplantation, in which the number of livers, hearts, and kidneys is reasonably finite so that allocation decisions must be based on that finitude. Considerations of efficiency and equity, while often in tension, are of paramount concern and can be directly related to QALY and CEA determinations. But dollars are not nearly so rare as donor hearts. To rely on a quantitative, unemotional method of determining value and for whom seems both cold-hearted and potentially ungenerous when there is little compelling reason to be that way.

AGE

Having considered QALYs and CEA as a method of creating cutoffs and showing that, by quantifying differences based on subjective preferences for various health states integrated with the costs of diagnosing and treating them, they do little to resolve the cutoff problem, I now turn to age. In the previous chapter, I briefly introduced the use of an individual's age for purposes of limiting the availability of healthcare interventions. I will now discuss this issue in greater detail and demonstrate its flaws. Unlike the hypothetical and abstract information on which QALYs are based and constructed, age has the attractive advantages that it is easily quantified, it is a feature everyone possesses, and, roughly speaking, it correlates more or less with accumulated medical conditions. In modern, industrialized nations like the United States, older people die more than younger and tend, as a population, to be on average sicker: hence, the allure of age as a healthcare cutoff benchmark and its utility as a proxy of illness.

Ezekiel Emanuel wants to die soon. In the year 2032, it's curtains for the well-known bioethicist. The 58 year old (as of 2015) wants to die when he's 75, thus outdoing Daniel Callahan's "three-score and ten" by 5 years. Professor Callahan chose the Biblically famous marker of a complete life to indicate when it would be reasonable to cease providing anything other than comfort and palliative care to those who were ill.[34] Emanuel announced his intentions in the popular press, thus expanding the audience for what would otherwise have been a very restricted group of readers had he published his essay in an academic journal. Like Callahan, Dr. Emanuel claims that he would have achieved anything and all that one could wish for by that age—a family with grown and now independent children, meaningful professional accomplishments, and sufficient numbers of satisfying experiences—and that to ask for more would be almost superfluous or gratuitous. Because of his interests in healthcare delivery and its costs, he relates his view to the explosion in medical expenditures in the elderly with the associated steadily diminishing returns in terms of quality of life.[35] Since he is also an opponent of the practice of physician-assisted suicide, he, of course, does not advocate for helping debilitated seniors on their way, and he also does not advise suicide to others except as a personal choice.[36] For himself, he would choose to live any time after age 75 the best he could but would refuse life-sustaining or extending intensive therapies and opt for simple (and cheap) methods to maintain his quality of life until that were no longer tenable or tolerable.

While he does not suggest that his view should be a mandate for others, it can be assumed that his very public persona and the venue in which he chose to present his views is meant to serve as a stimulus for a civic (and, it is to be hoped, civil) debate on the merits of providing such a disproportionate share of our healthcare budget to people who (he believes) cannot benefit from it nearly as much as those who are younger. He thus continues the ongoing discussion about what sorts of attributes about people, their diseases or conditions, their social situation, and the like can or should serve as targets on which to base healthcare rationing. But he, like many others, seems to employ age as a useful marker or indicator of functional ability rather than simply an ordinal symbol for how long one has been alive. While it is no doubt true that diminution of physical and mental or cognitive capacities decreases roughly proportional to one's age, there are ample examples of people in their 40s who are paralyzed or who suffer disorders that lead to permanent loss of intellectual aptitude. Similarly, there are many people—and Emanuel very well may be one of them if he permits himself to live long enough—who retain their wits and mental acuity well into their dotage. Surrogate markers for function are not nearly as useful as the function itself; we only use them when access to the actual function is difficult or impossible to ascertain and the correlative connection between the two is extremely close and precise. We can determine quite well the things that matter to most people—their ability to be mobile, have reasonable functional independence, and to be aware and interact with their surroundings (including other people)—and we really have no need to utilize a surrogate such as age. Nonetheless, these simple facts don't stop people from forging ahead.

Why would anyone think that age would be a reasonable and justifiable—both on medical-scientific and moral grounds—focus for rationing? As suggested by Emanuel's essay in the lay press and documented extensively elsewhere, there is little question that the elderly are not only getting older as a percentage of the US population as well as a subgroup, but are consuming increasing amounts of healthcare services along the way. While there is little doubt that modern, First World medicine has contributed in a significant way to people being able to live longer, these people are doing so at the expense of accumulating larger numbers of chronic medical conditions which themselves are of escalating complexity. With this comes an ever-accumulating quantity of medications needed to manage these multiple illnesses—many of which may be clinically silent—and, not surprisingly, produce surging costs. Moreover, while there is reason to believe that most of these illnesses are manageable, they are often incurable, and the efficacy of treatment per unit cost yields somewhat diminishing returns as persons age. These observations should not negate the fact that there are legions of senior citizens in the United States and other wealthy industrialized countries who enjoy both a very high standard of living and prolonged and excellent quality of life. Yet, many do not. Finally, because so much is spent in the last years of life (especially the final year), there is correspondingly less emphasis and dollars devoted to the young who may be able to take better advantage of the resources. Therefore, it seems to make sense to redirect money to children and non-elderly adults and hence restrict the interventions available to the old. If this view is acceptable, what could be the problems with it?

The first, and perhaps the most substantive, objection would be a moral one: to justify intentional discrimination against the aged, as reflected in restricting access to some kinds and/or amounts of healthcare interventions, would require good reasons to do so. In a wealthy country such as the United States that could be prepared (and afford) to be generous in its distribution of healthcare and its benefits, draconian restrictions for the elderly, *simply because they were old*, would be difficult—if not impossible—to justify.[37] Nevertheless, one reason advanced to utilize the elderly to save healthcare expenditures is that old people have already had their fair share of society's resources when they were young, and they have thus "used up" a substantial amount already. Furthermore, because they have fewer years left to live (on average), their ability to efficiently use the advantages conferred by effective healthcare interventions would be less than for younger people. Of course, medicine is increasingly effective at permitting people who get sick at young ages to live to become old, so one would have to account for those individuals who consumed much more than an average amount of healthcare resources earlier in life for, say, a successful treatment of cancer.

This argument might be somewhat acceptable if there were a societal consensus that this would be how to treat older people, but this is lacking. While Western societies may not (in general) possess the same kind of veneration for the elderly that is so much a part of some Asian cultures, we certainly don't ignore old people altogether. It seems to me that the best defense of limiting healthcare resources for the elderly might be because of a postulated limited ability to benefit from *some* (by no means all) interventions simply because they have fewer years to live than if the same resources were expended on the young. However, this only makes sense if there is a finite amount of money for everyone and choices such as this must be made. A good example of an analogous situation might be the case with solid organ transplants: it would be preferable to give a liver to a 45-year-old patient rather than a 65-year-old patient. If the transplant were successful, the young person would have more years to live with the organ than would the older patient. And this argument only works if we can show that the organ will last longer in the 45-year-old than in the 65-year-old (in general) because the former would naturally have longer to live than the latter, all things being equal. But, if the average transplanted liver allowed a patient to live only 10 more years, assuming the older patient was otherwise as healthy as the younger, they both could benefit equally from the surgery, assuming they both also valued each year of life equally. But the data—at least for liver transplants—suggest that patients may live longer than 10 years, thus favoring or privileging younger over older recipients.[38] Finally, as I mentioned earlier, while it is certainly true that *as a population* old people (which is in itself a term that needs to be defined) are sicker *as a group* and use more healthcare resources than the young, that observation cannot be plausibly applied to *individuals* (I will discus this point in greater detail in Chapter 4).

It is a trivial, but nonetheless important, fact of life that we all age, and we all die. Indeed, age is probably one of the only—and certainly the most recognizable—universal, shared, continuously changing variable characteristics of human beings. Other traits are either almost always (mostly) fixed at conception or birth, such as (biological) gender, and others change for only a period during one's life, such as height. Even those who are unfortunate to die at a relatively young age are older than they were at a previous time. However, this only becomes relevant to lives that pass through socially and, to a certain extent, biologically determined phases. These include infancy, childhood, and adolescence during which we physically, emotionally, and cognitively mature. Next comes early adulthood, when we go out into the world and set ourselves up as more or less independent. At this stage, we may also explore and establish relationships with others, including prospective mates to start a family, including offspring. This is followed by the middle years in which we watch our family grow and age, finally ending with the senior years, which, in advanced industrialized nations, is usually associated with retirement from the workforce. Each period is distinguished by characteristic abilities and capacities (often succeeded in the next by their diminution or deterioration). Modern healthcare has mitigated many of the most significant sources of suffering and loss, especially in the last years of life, but for many this description still rings true.[39]

Norman Daniels has given one of the most complete accounts of justifiable healthcare rationing on the basis of age in his "prudential lifespan" proposition. He argues that rational agents deciding under conditions of a "thin" Rawlsian veil of ignorance about themselves (but not about the society in which they live) would design institutions to distribute healthcare resources in such a way that they account for prudential considerations over a lifetime. One's need for healthcare and what one can accomplish by its efficacy are dependent on the range and kinds of opportunities available. He believes that a prudent individual would most likely wish to spend more of his resources on his younger—and more productive—years and less on his old age (whatever it is decided that might be).[40] Importantly, he employs the conceit that one should consider how resources are utilized over an entire *individual's* life. Thus, there is equality between lives because the amount spent is the same, just differentially allocated depending on the age of the person. This strategy should be separated from standard sorts of age rationing arguments that prioritize *groups* of people over others. By his appeal to single lives rather than cohorts of similarly aged people, he avoids the charge of age discrimination (age being considered a morally irrelevant characteristic comparable to skin color or gender). As he explains: "The 75-year-old and the 55-year-old will not be treated differently over the course of their lives. Before each is 75, he will be entitled to the life-extending treatment in question; afterwards, he will not. Thus treating someone now 75 differently from someone now 55 does not constitute unequal treatment of the whole person over his lifetime."[41]

Daniels's prioritizing of the claims of the young to more healthcare resources over the old is predicated on the assumption that there are strict limits to how much there is to spend on healthcare; otherwise, there would be no need to restrict what would be available to any age. The only constraints might be those imposed by patients on what they could conceivably want or need and physicians on what they thought reasonable to provide. Indeed, while there are some limitations on the amounts and kinds of interventions that can be obtained (at any age), the elderly in the United States have almost inexhaustible access to interventions (at the present time). The same is true at the other end of life, as the annual sums expended on neonatal intensive care will attest. We act as if there is no fiscal ceiling. Of course, we also do not have rational plans for prudent expenditures, irrespective of the age of the patient and his or her history of prior healthcare cost use. That being said, we do have limitations on what we can (and should) spend on healthcare, hence imposing a finite maximum on the available funds and thus necessitating some sort of rationing.

The "prudential lifespan" method is not a direct argument for age-based differential allocation of healthcare resources. All Daniels is saying is that the prudent individual, deciding for her own life, would quite reasonably resolve to distribute healthcare dollars weighted toward her younger, more productive years so long as there would be funds remaining to provide the sorts of interventions that might be more useful to her elderly self. Under certain conditions of constrained or scarce resources, society (as well as the prudent person) could decide to more heavily favor expenditures for some kinds of costly interventions for the young over the old. For example, this could include less emphasis on expensive life-prolonging treatments that may add weeks to months to the life of an older patient but at significant financial and disability costs, with greater prominence given to those interventions that could maintain or improve quality of life with consequent preservation of the opportunities to enjoy one's remaining time.

Nevertheless, there are two important questions left unanswered in this view. The first is whether it would be reasonable and morally justifiable to ration money (i.e., some healthcare resources) on the basis of age if money were limited; and second, how we would go about defining where the cutoff point(s) might be. What age(s) would be classified as young and old for the purposes of resource allocation? And could we reasonably assume that the money saved by restricting resources for the old would be utilized in a manner so as to produce as much, if not greater, good for society (for example)? As Daniels (and others) have noted, age is employed by US society quite readily to demarcate significant borders for access to various benefits and entitlements. For example, even though there is growing evidence that the brain does not socially or cognitively reach final adult maturity until well into the third decade, people can vote in all elections at age 18. At this same age, they can also have all the other rights associated with legal adulthood, including entering into contracts. In arguing that this age is somewhat arbitrary and unattached to biological facts are two observations: first, in a nod to neurophysiological reality, the legal age for drinking alcohol is 21 (although generally not for buying tobacco products, which is variously 18 or 19 years),[42] and, second, the voting and age of majority was lowered to 18 years due to political pressure during the Vietnam War (along with eliminating the draft[43]).[44] While these age boundaries were created for practical and political reasons with only a limited basis in neurobiological reality, applying a similar approach to age for the purposes of healthcare rationing would be fraught with social and moral peril.

I would be surprised if self-interest did not have a major impact on the outcome of such deliberations. Even within the confines of the notion that the transfer or allocation of resources would be within one's own lifetime and not between individuals (and generations of different people), I suspect it would be difficult for many—if not most—people to grasp the concept of these prudential sorts of distributions. They might well view such transfers as from what was owed to me by others who did not *deserve* such benefits. This would be especially true if there were means-based allocations such that less well-off individuals would receive resources much greater than their contributions, either in the past or prospectively for the future. Still, my goal is not to either attack or defend the use of age as an ethically justifiable criterion for rationing of healthcare resources (although I think it imprudent). Rather, I simply present this discussion to demonstrate that many people have employed it in such as fashion. But they do so by focusing on the easy part: defending the transfer of goods and services between the young and old either without saying how people qualify for membership in these categories or by describing in detail why a cutoff at a particular point was imposed. Moreover, in general, the problem of those people close to either side of the boundary is ignored.

At the same time, it is worth noting that favoring the young over the old in the allocation of scarce resources—although not necessarily resources in general—accords with our emotional and moral intuitions. And it is at least plausible—although highly unlikely—that older people might be magnanimous in forgoing claims on such a large percentage of the nation's healthcare budget once presented with the facts of future fiscal calamity (recall the story I related in Chapter 1 about my retired neurosurgeon colleague querying his neighbors about ventilator allocation during an influenza pandemic). There are at least four problems with this suggestion. First, younger seniors might not be nearly as magnanimous, especially for children who were closer to them in age. Second, there is also no way to tell how big the difference in ages would have to be for it to be significant (in either direction). Third, this only applies to a decision about the allocation of a scarce, life-saving resource (say, a ventilator) and not something of considerably less value, such as an item that might be thought elective or trivial or one that is needed but could be foregone without irreparable harm or suffering. And finally, it is distinctly possible that the views of seniors would be influenced by their own history, relationships, and health, with the latter perhaps being most influential. If an older person had numerous chronic conditions and debility, he or she might more readily relinquish any claim to life-preserving resources if a choice had to be made. Most importantly, perhaps, is that the various attempts to incrementally reduce Medicare benefits, increase the age of eligibility, or radically change the program to one utilizing private insurance have all met with a storm of protest.

However, Callahan, Daniels, and Emanuel (and others following a similar vein of thought) have all ignored the inescapable problem of cutoffs. Unless, that is, they decide to take the approach of the law, which has generally ignored the subtleties and ramifications of making somewhat arbitrary boundaries based on continuous variables. The law is not deaf to the fuzziness of these boundaries and their sometimes poor relationship to facts of life (including neurocognitive development), but a line must be drawn somewhere and it must be simple to understand and serve as an obvious delimiter of access to certain rights, privileges, and other goods. The law may be a blunt instrument, but should healthcare and decisions about who is entitled to what be as blind and indifferent to these differences between people? Yet the most important problem with strict cutoff points utilizing age is the very real fact that there is no salient difference between people very close in age if years lived is the criterion or characteristic we consider. The minute someone turns 21, he can legally purchase and consume an alcoholic beverage, but that does not mean that he is psychologically or biologically ready to do so. Age is used as a convenient surrogate for neurophysiology (in the case of determining maturity for would-be drinkers), but it is a poor one. Medicine is interested in a patient's age, but only as one indicator among many. Just as one's ability or virtue should not be judged by one's gender or skin color, health status should not be assumed by one's age. Any attempt to utilize age as a surrogate for healthcare need can only be viewed as arbitrary and hence oblivious to important moral distinctions between people. It is this that marks it as blatantly unfair.

In the end analysis, though, the basic justification for limiting healthcare resources for the elderly—if one must restrict them somehow—is a belief that older people may need less healthcare than younger people because the former derive less benefit from it either because they have less time left to live or that, in the elderly, diseases that even occur in the young may be more difficult to treat. The latter suggests then that older people may "deserve" intensive healthcare less than younger people because they are older. Of course, seniors are also closer to death—either natural or otherwise—and everyone has to die of something. It might also be assumed (incorrectly, I believe) that older people value a year of reasonably decent (not debilitating) health less than a younger person. While it may be a valid point to suggest that a (much) younger individual could derive more benefit from a curative treatment than a (much) older person if there were severe limitations on the amount of the treatment available, such is not the case in most of the common situations I am discussing. There is little question that a wealthy country like the United States has sufficient capacity to support curative treatments for *both* the young and the old. Similarly, we might examine the utility of providing marginally beneficial interventions for *anyone*, regardless of their age (I will discuss this more in Chapters 3 and 7).[45] Another relevant question might be directed at what kinds of needs would be more important to meet compared with others: we perhaps should not try to treat metastatic lung cancer as aggressively as we do high blood pressure. Furthermore, while the older person is the more likely than the younger to have accumulated one or more acute and/or chronic conditions, and there is a correlation with age, one's years are not a substitute for the individual needs that people have. Finally, we could begin to think about the expected years remaining to a patient as a softer indicator of how vigorously (and expensively) we should pursue treatment/cure/management of whatever is ailing them, perhaps substituting more palliative interventions that might improve their quality of life but not aim to extend it.[46] This is what I wish to discuss next.

LIFE EXPECTANCY

Closely related to age is life expectancy, although there are some major differences. I have already presented some details about CEA and the derivative, QALYs, in the context of the quantification of subjective preferences and the difficulties this approach presents for establishing justifiable cutoffs. In this part of the discussion, I will also fold in considerations of disabilities and quality of life, particularly *disability-adjusted life years* (DALYs) because these issues and QALYs have a great bearing on the overall focus on the amount of time people may be expected to have remaining to live and what limitations they may have with their ability to do or accomplish tasks secondary to any barriers imposed by health problems (distinct from the normal ravages of age). Like years accumulated (as marked by an individual's age), the years remaining in one's life could potentially serve as a metric to impose cutoffs to limit access to, or the amount of, medical services. In essence, it would represent a version of Daniels' prudential life span approach together with variations of Harris's fair innings view. How much benefit one would derive from a given intervention would depend on where one was positioned in life, irrespective of what one might have achieved so far or what one might still have remaining to achieve of one's goals and plans. Potentially, if a given treatment would offer 5 years of healthy life, a decision would have to be made if it is better to spend the money for a 30-year-old to enjoy the additional life, or a 60-year-old. This is a choice that could only be described as tragic.[47] Most important is the insensitivity to individual differences and the vagaries of discrete lives: it treats all 60-year-old people alike, equally successful (or not), each life equally fulfilled (or not), and hence ignores needs that are attuned to particulars not populations.

To a very great extent, and irrespective of how one would actually quantify the amount of time, any sort of analysis based on different weighting of years of life depending on when in life they were lived is fundamentally a value judgment about the intrinsic worth of that amount of time. In essence, we are asking whether a year of life to an 80-year-old is worth the same as a year of life to a 25-year-old. This also begs the question as to which individual that worth is assigned. It may be trivial to say that the (average) older woman values her life just as much as the (average) younger woman (if, indeed, this is actually so). But it becomes much more complicated if we ask whether society or our culture values the same time similarly. If there are differences in the latter, it has profound implications for the distribution of resources (such as healthcare dollars) to the younger versus the older, assuming that a choice must be made between the two. It is a measure of worthiness to the culture and country to match one group of suffering individuals against another, to judge that the distress, pain, and misfortune experienced by some is somehow qualitatively different from that of others and that it should somehow generate a different response. It would be indecent to pit the pain of one generation against that of another.

Throughout this book, I argue that this is a false choice and dichotomy in a wealthy society that is disposed to expend significant portions of its resources (although not as much as we currently do) on healthcare. I suggest that these sorts of tragic tradeoffs may be unnecessary and most certainly add substantive complications to prioritization and distributive dilemmas.[48] Rather, the question becomes whether such generosity should be devoted to interventions that have little chance of success or of meeting substantive (health) needs or that can lead to a decrease in suffering (however that may be accomplished). Thus, the debate about whether to aggressively treat the advanced, metastatic lung cancer of an 80-year-old man with less vigor than the same disease in a 40-year-old is meaningless because both have similarly little probability of achieving a consequential goal for any concerned parties: the patients, their families, or society. It seems to me that the main issue—given sufficient resources to meet the fundamental healthcare needs of all—is to focus on the relief of suffering.[49] Saving lives per se, without due consideration for the kind of life being saved, would seem not only shortsighted, but foolish. I will have more to say about this in the next chapter.

While it is certainly true that the average life expectancy for any *population* of people can be calculated with relative ease and quite accurately from standard census data (in an advanced industrialized nation with reasonably mature institutions capable of gathering and analyzing representative information), it is extraordinarily difficult to make a similarly precise prediction for any given *individual*.[50] It is undoubtedly correct to state that a child born to parents of a given socioeconomic group and with a certain skin color and gender in the present-day United States has some x percentage of living to say, 80 years, whereas a similar person growing up in a more/less privileged household with less/more education and the like has a much lower/higher chance of doing so; it is merely a probabilistic calculation. Likewise, whereas the average life expectancy if one reached age 20 was certainly less than 45 years in colonial America (this accounts for the enormous infant and child mortality before 5 years of age), there were certainly numerous instances of people who lived considerably longer, indeed to an age that we today would consider reasonably "normal."[51]

So, how much is a year of life in good health worth in the United States? Put another way, how much would the average American pay for one QALY? At first, this question might seem unseemly by equating a human life with filthy lucre, but it is unquestionably true that it costs real dollars to keep someone alive and as healthy as they can be, all things considered. Whether it is paying for clean water and effective sewage systems and waste treatment facilities, or for picking up the garbage, cleaning the streets, and minimizing industrial and other forms of pollution, the benefits of modern health-supporting activities are by no means free. While it is also true that a significant portion of the increase in life expectancy in the developed world has come about due to improved sanitation, better nutrition, and other advances in the social determinants of health, there is little doubt that the invention of antibiotics, vaccines, and many other technological breakthroughs that are the hallmarks of 20th- (and now 21st-) century medicine have also made major contributions. Indeed, people are now living both longer and better in large part due to greater successes in managing the array of accumulated chronic disorders that afflict many—perhaps most at one time or another—people in the First World. Of course, the ability to live a reasonable life with hypertension—and not be felled by a stroke at the age of 63 due to malignant hypertension, like Franklin Roosevelt—is not cheap. And, in the United States, due to the failure to impose price controls on many aspects of healthcare interventions, especially pharmacotherapeutics, there is a constant increase in the cost of both living and living well.

While the source or genesis of the figure is both debated and somewhat mythical, it has historically been cited that, in the United States, a QALY is worth about $50,000. Many people have suggested that this number originated in some early calculations about the benefits of renal dialysis in the 1970s, but that may be more healthcare economics legend than real.[52] Nevertheless, this appealingly round number has persisted; even if it were true, it is wildly out-of-date and accounts for neither inflation (both standard and healthcare-related) nor data derived from what people actually think. The question is not really the amount any given life is truly worth—since one should not be able to actually value a person's life in that manner (after all, for most people who want to go on living, their lives are invaluable). Rather, it is how much the people in a society (and necessarily a democratic one) would be willing to pay for a year of good health for others and whether all those "others" should be considered equal in this evaluation.[53] In the same way that it is difficult to obtain accurate hypothetical answers to surveys that inform the generation of QALYs for health states in the first place, it seems that it would be similarly challenging to assess the price people would put on a QALY. Nevertheless, this has been attempted, not with surveys but by complex economic analysis. The results from one such investigation calculated a range from $109,000 to $297,000 (in 2008 dollars).[54] Whether people would be willing to support these numbers—more or less—via taxes or some other payment mechanism is debatable and unknown. There is also little question that pure CEA using QALYs fails to take into account other major social values about the distribution of healthcare and the money needed to support it.[55] In many ways, it is quite important to at least get an approximation of the so-called "threshold" number because it can serve as an indication of the stinginess or generosity—within the limits of budgetary constraints—that a society deems worth spending on healthcare, as well as on what kinds of healthcare receives more or less priority (lifesaving interventions, palliation of chronic conditions, and so on).

DALYs were created as a companion measure to QALYs, "as a way to estimate and compare the burden of morbidity and premature mortality caused by widely varying conditions and states within and among countries. DALYs are calculated as the present discounted value of future years of healthy life lost to morbidity/disability and future years of life lost to premature mortality."[56] They are most useful in calculating the burden of disease(s) in populations. By employing a variety of different survey mechanisms (analogous to those used for computing QALYs), investigators can come up with various weighting schemes to determine an estimate of how people (and the populations they belong to) view various states of health. As Murray et al. describe the approach,

These surveys used pairwise comparisons and questions on population health equivalence, which ask respondents to assess improvements in health produced by various interventions that change disability or prevent premature death, to generate disability weights on a scale from 0.0 to 1.0, with 0.0 indicating ideal health and 1.0 indicating a state of health equivalent to death. Years lived with disability were computed as the prevalence of a sequela multiplied by the disability weight for that sequela. Because years of life lost and years lived with disability were measured in units of healthy life lost, they were reported with the use of a comprehensive summary metric—disability-adjusted life-years (DALYs)...disability is synonymous with any short-term or long-term health loss.[57]

These techniques have informed the regular reports from the World Health Organization on the Global Burden of Disease (and related disabilities).[58] DALYs attempt to account for time lost (not gained) that can be attributed to physical and/ or mental impairments, as well as for early death that can be due to accidental or disease causes.[59] There are various ways of weighting various factors, but it is interesting to note that there has been a major pushback against using age as a significant factor in creating comparable DALYs.[60] While this metric has proved quite valuable for analyzing different groups of people both within and across national boundaries, it is unclear how useful the metric can be for determining cutoffs for funding purposes. DALYs are most helpful is analyzing how well or poorly a population is doing owing to the prevalence and incidence of various diseases, as well as the degree to which institutions are meeting the needs presented by these illness-related challenges. However, they are also put to use in some forms of CEA to measure the impact of various interventions and their relative financial consequences.[61] At a large population level, public health officials would naturally wish to gain the most relief for the finite amount of money available to combat those diseases that were found to cause the most suffering and diminution of QALYs (i.e., DALYs). While these sorts of investigations can also provide valuable information about subpopulations within highly developed countries such as the United States and hence can serve to direct attention to poorly served groups of people, in the absence of a concerted effort at the national level to address these deficiencies, they may be of only academic interest.[62]

But the ultimate question raised by the focus on age as a cutoff—irrespective of the methodological obstacles that would be insurmountable—is a moral one. Whether one aims at years lived or years left to live as the target for limiting healthcare expenditures, it nonetheless establishes a statement of value on the worthiness of a life. By establishing that giving 5 years of life to an elderly person is worth less to society than when the money is spent to give those same 5 years to a young person, we make a statement about life itself. It is not too far a stretch to imagine making these same judgments about the value to those 5 years for a 30-year-old with Down syndrome, quadriplegia, or sickle cell disease. The real tragic choice is forcing these decisions when they are unnecessary.

CITIZENSHIP OR RESIDENCY STATUS

There are many people in the United States who would like nothing better than to refuse to provide any medical care to undocumented immigrants.[63] Hence, immigration or residency status could be employed as a cutoff point. While there is little doubt that much of this sentiment is derived from bias against populations of people, it is also reasonable to surmise that a superficial analysis would suggest that one could conclude that eliminating the many millions of people in this country who would fit into this category from consideration for healthcare services could save significant amounts of money (however, the fact that these individuals can still seek emergency and charity care when desperately ill or injured, and that these services can cost even more that preventive care, is a not a consideration for many). I will only briefly consider this subject because I have discussed it in greater detail elsewhere.[64] Yet, it is worthwhile mentioning it in this context due to its political and social significance. The United States is a country largely created by immigrants. Notwithstanding that fact, we have a long history of recurrent negative opinions against the newest immigrants, often expressed most vociferously by those who are recently assimilated.[65] It is astonishing how quickly people whose parents or grandparents were immigrants come to regard the latest wave—irrespective of their origin, be they Irish, Italians, Eastern European Jews, Asians, and now Latinos and people of Middle Eastern origin—as foreigners unfit to live here. As the United States has slowly and fitfully crept toward a more encompassing view that a core duty of government is the welfare of the country's residents (and not the sole responsibility of the charitable sentiments of others), programs that support the less well-off or socially marginalized have become favored targets in which to restrict access to the latest Americans. Whether it is California's infamous Proposition 187 in the 1990s[66] or more recent attempts to deny access to basic human services to immigrants, documented or undocumented, the animus may appear to be new but it has a long and sordid legacy in America.

At least theoretically, it should be straightforward to determine whether someone is a citizen or legal resident of the United States (we will ignore the woeful state of the record-keeping for the sake of this argument). If that were actually so in reality, then it would also be simple to declare that access to some form of taxpayer, government-funded healthcare system would be denied to anyone here either illegally or without the proper documentation or even to visitors on tourist visas (if they wanted to be truly mean).[67] The advantage of this form of cutoff perspective is that immigration status, unlike age or QALYs or almost any other characteristic about people that has been discussed as a metric to use for restricting healthcare, is a binary state: one either is or is not legally a resident in the United States. Hence, it would also be quite simple to declare that those with the correct and verifiable identification would be eligible for services, and those lacking authentic documents would be left out. Of course, this is mostly how it works now with Medicaid, Medicare, and the like. And there is little question that if states and the federal government were required to cover healthcare costs for the 12 million or more undocumented people in this country, healthcare budgets would expand significantly.

There could be other characteristics about people that could be employed to distinguish them as potentially "undeserving" of healthcare within even a centrally controlled and dispensed system. It has often been stated that one of the main reasons undocumented immigrants should not receive any public services—irrespective of any positive, beneficial effects they may have on American life and/or the economy—is that they are criminals, purposefully breaking the law by entering the country in an unsanctioned manner and hence should be treated like any other lawbreaker, citizen or not.[68] It has often aroused the outrageous fury of Americans when they hear of incarcerated prisoners receiving scarce resources, such as solid organs for transplant. Even though the US Supreme Court has consistently ruled since 1976 that prisoners must be provided with the standard of care—including transplants as they increasingly became the standard of care for such conditions as liver failure, idiopathic heart failure, and the like.[69] While few object to the more mundane and quotidian aspects of prisoner healthcare that almost exclusively goes on behind closed prison doors and rarely becomes known to the public, when there is a case that is publicized, the outcry can become fierce.[70]

Of course, although the population of people behind bars in America is huge and the number of undocumented persons is in the many millions, both are finite numbers. Even if the goal of any kind of scheme for rationing healthcare is solely to control overall costs, to restrict (or even completely bar) the availability of healthcare interventions for these people is penny wise and pound foolish. It does not take an advanced degree in health economics or even medical training to understand that prevention and primary care save much more than they ever cost. Providing emergency or episodic care only is shortsighted, in addition to be inhumane. Except for prisoners, we already do this, and the costs to hospitals and other providers for furnishing urgent and other kinds of interventions are enormous and only going up. Including these populations in a general scheme of overall healthcare that incorporates similar restrictions for clinically similar cases would make the most financial and moral sense.

CONCLUSION

In this chapter, I introduced some common (and a couple of not-so-common) targets and methods that have been used (or thought about) to ration healthcare. They all suffer from one or more fatal flaws—especially moral—that doom them to being poor candidates for the sort of systemic rationing I have in mind to accompany wholesale healthcare reform. Even the quantitative approaches are afflicted with the cutoff problem. If one wishes to restrict access to certain kinds of healthcare interventions on the basis of age, assuming that one agrees with the premise that old people as a group benefit less than others from healthcare, then one has to decide how one would qualify to be classified as "old" or too old for whatever it is that would be considered off-limits. No matter what age we chose, it would undoubtedly be arbitrary and would be extraordinarily difficult to defend, especially to those people who found themselves immediately (or not so immediately) adjacent to the boundary. It would be impossible to plausibly claim that there is a substantive moral (not to mention physiological) difference between (for example) a 75-year-old man with advanced lung cancer for whom we might restrict access to certain kinds of interventions *because* of his age (and not because of the lack of efficacy of the interventions) and a 74.5-year-old man with a similar condition. One could argue that we commonly impose firm age cutoffs of this sort in our daily lives without much protest;

the ages of legal majority for voting, drinking alcohol, use of tobacco products, eligibility for Medicare and Social Security, and the ability to operate a car are some familiar examples. We seem to have accommodated the arbitrariness of strict boundaries of this sort without too much fuss (although the political calculations during the Nixon administration on voting age and the draft may be an exception, the result was still just another firm cutoff). I would suggest that the impact of age cutoffs for access to healthcare is considerably greater and more central to well-being than the legal age of being able to buy a drink. Indeed, the effects of having access to Medicare benefits can be life-changing and life-saving but are generally unavailable to those people under 65 years of age, thus speaking to the discretionary, but enormously significant, influence of arbitrary cutoffs of this kind.[71]

At the same time, even those characteristics that seem cut and dried and binary offer messy complications. Take prisoners for example. While it would be relatively simple to say that all convicted felons, no matter what, should not have access to anything other than emergency care (assume for the sake of this point that the Supreme Court would permit this kind of meanness), it gets much more complicated when one starts delving into the particulars. When one starts to discuss the situation with people, subtlety and nuance begin to be appreciated. First, not all prisoners are the same. While it is no doubt true that stories about murderers getting heart transplants arouse ire in many, most people in prison are not murderers. Indeed, the conviction and sentencing free-for-all in the 1980s and 1990s put enormous numbers of nonviolent drug offenders behind bars for very long terms.[72] Thus, there may be degrees of indifference or even hatred toward prisoners depending on the crime for which they have been convicted.[73] Second, there are huge numbers of people who were former prisoners, and they may be expected to have some degree of empathy for their former inmate companions. Third, most imprisoned people get out; to refuse them healthcare while they are incarcerated could reduce the chances of them ever leaving jail. Fourth, publicity surrounding wrongful convictions is constantly in the news, so that many (perhaps most) people are well aware that there may be significant numbers of prisoners who shouldn't be there because they are innocent. And finally, the large prison population in the United States also means that there are even larger numbers of relatives and friends on the outside who presumably care about the welfare of their loved ones on the inside and who might feel that the latter would be wronged by being denied beneficial healthcare.

Thus, even the most simple and perhaps benign traits or characteristics *about* people fail the test of being able to be employed justifiably as cutoff methods for rationing healthcare. Arguably the most amenable and successful—the QALY—also suffers from fatal flaws, mostly due to its strict utilitarian animus that assumes that all QALYs are equivalent so long as they contribute to general utility. While there have been attempts to moderate the blunt "soullessness" of the QALY by incorporating concerns for equity and personal needs, on a system-wide basis they must continue to be numerical in nature. Moreover, even though many advocates of QALYs shy away from endorsing strict thresholds for what a QALY should be worth, such concerns are integral to the purpose of QALYs and again also cannot avert a sharp cutoff problem. In the chapters that follow, I will explore an alternative that avoids sharp cutoffs by using a more reasonable target for rationing healthcare and by using a form of adapted procedural justice to soften boundaries and personalize them for individual patients and claimants. What I will suggest is a reasonable and fair approach to determining what should and should not be included in a comprehensive healthcare benefits plan that is first focused on medical needs and then on efficacy of interventions and clinical appropriateness.

The United States is fortunate in a number of ways. One of the most salient to healthcare reform is the enormous wealth generated in this country that *could* be devoted to caring for (and about) the health of those who live here, should we choose to do so in a manner that was reflected by the overall health of the populace. The fact that this nation is so rich makes the argument about healthcare rationing almost superfluous. If we maintained the same level of spending we do now, but allocated those trillions of dollars more intelligently and fairly, many of the inequities and poor outcomes of which we should be most ashamed would disappear. Indeed, as I will argue (and have argued previously),[74] the cutoffs we make could be ones that are both medically and morally justifiable, rather than those discussed in this chapter, in which entire populations of people are determined to be worth less—or deserve less—than others. This is indubitably a moral judgment, and one we should avoid making.

3

NEEDS, WANTS, PREFERENCES,
AND DEMANDS

In the previous two chapters, I introduced the cutoff problem and discussed some characteristics about people (and presumably the disorders we are prone to develop) that have been proposed as possible targets to develop restrictions on the availability of healthcare interventions. I have argued that measureable features that individuals possess, such as their age, and that correlate more or less with consumption of healthcare resources for their illnesses, fail as cutoffs for both practical and moral reasons. At best, they serve as surrogates for what we really should be interested in. Discrete, binary metrics, like immigration, citizenship, or prisoner status, while attractive politically as a focal point to refuse access to healthcare, cannot withstand ethical scrutiny. Continuous variables, like age, fall short because of creeping boundary issues and the arbitrary unfairness of cutoff points for those at the borders, as well as for the problems of poor individual association between years lived or remaining and disease amount and severity. All suffer from the critical inadequacy of pitting the claims of one group of sick people against another: old versus young, free versus incarcerated, citizen versus immigrant, and the like. In a land of great wealth, such competition for important resources that can contribute in such a material way to personal and population welfare is not necessary, in contrast to that for critically and finitely scarce resources such as livers or hearts. But could there be other, perhaps clinically relevant characteristics, that might be more fitting and that could presumably be more morally justifiable?

While I did not discuss this in detail, many insurers (both government and private) utilize some form of what is referred to as "medical necessity" to determine if an intervention and/or a condition qualifies for funding consideration and approval. This can be somewhat of a nebulous and ambiguous term, and I will analyze it more later in this chapter. Cutoffs can also be arbitrarily specified in some systems by setting a defined amount of money available to pay for healthcare services and ranking the importance and cost effectiveness of interventions (as well as factoring in the incidence and prevalence of various conditions); what is covered are those conditions and their paired interventions that are on the "list" until the money runs out. In this chapter, I wish to examine a different aspect of individual (and population) health that I will argue will serve as a better characteristic to utilize as a feature to determine cutoffs. As part of this discussion, I will then propose a method that could be used to locate the cutoff lines or points that has a far better chance of being fair and thus gaining the public (and moral) legitimacy required to be practicable and plausibly achievable.

My goal in this book is to consider how we can equitably and reasonably draw a line on permissible interventions and those that would not be covered in a comprehensive, universal, single-payer national healthcare plan.[1] To make such a distinction, we will have to differentiate in a justifiable way what is reasonable to offer and what is not. This will depend on a number of factors, not the least of which is the amount of money we wish to devote to healthcare. Since there are both financial and moral reasons to undertake comprehensive healthcare reform in the United States, the two must be balanced against each other to achieve the best realistic outcome.[2] The former is well known because we are on target to approach annual healthcare costs of 20% of gross domestic product (GDP) in the next decade; this is unsustainable, especially with the pitifully poor return we get for our investment.[3] The latter is connected to the facts that significant numbers of people go without healthcare or have substandard medical care due to lack of insurance and that there are massive inequities of both access to and delivery of healthcare. I have previously argued that some form of fair rationing system must be implemented within a structurally altered system that is capable of delivering quality care to all. I have also suggested that a wealthy country like the United States could afford to be quite generous in what it offered as part of a comprehensive healthcare package, for both medical and practical political reasons.[4] However, generosity does not mean that people would be able to have whatever they want. There must be some limits on what is available because reforming health insurance by improving efficiency, trimming bloated administrative costs, and minimizing waste will not be sufficient. The question, then, is what should be restricted, and how can we decide what is on and off the list?

Where do we make rationing kick in? Do we only employ rationing to save money, or can it also be viewed—within the confines of national health insurance of the type I have specified—as leading to saving or improving lives? The latter question (which I hope to affirmatively answer) sounds counterintuitive: how can restricting access to certain kinds, types, and amounts of healthcare interventions such as diagnostic tests, treatments, and the like actually improve patients' lives and even save them? Isn't more always better? Of course, the answer is "no," and there is a great volume of data to show that significant percentages of both diagnostic and therapeutic interventions are wasted, in the sense that they do not contribute to improving outcomes and well-being and often cause direct and even grievous harm.[5] Much of what we do in healthcare is not needed by the people who are on the receiving end, perhaps because we have evolved an adulterated and weakened sense of the concept of "need." In this chapter, I wish to discuss what we should mean by healthcare needs and suggest ways that we could practically restrict healthcare interventions to those things that people really needed and, by so doing, improve health and save money. In this way, I hope to closely relate a tolerable understanding of healthcare needs to what would be reasonable to provide in a national healthcare insurance system.

If the aim is to transform the American medical system from one in which interventions are not commodities based on price and market demand (and the ability of people to afford to purchase them), then it should be considered as something beyond that simple notion, perhaps because of its singular and central importance to what people can make of their lives and its capacity to make peoples' lives more tolerable (by reducing suffering). If this is reasonable, then it seems most natural that permissible (and hence funded) interventions would be based on medical or healthcare need. If this premise is promising to explore, then the next step is to analyze what is meant by medical need.

Few people of good will—excepting perhaps the most selfish, misanthropic, or miserly Dickensian skinflints—would begrudge the provision of something that could meet a true need of a fellow human being if it were in their power and resources to supply the needed item. Be it food, shelter, or clothing, most of us think it not only reasonable but mandatory that our basic needs be satisfied if we are to have the opportunity to lead some version of a good life. However, this simple observation raises two significant questions: what qualifies as a (healthcare or medical) need, and who should bear the responsibility for satisfying it?

The language and literature—both academic and nonacademic—is replete with what we might call "needs talk": this or that need is unmet, people need more or less of something. The implication is that for an individual or group to have a need it must be definable and perhaps urgent in the sense that failure to address it in some sort of effective manner could lead to an avoidable harm and that there exist means by which to satisfy these needs. I am certainly not immune to the attraction of employing the needs idiom: I easily fall prey to needs talk as, for example, when I argue with an insurance company that my patient *needs* such-and-such a drug or a diagnostic procedure (MRI, PET scan, etc.). If I held that it was not necessary, or perhaps negotiable or optional, then the company would quite understandably deny payment. The only effective argument that persuades them to approve the intervention is one that is based on *need* (and that is covered under the terms of the policy).

Where does the need for (modern) medicine fit in with other needs that we have? Healthcare is a quintessential creation of humans, invented to address the fundamental susceptibility to illness and suffering (due to illness) shared by us all. If it is needed, in the sense of something that can have a positive impact (in a beneficial sense) on someone's life, then it is a secondary one, conditional on the provision of other, more fundamental resources (such as oxygen/air, water, sufficient nourishment, etc.). Furthermore, it is reasonable to assume that there would be some kinds of medical needs that have priority over others, perhaps defined by the fact that the lack of meeting them results in more suffering either for individuals or groups/populations than others. In addition, the interventions that we have for certain conditions (or needs) are more or less effective, and there may be one or more ways of addressing a need, some of which may be better or less suited to do so (either by strict efficacy criteria or for what meets a patient's best interests more or less). And, of course, some ways of meeting needs are more or less expensive even for similar outcomes or results.

In a wealthy society, where the provision of resources for basic or primary needs would (one would hope) be taken as a given, meeting medical or health needs would also seem to be a matter of course. If that society believes that addressing at least some of these needs is a matter of right (for individuals), then the questions are how many of those needs is it reasonable to think the society should meet, and how should we define an order of priority? If one also takes the view that the budget for meeting medical needs should be based on what meeting these needs would sensibly cost (rather than vice versa), then the list of credible and significant needs is of paramount importance. But what measure (or measures) should be used to construct this ordinal list? Finally, there must be some sort of difference (although probably not categorical) between needs of this type (i.e., ones that are reasonable to put on the list) and mere desires or wants.

One could take a more-or-less purist libertarian view and hold that people who have health-related problems or needs do not have a justifiable claim on their fellow Americans to provide help to meet those needs. Rather, they should be reliant on their own wherewithal to acquire the means to satisfy their own needs. Indeed, perhaps the most orthodox (or extreme) conviction of this sort might actually maintain that there are no true needs, simply preferences, the satisfaction of which is central to the function of a market (for example). And those individuals who cannot acquire "satisfiers" by themselves for one reason or another, must appeal to the charitable sensibilities or sympathy of others and not look to some central authority—such as government—to supply what they lack. For those who may be judged to have their poor lot in life due to their personal behavior, and hence may be thought to deserve their misfortune, they have only themselves to blame. For people who find this point of view appealing, the idea of a nationalized health system that applies to all (even with the option to purchase "extra" resources for oneself) is anathema. Not surprisingly, I reject this philosophy as unworthy of a liberal, compassionate democracy that professes to care for its population. Nevertheless, it is important to note that a sizeable minority of people in the United States believes in some version of this, and their opinions must be acknowledged.[6]

The overwhelming success of modern, scientific medicine (coupled with the even more spectacular results of the past century of improvements in nutrition, public hygiene and water supplies, etc.) has generated a new class of patient, most commonly observed in the developed, industrialized world: one living with one or more chronic diseases. An excellent example (there are many) would be diabetes. Diabetes comes in two general categories: type 1 is almost exclusively diagnosed in childhood, most frequently with an explosive clinical onset, and is characterized by the complete lack of production of insulin due to the destruction of the hormone-producing beta islet cells in the pancreas, presumably by an autoimmune mechanism.[7] Type 2 disease, on the other hand, which used to be known as "adult-onset diabetes," is now increasingly being diagnosed in the young due almost entirely to the epidemic of obesity. It is distinguished by the resistance of the body to the effects of insulin.[8] However, both kinds of diabetes may require insulin treatment, and therein lays an interesting story and lesson about the acquisition of medical efficacy for a clearly understood need and how the two are intimately related.

Prior to the epochal efforts of Frederick Banting and Charles Best, who purified insulin from the pancreas isolated from animals (dogs and oxen) in the early
1920s, the sole (and ineffectual) treatment for type 1 diabetes was a form of prescribed starvation to deprive the body of sources of glucose.[9] Shortly after perfecting
their technique, they purified some of the mixture isolated from a bovine source and
administered it to diabetic children with amazing and gratifying results.[10] Literally
overnight, a previously always-fatal disease was transformed into one in which
patients could lead more or less normal lives. In the succeeding 90-plus years, major
improvements have been made in the treatment of diabetes, including the production
of human insulin by recombinant DNA techniques and the introduction of insulin
pumps to better regulate blood sugar in a more physiologically normal way. Patients
with diabetes now have a chronic disease, and many go on to live long and productive lives, albeit with a cost, including increased risks of kidney disease, blindness,
heart disease, and a host of other secondary effects of the disease.[11] Those with the
acquired type 2 form of the disease comprise one of the largest populations with end-
stage renal failure in the United States.[12] The initial giddiness of saving the lives of
children with diabetes was not tempered by the foresight of what that success would
bring. Technology—even with all of its ability to improve our lives—has a habit of
"biting back."[13]

The point of this story is that diabetes, like many forms of cancer, heart and lung
disease, and the like has been altered from a rapidly fatal, acute illness, to one that
is livable as a chronic condition. However, the price that has been paid (especially
with the burgeoning group of type 2, obesity-related, insulin-dependent diabetics) is
the enormous growth of people with chronic conditions. Indeed, many patients have
more than one diagnosis. It is estimated that in the next 20 years or so the number of
people with one or more chronic diseases will comprise at least 50% percent of the US
population.[14] Not surprisingly, caring for these patients and their conditions is very
expensive and will continue to increase.[15] This trajectory is unlikely to change short
of some major social and behavioral interventions. In addition, Americans' addiction
to the idea of technological progress and what might be called "gizmoitis" or the end-
less fascination and devotion to the new, irrespective of whether it actually represents
an improvement on what went before, also contributes to continual cost growth.[16]
Nevertheless, very few people would hold that we should not develop new treatments
or therapies or fail to provide those that already exist for patients with chronic heart
disease, diabetes, hypertension, or even many types of cancer, especially since most
of us know someone with these illnesses (or carry one or more of these diagnoses
ourselves).[17] Even so, as Hanson states the challenge:

> The seemingly limitless possibilities of high-tech medicine not only offer us
> new hopes for escaping our condition, they transform these hopes into needs. If
> there is a possibility of progress in the pursuit of these goods, the argument goes,
> then we have a need—if not a right—to what medical progress can offer. On this
> view, medical need becomes a function of technological possibility, which is now
> defined without boundary.[18]

If this is true—and there is every reason to believe it is—then how can we interrupt what seems to be an unalterable course or else face the alternatives, which are both financial ruin and continued worsening of already existing problems of inequity and unfairness? Is it possible that not everyone who is receiving treatment or interventions is benefitting in a substantive way and hence may not "need" what they want or receive? It would be difficult to argue that people with diabetes do not need insulin, as we know all too well what would happen to them without it. But all needs for medical interventions are not the same with similarly grave negative consequences as this. Hence, all claims by people to address what they believe to be their needs may also not be equivalent or of equal strength. It may be the case that not everyone who is a recipient of specific forms of healthcare actually needs it.

While I will present a brief discussion on needs theories in general, I do so only as a prelude to my more general examination of how to distinguish needs from wants or preferences and how this must be placed within a contextual framework of a modern, industrialized, and wealthy society. I will especially concentrate on applying the differences between these kinds of states that can (or cannot) be alleviated by healthcare. There is good reason to believe that we all have basic needs that must be satisfied for us to live even a minimally decent life. These include such essentials as a caloric intake that is sufficient and varied enough to meet our growth and developmental requirements. Similarly, we need certain amounts of water that are dependent on climate, and it is not unreasonable to qualify this need by adding that the water should not be contaminated with pathogenic bacteria (such as *Vibrio cholerae*, the organism that causes cholera). Medical or health needs merge into these basic needs by several routes, including the one mentioned in the previous statement about clean water; if contaminated water is all that is available, we must be prepared (if feasible) to meet the challenge (or need) represented by bacterial toxigenic dysentery which, if not treated rapidly and appropriately, has a high mortality rate, especially in the very young.[19] Hence, medical needs can be created by external factors such as infectious diseases or other forms of environmental contamination (including human-made) as well as "internally" from lifestyle choices such as cigarette smoking and the like that may only manifest themselves as we go about attempting to satisfy our most basic or primitive needs.

Let me state at the outset that I will argue from a premise or perhaps even a stipulation that there are categories of human need, especially in healthcare, that are objective and can be determined in a reasonably precise manner. This does not mean to say that there cannot or will not be disagreements, arguments, and debates about the blurry areas of need in healthcare. I am only claiming that we should be able to agree on most of what we think would meet the definite needs of human beings who are suffering from medical conditions. It is not unreasonable to believe that needs do not have to be reduced to their smallest component and specified in minutiae to clarify what needs are significant and how they should be met. Indeed, it may only be necessary to categorize needs in general terms and leave the exact specification of how they should be met to more local authorities and practitioners.

Perhaps most important, however, is the fundamental requirement to frame the debate within the larger context of what are (or perhaps should be) the proper and reasonable goal(s) of healthcare (and specifically medicine) in general.[20] It would be incorrect—and possibly incoherent—to argue that a healthcare system should provide certain interventions because they are needed by people if these interventions fall outside the boundaries of any intelligible and accepted goals of healthcare. For example, it is not unreasonable to say that perpetual "life" support for those patients declared dead by neurologic criteria (i.e., brain death) does not meet any intelligible goal of healthcare and hence should not be offered or available, irrespective of the costs involved.[21] It would be difficult to argue that such individuals *need* intensive care in the same way that someone with a reasonable hope of some form of recovery might need it.[22] This is not to say that a healthcare system should not attempt to meet all of the worthwhile goals of medicine, simply that what the system is able to offer within the confines of its budget should conform to these goals. It is likely, if not probable, that not all of these goals can be met, especially when resources are scarce (either by design or default). For instance, while we might like to provide liver transplants for all patients in liver failure who we have decided "need" one, there are plainly insufficient organs to do this, so straightforward rationing is called for. The same might be said when money is also (relatively) scarce: we cannot buy all that we might wish to and hence must make choices about what is more appropriate to purchase. Nevertheless, while we may not have livers or hearts for all who could plausibly benefit from transplantation, the ends of medicine would dictate that we not simply abandon such patients, but rather provide them with comfort and palliation. Their suffering can still be eased, which is a need we can almost always address. Expansively, the goal(s) of a healthcare system should be to embrace, endorse, and advance the ends of medicine while at the same time promoting the social goals that a liberal and technologically sophisticated society could reasonably desire, such as excellent and broad-based population health (as indicated by such metrics as life expectancy, infant mortality, etc.) purchased in an efficient and equitable manner.[23] But what do we mean when we say there is a *need* for healthcare or a *need* for specific treatment or diagnostic test?

(HEALTHCARE) NEEDS AND WANTS

In a just society, we may be presumed to endorse the view that people are entitled to have certain of their needs met, irrespective if they have the means to meet them themselves (of course, this assumes that there is an initial endorsement of the basic tenets of a just society). Other than the somewhat prosaic or commonplace usages of the word "need," what does it really signify when we (or others) say that we need something? We tend to employ the same words when we are expressing a desire or preference for something that we could reasonably do without, such as "I need a haircut," or "my car needs a tune-up," or "I need to buy my wife a present for her birthday." In all of these sorts of statements, we are conveying the impression that this is something that we very much want to do or have, that we feel some sort of urgency about carrying it out, and that we most certainly have a goal in mind (having a presentable appearance, making sure my car is in good running shape, and that I can show my wife that I care about her, etc.).

However, in each case (and innumerable others that come easily to mind), we are professing a wish or a want that, no matter how important it may be to us, could arguably go one way or another without our lives being significantly harmed in a substantive way. Without going into tremendous philosophical detail about what content our desires must have to count as personal or legitimate, I think it is credible for this discussion to claim that wishes, wants, or preferences have an element of choice about them (we could carry them out or not) even though we might suffer some form of harm—perhaps even a kind that we might momentarily consider to be grievous—if we failed to accomplish or satisfy these desires, or experience some improvement or maintenance in our state of well-being if we are successful. But in neither instance do we feel that desire fulfillment is absolutely mandatory, *no matter what*. Simply because we say that we must have or do something or believe that the failure to accomplish a task or acquire some object will be terrible for us, others who can look at our situation objectively and dispassionately may not agree. It is common for children to state that their lives will be ruined if such-and-such does not occur, frequently referring to events their parents view as trivial and with greater level-headedness and farsightedness. This is not to say that not having a "need" or desire of this sort met would not be sad or produce unhappiness. And, in some rare cases, it could trigger or magnify the symptoms of an underlying psychiatric disorder. It is just that, in the overwhelming majority of cases, others examining this "need" could consider its necessity as dubious. In addition, wants of this kind do not have the same kind of urgency about them or in them that true needs have (see later discussion), even if that urgency is not always temporal in kind (meaning that satisfaction of true needs does not necessarily have to be immediate to communicate their importance).[24] Moreover, desires and wants are subjective, often personalized individual expressions and difficult to quantify or generalize to others. Finally, and somewhat related to the concept of choice, is that not all rational people placed in the circumstances that make me desire something will desire the same thing or what I want; they may have different desires (they like their hair longer than me, or they don't wish to spend their money on maintaining their car, etc.). This implies that there is a certain arbitrariness about desires that is often (though not always) lacking in "true" needs. What then may we consider to be these "true" needs or material (or other) things that people can't arguably do without?

Adam Smith, writing more than two centuries ago, encapsulated his idea of needs as necessary things to have to remedy or satiate conditions that must be dealt with:

> By necessaries I understand, not only the commodities which are indispensably necessary for the support of life, but whatever the custom of the country renders it indecent for creditable people, even of the lowest order, to be without. A linen shirt, for example, is, strictly speaking, not a necessary of life. The Greeks and Romans lived, I suppose, very comfortably, though they had no linen. But in the

present times through the greater part of Europe, a creditable day–labourer [sic] would be ashamed to appear in public without a linen shirt, the want of which would be supposed to denote that disgraceful degree of poverty, which, it is presumed, no body can well fall into without extreme bad conduct.. . . Under necessaries therefore, I comprehend, not only those things which nature, but those things which the established rules of decency have rendered necessary.. . . All other things I call luxuries; without meaning by this appellation, to throw the smallest degree of reproach upon the temperate use of them.[25]

Della Nevitt (a modern day economist) distinguished between needs versus luxuries (or mere preferences or wants) by stating:

There is no clear dividing line between "luxury" and "need" goods or services. Both are sub-sets of the wider set of demands and can only be fully defined in relation to the society under examination although certain goods such as salt, water or oxygen are incontrovertibly "necessities" in the sense that no living creature can survive without these essential goods. However, the modern use of the word "need" has little to do with survival and relates to a concept of goods which are demanded by many people and "should" be made available to everyone, either through a government non-market scheme which distributes the goods directly to those classified as a need, or by income distribution and/or redistribution. Luxuries, on the other hand, are things which many people demand but in respect of which the government has not intervened in the market. Goods and services can of course be transferred from a "luxury" to a "need" category and vice versa.[26]

This is the view of economists (at least classical ones), where needs are analyzed within a framework of consumer preferences within a market, even though many will (perhaps reluctantly) admit that basic biological "needs" are categorically different from those products (natural or not) that could be conceivably forgone. But I think we must be more specific in clarifying these distinctions and placing them in both individualized and group contexts.

It is quite common to illustrate the concept of needs by the following statement:

"Sarah needs X in order to Y so that Z does/doesn't happen."[27]

This means that Sarah requires the provision of something X because she has a goal of Y which allows her to either accomplish or avoid the state of Z occurring. While this is a basic needs expression, it could easily be applied to wishes or desires as well. For example, we could fill in the blanks by saying that:

"Sarah needs *to get her car tuned up* in order to *keep it in proper running order* so that *it doesn't break down on her way to work in which case she would have to take a bus*."

Compare that to a somewhat different statement of Sarah's predicament:

> "Sarah needs *to get her car tuned up* in order to *keep it in proper running order* so that *it doesn't break down on her way to work, in which case she would be late and her boss would fire her.*"

Stated in this way, needs are conditions of want or absence (of something) that are required to be satisfied in pursuit of some goal. What seems to distinguish them from mere desires, in addition to the points I raised earlier, is the degree of importance or even necessity of attaining the goal coupled with the consequences to the primary goal-holder (and possibly others as "bystanders") of not satisfactorily realizing the goal. In this way, we might ask the defining question as to whether the achievement of the goal (its acquisition of something "beneficial" or avoidance of some harm) by satisfying a related need is causally associated with the maintenance or improvement of substantive well-being. Thus, needs statements of this type express an instrumental (and consequential) concern.

By changing the goal expression at the end, we have changed a trivial harm (having to take a bus) into one of major importance for Sarah (she would lose her job if she were late for work). We could make the harm she potentially could experience even more onerous if we also stated that she got this job after being unemployed for 2 years, she supports her aged mother and two young children with her salary, and the like, all of which go to enhance the significance to Sarah of needing to get her car tuned up. Avoiding having to take a bus due to a broken-down vehicle does not seem to carry the same moral strength—and it certainly doesn't evoke the same kind of sympathy we would have—of the latter case. While this may be true enough, it seems somewhat subjective. There could be many other terms we use for various consequences of Sarah getting her car fixed (or not) that we might tend to view either way. We require a more concrete or objective method (to the extent this is possible). In addition, the more significant we make the consequences of failing to achieve the goal (by satisfying the need), the more of us who would probably agree that it actually is a substantive need and not merely an expression of a desire or preference. It is this ability to convince others of the validity of having a legitimate need that should be satisfied if at all feasible that is the key point. If these hypothetical reviewers—perhaps performing the function of Adam Smith's "impartial spectators"—could reasonably and sympathetically agree that the need is well-founded and justifiable, and a harm of sufficient magnitude would be prevented if satisfied (or an equivalent good provided), then it would be rational to find it acceptable.[28]

We may then transform the (instrumental) needs formula statement and apply it to the healthcare realm thusly:

> A needs (healthcare intervention) B to satisfy/in order to C so as to D where D is some larger life event or plan or goal that is dependent upon receiving a health-related intervention.

This statement could also be amended to include an avoidance-of-harm clause:

> A needs (healthcare intervention) B to satisfy/in order to C so as to D and avoid E, where D is some larger life event or plan or goal that is dependent on receiving a health-related intervention and E is some negative consequence that might occur should the need not be satisfied.

The immediate or proximate goal is directly related to the specific intervention (C is related to B), which then must be connected to the larger life goal/plan that a given patient has (D).

For example:

> Jane needs quadruple bypass surgery to relieve her angina so she can dance at her daughter's wedding, or
>
> Henry needs metoprolol to control his hypertension so he can live longer/work, etc.

This expansion provides more clarity and cohesion with the goals of healthcare as I have outlined them. Cohen seems to refer to this approach when he states that true instrumental needs further fundamental goals that "are valuable in *themselves*" (emphasis in original).[29] He includes such things in this category as survival or life, although he does not specify whether this should be qualified by defining what kinds of life are valuable in themselves (assuming that not all biological human life is such). But this view permits an analysis of both reasonable health-related goals and reasonable life plan–related goals. Moreover, it is in this way—both in the beneficial goals to be achieved or harms avoided—that carries the moral force of these sorts of needs. The actual thing that is needed by Jane may be (relatively) trivial in this sense; it is what it is needed *for* that carries the weight.

It is also worthwhile noting that needs are not always identified and expressed as being needed by the person who needs them. For example, young children and the intellectually disabled may be incapable of stating their needs. Obviously, they may still have them, including the need for water, nutrition, and the like. It must be left to others to know or specify both what they need and how urgent the need is, as well as perhaps assigning responsibility (to some extent) for meeting these needs. For many of these people, societies designate certain individuals for identifying and meeting the needs of these dependents. For instance, parents (or parent surrogates) are the default identifiers of and meeters-of-needs for their children, and they are held accountable when they fail to do so in a manner deemed sufficient. By the same token, prison guards and wardens are appointed to the analogous guardianship positions for their inmate charges. And caretakers of nursing homes are supposed to meets the needs of their patients, both those who are cognitively intact and those who are not. Simply because someone cannot give voice to his or her needs does not diminish their significance or "neediness," but it does make these people notably vulnerable to having their needs ignored, misinterpreted, or undermet. One other difference between people who can competently express their needs and those who can't is that the former can prioritize them and make decisions about whether to sacrifice meeting a need to accomplish a desire whereas the latter require others to rank their needs for them.[30]

While some see needs claims on others to be problematic due to their more-or-less subjectivity (see earlier discussion), one way to delimit the degree of personal partiality or their individualistic qualities is to rely on how others view these needs. For example, many of us might believe that it is unreasonable for a publicly supported (no matter how generous) healthcare system to pay for certain kinds of cosmetic surgery on the basis of someone stating, "I need a nose job because I don't like the shape of my nose."[31] On the other hand, we might reach a different conclusion if the statement was "I need my nose reconstructed after the automobile accident when my face was smashed against the dashboard when the airbag failed to inflate." One could also argue that there is subjectivity in how we view others' claims of need, and there is no doubt that the manner and kinds of opinions that could be offered could be rife with bias or bigotry, particularly if a dominant group attempted to arbitrarily exclude the needs of a marginalized population.[32] However, these kinds of activities could be limited (or even excluded) if appropriate regulations demanded reasons justifying the action, in which only certain kinds of reasons would be acceptable. I will discuss this in greater detail further on.

Let me return to Jane's hypothetical case. Both the goal of the surgery (to relieve angina pain) and her life plan (attend and dance at her daughter's wedding) not only sound reasonable and connected, but also achievable. If we said that Jane "needed" bypass surgery to relieve her pain and hence make her eligible to be an astronaut on the space station, we might hesitate and suggest that her latter goal is unrealistic (that doesn't necessarily mean that she wouldn't get the surgery, just that she should be encouraged to develop more realistic life goals that align better with her medical condition). Or, suppose we said that Jane "needed" (wanted?) chemotherapy for her metastatic lung cancer not to relieve pain but to be cured so that she could go back to work for another 10 years; we might have to think more about this and perhaps even deny her, stating that this "need" was not realistic or reasonable because her goals for the "need" were unreasonable. Or, another example might be that Jane needs her mother (who is in a permanent vegetative state due a previous cardiac arrest and prolonged cerebral anoxia) to receive CPR if she experiences a cardiorespiratory arrest so she can remain (biologically) alive for the miracle of recovery that Jane is praying for. This is not a real healthcare need because it does not meet the goals of healthcare of relieving suffering and promoting well-being. If Jane wanted comfort measures for her mother and not heroic interventions, that could better align with what medicine could and should reasonably provide. More important, dispassionate observers would likely view the latter as a more reasonable need that should be met rather than the former. In some very important ways, these suggestions are complementary and draw on Daniels's theory of "just healthcare" in which the goal is to attempt to restore or maintain as much of a "normal opportunity range" as is feasible.[33]

One useful approach has been to categorize needs on the basis of the interests they serve (usually personal interests). For example, *instrumental needs* are ones that are required or are a necessary condition for attaining a given goal or objective, which is contingent upon the presence of the instrumental need. For example, I might say that I need clothing to stay warm in winter in northern latitudes. The goal or aim is to maintain body temperature (warmth) or else I will develop hypothermia and die, and I need certain kinds and amounts of clothing in order to do that. The other way to look at it would be that the *absence* of clothing leads to hypothermia.

Fundamental needs are first-order, noncontingent necessary adjuncts or ingredients to one's life, the absence of which will result in definitive harm (or, presumably, the lack of a definitive good). Sometimes the two can overlap. One could say that food of a certain type, variety, and caloric content is a fundamental need (otherwise malnutrition would result), but fancy French cuisine with many courses and fine wines to accompany the meal with dessert is an instrumental need to becoming a gourmet restaurant critic as one's life work. Thomson makes the point (as do others) that the lack of whatever it is that may satisfy a fundamental need would result in "serious harm" to an individual (he doesn't say anything about whether that harm is reversible or irreparable as a categorical distinction).[34] Wiggins and Dermen make an additional distinction between the "elliptical" meaning of needs (needs contingent upon some goal or end) and a "categorical" sense (absolute needs such as clean and sufficient quantities of water, food, etc.).[35] Similar to this is Norman Daniels's characterization of healthcare needs by the degree to which they affect (negatively) a person's ability to take advantage of the opportunities available to formulate and carry out the range of life plans afforded by the society in which he or she lives:

> The impairment of the normal opportunity range is a (fairly crude) measure of the relative importance of health-care [sic] needs, at least at the social or macro level. That is, it will be more important to prevent, cure, or compensate for those disease conditions which involve a greater curtailment of an individual's share of the normal opportunity range.[36]

Of course, this does not tell us anything about how little a derangement or diminution of opportunity range availability that may be causally related to (symptomatic) diseases, (asymptomatic) conditions, or (physical and/or psychological) disabilities would count as a true need that would command the concern of healthcare providers. For example, if a patient has a minimal or little chance of recovery and the decision is made to turn off the ventilator that he "needs" to stay (biologically) alive, or she is prevented from having access to the ventilator in the first place, has this person been deprived of having a fundamental need met? Or can one say that this kind of need may be fundamental, but its "fundamentalness" is contingent on other conditions being in place (e.g., some reasonable amount of consciousness that enables a person to be aware of her surroundings and able to interact with them and hence experience pleasure—or pain). This contingency means that this version of fundamental needs *differs* from that of Thomson. This distinction means that these kinds of healthcare needs are therefore not fundamental in his sense because they are neither inescapable nor non–context-dependent nor noncontingent. They are dependent on the state of technology and medical science and the availability (and/or ability to pay) of that technology. As he states of fundamental needs, "what one needs, one cannot forgo."[37]

Two of the leading needs theorists are Doyal and Gough. They outline the necessary conditions that must obtain to set the basic needs of all people and thus are universalizable between cultures.[38] They call the things or conditions that help meet the needs "satisfiers." Like Thomson, they distinguish needs from wants by the former's relationship to serious personal harm that results when the need is not satisfied. They take for granted that these are above the truly basic biological needs of humans *qua* humans. These include (a) basic health, (b) personal autonomy (to achieve agency status whereby one can act on one's intentions and make plans and carry them out), and (c) adequate opportunities to exercise agency. It seems clear that the first two are the central ones, and the last is more a requirement of the society in which one lives. It should also be apparent that (a) and (c) are very close to what Daniels views as the specific moral value inherent in good health (and hence healthcare, which can contribute to maintaining or restoring health) due to what it offers to the individual as far as the ability to carry out life plans.[39] Similarly, this view seems to be shared by Nussbaum and Sen in their capabilities approach.[40]

Some needs are not dependent on advanced technology, such as those for clean water, shelter, adequate nutrition, and the like. However, other needs have evolved along with our technological development and in some ways can be determined by its level of sophistication. In other ways, these kinds of needs are also somewhat subjective and open to debate (whereas the need for adequate nutrition is not). For example, prior to the mid-to late 1940s, one could not say that a person with pneumococcal pneumonia "needed" penicillin because it was not widely available until after World War II, and even then only in wealthy countries whose industrial infrastructure was not destroyed during the war. Likewise, one could also not say that someone with unstable angina "needed" an endovascular stent in her coronary artery before the time when they were in wide use and available (again, in the United States and similar nations).[41] This observation suggests that how we define what is permissible to be recognized as needed depends on a number of contingent facts about the situation and its participants. First, there are technological factors that are features of a given society and epoch, such as its level of technical sophistication and development, infrastructure, and the like. Second, cultural and social characteristics and norms undoubtedly play a role in shaping the desires, wants, and needs that people have. And third, the wealth of a society and its constituent members, and how they wish to spend it and on what, contribute both to molding preferences and needs as well as providing the financial wherewithal to satisfy them.

Finally, it is important to emphasize the important point made by Frankfurt (and others) about the significant relationship to the avoidance or reduction in harm that can come about by virtue of having needs met.[42] Indeed, it is this tie that gives moral grounding to needs and their claims, especially their claims on others. While Frankfurt tends to be somewhat dismissive of the acquisition of benefit that some might believe they would obtain should they have their "needs" met, preferring to focus on the negative consequences of unsatisfied needs, I think he may be in error here, especially when it comes to healthcare needs. It is no doubt true that many kinds of specific interventions help people specifically by avoiding harmful effects such as death, disfigurement, or pain. But there are others that are prophylactic in nature, such as immunizations, the goal of which is to avoid potential harm (when it has yet to occur). And still others are palliative in that they serve to reduce the amount and presence of suffering already incurred as well as minimize future ills. Still others seek to bestow benefits to populations such as clean air and water, proper sanitation, and vaccinations against preventable infectious diseases. While it might be possible to construe all of these sorts of medical interventions in the language of harm, it somehow seems more natural to view at least some as beneficial in that they have as their goal making peoples' lives better, rather than keeping them the same. This does not mean to say that all needs that people define as such could be reasonably seen to improve their lives (and possibly even avoid some form of harm as well) have the same urgency or necessity (as Frankfurt would call it) as others. This evaluation necessarily takes place within the context of the proper or reasonable goals of the medical enterprise and medical practice. I have briefly mentioned this topic earlier, but now I need to flesh it out a bit more and its relevance to help clarify the distinction between needs and wants or desires *for healthcare.*

Needs for Healthcare

I am attracted to the idea of Eric Cassell that the proper goal of medicine (or healthcare) is—and should be—the relief of suffering.[43] In his view, suffering is a much larger experience that people have, often in response to, but distinct from, the physical perception of pain. It is more existential in nature, and "although bodies may experience nociception [the physical correlate associated with noxious stimuli, both external and internal], bodies do not suffer. Only persons suffer."[44] This statement directly implies that only individuals who are conscious in some consequential sense—meaning that they can suffer in this important way—are worthwhile objects of our healthcare (or medical) efforts to address their suffering because only they have the capacity to suffer.[45]

As a corollary to this, the capacity for others to suffer is what drives our empathy, compassion, and concern, and, as healthcare providers, motivates us to intervene and inspires devotion and duty. Hence, certain kinds of unconscious people, such as those in a permanent coma or permanent vegetative state, cannot suffer in this psychologically and morally significant way and therefore cannot benefit from healthcare.[46] This also entails that such individuals cannot be harmed by the lack of healthcare interventions.[47] By the same token, conscious persons—even those who are minimally so but who retain the capacity for suffering—can benefit from (and perhaps need) the relief of their suffering that medicine can provide, whether it be by curative or palliative means.[48] Either way, the goal remains the same. Accordingly, treatment without addressing the suffering of a patient fails in achieving this goal.

Moreover, it should be said that those people who can express themselves in a way that can define and indicate their suffering—especially in an autonomous manner—should be able to have significant, if not total, control of the manner and the degree to which their suffering can be alleviated. Thus, in this framework, people *need* to have their suffering assuaged.[49] But, significantly, people who cannot suffer in this fundamental way do not—indeed cannot—have the same kind of (healthcare) needs as those who have suffering that can be treated. Hence our obligations to them do not include addressing their "needs" (usually as defined by others, such as their surrogate decision-makers) that do not exist.

There are other views that can offer more specification or detail as well as somewhat differing notions of needs within the broader outline provided by these general goals. For example, W. R. Sheaff frames his conception of healthcare needs around his definition of health, in which it embraces an individual's natural functional capabilities.[50] In his view, the goal of healthcare is to restore, to the extent possible or feasible, these function(s). He then distinguishes "needed" healthcare from that which is not needed, "trivial," superfluous, and is presumably the expression of mere wants or desires in this way:

> Some health care is not practically iatrogenic but equally has no practical effect in extending the patient's painless use of his natural capacities. In that sense it is "trivial." The standard example is surgical treatment of a painless, non-function-impairing condition (e.g. liposuction, breast enlargement). Triviality is not an argument against all cosmetic surgery; only for distinguishing its trivial form from its nontrivial uses. Cosmetic surgery that improves an individual's capacity for social interaction by removing an obvious disfigurement or removes severe emotional distress counts as non-trivial because it meets a natural need or restores a natural capacity (for social contact, say). (p. 95)

It seems to me that an obvious problem with this expansive view of needs (meaning those that should be met in a reasonably generous healthcare system) is the last statement that allows for self-defined and manifested emotional distress to be an arbiter of dysfunction. Therefore, if someone thinks the shape of his nose is so hideous that he cannot go out in public, Sheaff would presumably say that the system should pay for his nose job as opposed perhaps to the psychotherapy that might be beneficial. Of course, it might be cheaper to perform the surgery, all things considered, than to support the kind of therapy that might be required to reconcile him to his physical features. That is not to say that there are not patients who are or can be severely debilitated from these kind of psychological reactions to perceived deformities. Sheaff does draw a fairly rigid line at interventions that he calls "Superman" technologies but which others generally refer to as enhancements.[51] He does so because he says that these interventions do not meet general healthcare needs because they extend or expand our natural capacities or functionalities as oppose to restoring them from some sort of diminished state (as caused by disease, congenital infirmity, or injury).

He compares these technologies to devices like trains that enable us to go places faster: nice to have but not an essential need.[52]

David Ozar lays out an interesting theory of basic healthcare needs as depending on one's physical state and how near to harm (both grievous or life-threatening and less immediately ominous) one is and relates them to basic needs for other life-sustaining resources (food, water, clothing, shelter).[53] He describes several states in a hierarchy of needs: utter lack of means, bare survival, subsistence, and then minimal security (the last situation is achieved when someone can meet the basic needs as well as have resources left over to devote to the pursuits that allow for the expression of "humanness" such as non-basic needs goals.[54] He thinks that basic healthcare should meet the needs of people to permit them to rise to the (health) level of minimal security (this is very similar to Daniels's view of the value of healthcare and its instrumental importance in restoring/preserving health that is needed to take advantage of life opportunities to create and pursue goals that one considers worthwhile).[55]

In a very thoughtful recent analysis of healthcare need, Andreas Hasman et al. and Tony Hope et al. criticize earlier theorists of medical need for their lack of specificity in what exactly they mean by need and how it could relate to the delivery of healthcare interventions, especially in a system with rationing of one sort or another in which prioritization of needs is required.[56] They also make the point that it is reasonable to acknowledge that some needs are greater than others, if for no other reason than a hangnail is not as demanding of our attention and sympathy—or does not cause the degree of suffering—as a burst appendix that requires immediate surgery to save someone's life. Thus, they view healthcare needs as "graded" rather than simply present or absent. Moreover, they assume that interventions must be effective at some level in meeting a need (presumably similar to Gough and Doyal's "satisfiers" described earlier) to be considered as something that could then be paired up with a given condition (recall Oregon and the condition–treatment pairings).[57] They describe three different ways of defining needs based on how one views the condition that suggests that someone needs healthcare: The "poor initial state interpretation," in which the gravity of the patient's illness, pain, suffering, or overall condition generates the need, and the satisfier can improve the patient's condition. Second, the "normal functioning range interpretation," which is also favored by Daniels in that the need is generated by a condition that prevents a patient from being within the normal functioning range. And third, the "significant gain interpretation," which is tied to how effective a satisfier is in meeting the need and relieving the condition. The key to choosing one of these views (or some combination) is to use them in setting priorities of the importance of needs to determine allocation of resources.

However, I see several problems with this analysis: first, they fail to see that people may still have needs even if there are no effective satisfiers to meet them. Second, they do not really discuss what an effective satisfier is or the minimum efficacy required, which is of course related to considerations of resource scarcity, although one could maintain that marginally effective satisfiers should not be offered no matter how generous or rich the insurance scheme is. And third, they do not really develop a reasonable strategy or method to actually accomplish their proposal. Definitions are well and good, but the practical application is the proof of principle.

It is worthwhile at this point to also mention some criticisms of Daniels's view of health as they relate directly to the concept of health needs. His argument is heavily dependent on the *biostatistical theory of health* developed by Christopher Boorse.[58] Boorse proposes that health (and hence its absence, disease) can be located and defined in a value-free, objective manner by appealing to what is empirically normal about the way that humans function. He defines "normal" as that which is statistically average or within acceptable or reasonable bounds of efficient functioning; departures from this statistical range would thereby be classified as abnormal and thus disease(d). For example, a left ventricular ejection fraction (that percentage of the blood filling the main pumping chamber of the heart that is expelled into the arterial circulation upon each contraction or beat of the heart) of less than a certain value, especially if accompanied by such symptoms as shortness of breath with mild exertion, would constitute such a deviation from "normal" that we would label it as heart failure. Of course, there are some diseases that represent such obvious and common disorders or abnormalities (and might almost be described as universals) that there would be no debate because they transcend all major differences between people; a good example might be bacterial pneumococcal pneumonia.[59] However, for almost everything else, what is normal must be related to what Boorse calls a reference class, thereby recognizing that what might be normal for a baby would be highly abnormal for an adult and the like He settles on three of these reference classes: age, gender, and race (for a given species). By this method, he is able to describe the following criteria for health:

1. The reference class is a natural class of organisms of uniform functional design; specifically, an age group of a sex of a species.
2. A normal function of a part or process within members of the reference class is a statistically typical contribution by it to their individual survival and reproduction.
3. Health in a member of the reference class is normal functional ability: the readiness of each internal part to perform all its normal functions on typical occasions with at least typical efficiency.
4. A disease is a type of internal state which impairs health i.e. reduces one or more functional abilities below typical efficiency.[60]

While seemingly elegant in its simplicity and appeal to our intuitions, there are several problems with this approach. The most common criticism has been to question the meaning and plausibility of the reference class used by Boorse.[61] Another significant flaw is his appeal to statistics, a weakness that is inherent to any attempt to cope with the unavoidable and necessary variability that is part of human biology (and pathology) and that I will explore in greater detail in Chapters 4 and 5. It suffices to say at this point that it is extraordinarily difficult to draw a line of statistically normal that is both reasonable and justifiable—especially when it is applied to distinguishing between those who are or who are not sick, or those afflicted with a condition we are willing to label a disease and those who are simply different in some way. Nevertheless, at least one of Boorse's critics suggests a solution to this puzzle, advancing a Rawlsian approach of "veil of ignorance" consensus-building to agree upon a set of baseline principles; this idea accords well with what I will propose later in this chapter.[62] Most important is the recognition that, in the real world of messy problems and perhaps even messier solutions, the idealistic goal of defining what is or is not illness must account for the heterogeneity of values, beliefs, and even prejudices held by providers and receivers of healthcare.

A comprehensive understanding and theory of healthcare needs must encompass not only the definition of a problem but also the way(s) in which that problem can be approached for amelioration. It stands to reason that personal states may vary in severity as well as whether they could even be viewed as diseases or conditions that others (not afflicted by/with them) would judge as such.[63] Even those problems that truly cause individual suffering—for example, the person with a nose that he thinks is hideous and is a severe impediment to his social life—may be considered to be less worthy to be thought of as having a disease than others. Conversely, there are treatments or interventions that also may be viewed as questionable, such as quackery, "holistic" medicine, "alternative" medicine, and the like. These are methods and/or philosophies of practice as well as individual therapies or treatments. Are the needs that these sorts of practices identify (and hence legitimate) and the remedies they prescribe reasonable to consider as bona fide (for the purposes of funding via a health system)?

Another way of identifying "real" healthcare needs and their "real" or legitimate satisfiers may be to ask whether a given need–satisfier pair (assume for the sake of simplicity that there is only one satisfier per need, irrespective of whether it is legitimate or not) would or could pass a "commodification" test. What I mean by this is based on an understanding that healthcare and the goals it serves should exist outside of the marketplace in the sense that the kinds of needs it meets (sickness, disability, ill health, suffering) are not the kinds of conditions that a marketplace should exist to meet. Since we are all susceptible to illness and suffering, and medicine can play a unique role in ameliorating these conditions, one could argue that the treatment of illness should not be a standard commodity to be bought and sold under the laws of supply and demand. However, if the need is more a desire or want (elective cosmetic surgery, for example, that can be distinguished from restorative or reparative plastic surgery), it may not be reasonable that it be provided as part of a comprehensive package of healthcare benefits, but rather should be available for "sale." Nevertheless, some things should not be for sale.[64] While Debra Satz and Michael Sandel concentrate on obvious things such as organs, I would expand this to encompass all satisfiers of whatever we decide are true and legitimate medical needs. Thus, one's willingness to pay extra to get something that is available to all should be irrelevant to obtaining what would be a necessary good. Therefore "true" needs and their satisfiers would be those that we could agree (by a method that takes advantage of the "impartial spectator" conceit) should then be available to all who meet the criteria of having these needs. Those conditions that do not meet these consensus criteria of instrumental or fundamental importance (of the consequences of not meeting them in some manner) should be better viewed as desires, wants, or preferences.

Let us consider elective cosmetic surgery. This might be distinguished from restorative cosmetic surgery performed (for example) after mastectomy for cancer, although one could also imagine this being open to question as to whether such patients really "need" such surgery or simply desire it to make their lives go better. For someone to say "I need breast augmentation" with a strong justification such as "if I don't have it my personality and social life with be irreparably harmed," for the purposes of system payment, we have to decide whether this is truly a need that should be met. Current private insurance practice generally pays for cosmetic surgery after mastectomy for cancer, as it is accepted as a true need. We have determined that the subjective assertion that such patients' lives will go better if they have breast reconstruction is more meaningful and forceful than the other claims for similar cosmetic surgery in the absence of cancer, as for, say, breast augmentation for purely ornamental or physical enhancement purposes. Neither kinds of surgery will save the person's life, only—according to their beliefs—make it go better (or avoid the harms associated with the absence of the need being met).[65] Just because we may wish to draw a line demarcating some healthcare needs as meriting satisfaction (by a centrally controlled and regulated system of comprehensive health insurance employing rationing of some sort) from others that are less "deserving" does not mean to say that the latter are not needs in their own right. Simply because we decide that the insurance scheme will not pay for elective rhinoplasties in otherwise normal individuals who don't like the nose they were born with does not negate the belief of these individuals that they "need" a nose job and that a successful one would contribute positively in a materially significant way to their well-being. It is just to say that this sort of need may be below a mutually agreed upon cutoff line or threshold because of any one or more reasons, such as the condition affects too few people, it is not "serious" enough, there are other means available to bring one to accept one's anatomy, and there are significant numbers of people who do not consider this state an abnormal condition at all, as opposed to a normal variation. Rather than paying for a nose job in an otherwise normal individual, perhaps a comprehensive healthcare system should pay for psychotherapy if the individual is incapacitated by concerns about the size and shape of his or her nose. Indeed, if it could be determined that the patient was suffering due to a definable mental aberration or obsession about his nose, it would be perfectly justifiable to pay for some form of treatment to relieve him of this suffering and incapacitating dysfunction. Similarly, one could analyze other elective needs such as refractive keratotomy for nearsightedness.

At this juncture, it is worthwhile emphasizing a couple of important ancillary points: first, one can't really need something that doesn't or can't exist (e.g., some technology that hasn't yet been invented), but one certainly can need (or want) something that one can't easily obtain by oneself or have provided by others. Second, there is a difference between a person who desperately needs something that is available but for which the person does not possess the means to obtain it (say, some life-saving drug that is very expensive and the person is uninsured) and those who do possess the means and have similar needs. A simple and common example of a scarce personal resource would be money, but it could also be transportation (to get to a store to buy the drug for which the person has sufficient funds to buy) or even physical assistance (say, for a disabled person). Thus, there would be more than one need in these cases: the need for a drug (for example) and the need for the means to obtain it. There could be more needs in the chain as well. This claim would then place a premium on prevention of medical conditions over treatment for those that could have been prevented by simple means. Doyal and Gough also describe this kind of ordinal ordering system (pp. 157–158), as does David Braybrooke,[66] although the former refer to what I call "primary" needs as intermediate. They also include "appropriate health care" within their list. This is because they argue that their primary needs are some (high) level of health and autonomy both of which are baseline, enabling conditions from which all else follows.

However, since I am focusing on healthcare and analyzing what might be needs within this domain (realizing that the domain itself could be described a need), I will stick to my distinction between primary and secondary needs within healthcare itself. It is also possible that there may be a category that we could call "tertiary" needs, which could indeed blend into preferences or wants. Another way to look at this is that my primary (healthcare) needs are those that all humans (may) have and from which all humans suffer more or less similarly from not having them satisfied. Lesser needs may strike those who have them as no less important, but these affect fewer people.

Unfortunately, attendant on this shifting definition of what might constitute healthcare needs is who gets to define them and how co-extensive with widely shared desires and preferences they should be. In the United States, there is a clear antipathy to having "Big Brother" decide what is available (i.e., what needs will be addressed and thus paid for), although in practice this happens all the time with private insurance companies and public insurance plans, such as Medicaid, Medicare, and the VA system (however, it is not overt and publicized as such).[67] Mägi and Allander make some interesting suggestions in their analysis: there are three levels of assessment of need: the patient decides that she has something wrong that needs the attention of the healthcare system (or needs preventive and/or primary care services), and then the doctor decides a patient needs some intervention. There is also a third component, in that these two have to align with what some third party (the payer, assuming that the patient is not paying for this herself and the doctor is not dispensing free care) agrees is a need. Who should have the power to define what qualify as healthcare needs? There are two aspects to this question. The first is the systemic one about deciding what clinical needs are sufficient to be included in a standard (perhaps very generous) package of benefits. The second is more granular. How should the creators of the healthcare system go about deciding what criteria to use in determining what a healthcare need is that should be included in the benefit package? Who should be the "voters," and how responsive to the public should they be? Furthermore, how often should this package be reviewed to incorporate new treatments, technology, and the like? How should the local gatekeepers go about determining whether a patient needs something that is or is not covered? Presumably, there will be general criteria and a list of covered conditions and interventions (including diagnostic tests and treatments that are linked to particular established or suspected diagnoses) not dissimilar to the famous Oregon list or that established by an insurance benefit package (i.e., we will pay for breast reconstruction surgery after mastectomy for breast cancer but will not pay for a cosmetic augmentation mammoplasty). How to interpret and fit patients into the list of covered items will be left to physicians and other frontline providers.

Having presented a detailed analysis of some of the difficulties encountered in defining what is a need, and specifically a healthcare-related need, I want to turn to a discussion of how needs are addressed in the "real" world. This will require an examination of what is meant by the term "medical necessity" and its relationship to appropriate and inappropriate interventions, how they may be judged as such, and, finally, how this relates to need. I shall begin with a discussion of what might be viewed as an extreme end of the spectrum in a further attempt to clarify what could be thought to be reasonable needs and the methods appropriate to define and address them.

DEMANDS

In mid-December of 2013, 13-year-old Jahi McMath was admitted to Oakland Children's Hospital for a routine tonsillectomy and adenoidectomy.[68] Shortly after surgery, she experienced massive bleeding and then a subsequent cardiac arrest for reasons that have not been made public. She suffered severe and irreversible brain damage and was shortly thereafter declared dead by neurologic criteria (i.e., "brain death"). Her family did not believe the diagnosis and went to court to prevent life support from being removed and a death certificate issued. It was at this point that the case became public, and much brouhaha ensued. The child's body is now reported to be residing (maintained on a mechanical ventilator) in an undisclosed location in New Jersey under the auspices of the Terri Schiavo Foundation. This case is tragic on many levels, but the question it raises for my purposes is whether patients or families can demand to have whatever healthcare intervention they want—in this case, maintenance of intensive care for a dead body while awaiting her a miraculous recovery—and have the medical system comply? Can patients (frequently also labeled as "consumers" in the medical marketplace) both define their conditions and needs and command a remedy or a "satisfier" (as I employed the term earlier)? Consider another case.

Mr. Martinson was a man in his early 60s with known atherosclerotic heart disease, poorly controlled hypertension, type 2 diabetes, and moderate kidney dysfunction.[69] He was brought to the emergency department by the local EMS after he was found unresponsive at home. CPR was initiated in the field and circulation was restored; he had suffered a major heart attack. He was admitted to the cardiac intensive care unit and his condition improved, but his cognitive function was severely impaired due to the amount of time his brain was deprived of oxygen. Nevertheless, his was able to recognize his family and respond to them. His doctors were cautiously optimistic that he could improve further with aggressive rehabilitation. However, his kidneys were permanently damaged, and he required hemodialysis three times a week. Because he had experienced some arrhythmias (common after severe myocardial infractions of this type), he had an implantable cardiac defibrillator inserted. As he was being prepared for discharge, he had another heart attack, this time a "PEA" arrest (pulseless electrical activity) with a "non-shockable" rhythm.[70] Even though he was successfully resuscitated with restoration of circulation, he suffered even more brain damage and was thereafter unresponsive. During the next couple of weeks, he had at least one more PEA event. He remained a "full code" as his family insisted that "everything be done" to keep him alive. Even though he remained stable, his neurologic condition did not improve, and he entered a permanent vegetative state with no evidence of consciousness. He family, polite and respectful throughout, remained adamant in their refusal to permit him to die (he also still required thrice-weekly dialysis and, because he could not sit up due to his neurologic condition, he was unable to be treated at an outpatient dialysis facility). They even refused to permit his doctors to turn off his defibrillator. They were very religious people, constantly praying for his recovery and convinced that he would miraculously recover due to their prayers.[71] After a 19-month stay in the hospital, he was discharged to home with 24-hour nursing care and ambulance transportation to the hospital for dialysis, all paid for by the institution. He died peacefully about 2 weeks after discharge, never having regained consciousness; the family was very grateful for the care he received.[72] Should they have been able to have their demands met? Did this patient "need" dialysis and a defibrillator, or is it more realistic and plausible to say that he "needed" palliative measures to permit him a quiet death? Both of these questions raise the more important issue of who gets to decide what are reasonable needs (and the process by which these decisions are made) in a comprehensive healthcare program.

In many ways, a demand for something is very similar (if not identical) to a rather strident expression of a desire or want, often in the face of opposition from the person or persons or authority empowered with responding to the demand. But perhaps these first two cases arguably represent the far end of the spectrum of family demands for treatment and are so unreasonable that it is simple to dismiss them as irrelevant, despite the fact that family insistence for so-called "futile" care has been a long-time problem for physicians and hospitals.[73] This next case may be more emblematic of the complex challenges with blurry lines that are perhaps more frequently encountered.

Sarah was a 20-year-old woman who was diagnosed with osteosarcoma, a rare malignant bone cancer, when she was 19. The primary site was in her right distal femur (thigh bone), but she also had several nodules in her lungs that were almost undoubtedly metastatic tumor. Isolated extremity osteosarcoma can have a very good prognosis with cure rates up to 75% depending upon how sensitive the tumor is to chemotherapy.[74] However, patients who have metastatic disease at diagnosis do not fare nearly as well, and patients like Sarah have less than a 25% chance of long-term survival.[75] Nevertheless, she was young and otherwise in excellent health and it was felt by her, her family, and her doctor (me) that it was worth going for broke. And that is what we did. She initially did quite well, and the tumors in her lung almost disappeared. She had her primary tumor removed in its entirety. Unfortunately, shortly after she completed her almost year-long course of chemotherapy, a CT scan of her chest showed recurrence of her tumor on one side. Since there were good data suggesting that long remissions could be achieved in a reasonable number of patients with a surgical approach to removing the lung metastases (as long as they were few in number), that approach was taken. However, several months later, the disease recurred again. At this point, there was little we could offer (even experimental treatment was not an option because, due to her diminished functional status, she was not eligible for any open clinical trials) other than comfort palliative care for the time she had remaining. Notwithstanding assurances that anti-cancer treatment in this setting would be ineffective and almost undoubtedly harmful due to side effects, she and her family were unwavering in their demand for more chemotherapy. I refused to comply, and they transferred her care to another oncologist who was willing to prescribe more treatment. She died several weeks later after a failed 45-minute resuscitation attempt at a community hospital (the family had also refused to permit a "do not attempt resuscitation" order to be issued, and the local hospital had no idea that they were trying to revive a moribund patient with terminal cancer until it was too late). Should the patient and family's demand for therapy for which there was poor and/ or minimal data supporting its efficacy (merely anecdotal case reports) have been honored? Should we do so in all similar cases? Can our healthcare system survive if we continue to do so?

This section would not be complete without mentioning the case of Abigail Burroughs:

In 1999, Abigail Burroughs, aged 19 years, was diagnosed with squamous cell carcinoma of the head and neck. Despite chemotherapy and radiation therapy, the tumor was not eradicated. Cytogenetic analysis of the tumor revealed increased expression of the cell surface membrane receptor EGFR (epidermal growth factor receptor). At the time, 2 targeted EGFR treatments, genfitinib and cetuximab, were undergoing clinical trials. But Abigail did not meet inclusion criteria for the genfitinib trials, and the cetuximab trial was restricted to patients with colon cancer. Shortly before her death on June 9, 2001, she enrolled in a clinical trial of erlotinib (OSI774). . . . In November 2001, Abigail's father, Frank Burroughs, founded The Abigail Alliance for Better Access to Developmental Drugs to advocate for greater patient access to pharmaceuticals in early stages of development and testing. Ordinarily, investigational drugs may be used only within a controlled trial. Under the compassionate-use policy instituted by the FDA [Food and Drug Administration] in the 1990s, the FDA may approve the use of an investigational drug outside of clinical trials for life-threatening diseases when there is no comparable treatment alternative, clinical trials of the drug are under way, and formal FDA approval for the drug is being sought. . . . In 2003, the alliance and the Washington Legal Foundation submitted a citizen's petition to the FDA requesting broader availability of investigational drugs for terminally ill patients. Before the FDA acted formally on the petition, the alliance sued in federal district court, alleging that the failure of the FDA to permit the sale of investigational drugs to terminally ill patients violated patients' rights to privacy and due process under the Fifth Amendment.[76]

The district court dismissed the suit, but a three-judge panel of the Washington Circuit Court of Appeal reversed that decision and ruled in favor of the alliance. The full court heard the appeal and ruled against the alliance's suit.[77] The Supreme Court declined to hear the case, and there it ended.

These cases provide stark examples of the sorts of demands that desperate—and sometimes not-so-desperate—patients and families may make for healthcare interventions from physicians and other providers. Be it a CT scan to look for cancer or an operation or a drug to treat some condition for which there may be little or no clinical indication, insistent demands for intervention are a constant in clinical practice. And the details, as well as the stridency and actual numbers, have only increased with the advent of the Internet and the easy availability of medical "information" to almost anyone who seeks it.[78] Patients (or their loved ones) demand what they think they need, irrespective of whether something else would be better or more appropriate, and doctors acquiesce much more frequently than they would care to admit.[79] One might think that the sort of health insurance one had would influence the readiness with which demands are made, but that does not appear to be the case,[80] although decreasing the influence of moral hazard induced by insurance may have a somewhat dampening effect.[81] But because there are such demands, and because we are also discussing what would be reasonable to support as part of a comprehensive insurance plan, further examination of this issue is required. In the next section, I will introduce a possible practical approach to resolve issues of wishes, needs, and clinical appropriateness.

NECESSARY/APPROPRIATE AND UNNECESSARY/ INAPPROPRIATE HEALTHCARE

Necessity[82]

A number of years ago, I took care of a 20-year-old patient who had metastatic cancer. He had lived with one form or another of life-threatening illnesses his entire life due to a genetic predisposition to develop malignancies, and he ultimately died from his last bout with the disease. He was remarkably mature and well-adjusted, even to the point of having a well-honed sense of humor about his situation, albeit a somewhat grim and occasionally morbid one. One day I suggested that he undergo what I described as a "minor surgical procedure" that could help relieve some of his symptoms. I actually came on pretty strong, convinced as I was that he could benefit from it and my belief that he "needed" it. However, he then proceeded to inform me that while I may consider it "minor," since it was happening to him, it was "major" and maybe he might just do well without it.

What does this have to do with medical necessity? There is a cottage industry that helps doctors convince insurance companies that what they wish to do for/to their patients meets the definition of necessary care promulgated by the company at the time of the proposed intervention. Indeed, there are legions of companies that exist to improve the way that medical bills are described and coded to not only maximize the payment but the chances that a bill will not be rejected for an intervention being "unnecessary."[83] This can be a risky business because so-called "upcoding" can blend into fraud.[84] Importantly, though, what is necessary may often be in the eye of the beholder, either the patient and/or the physician taking care of him. Desperate people who are suffering from any number of complaints may believe that any form of relief, irrespective of how outlandish or unusual, should be covered by insurance because "it is necessary for them." And, of course, advocates for every disease or condition interest group in the country clamor for coverage for their particular self-defined "needs," irrespective of the costs, benefits, and relevance and without regard for others who may have equal or better claims to the resource pie. They all declare that whatever they want for patients with "their disease" absolutely needs X, that it is necessary for their well-being, survival, and more. But how can a universal healthcare plan cover everything for everyone that they self-determine they need and control costs? How can we distinguish between what we may reasonably consider necessary—a satisfier for a true need—or clinically indicated from what is inappropriate?[85]

Having established some reasonable criteria for what might qualify as healthcare needs as distinguished from mere wants or preferences, it remains to discuss which of those needs should further become eligible for funding under a comprehensive, nationalized healthcare payment program. In other words, how can a reasonable and justifiable cutoff be created? Conceivably, all reasonable needs could (or should) be met, but this would ultimately depend on the amount of funding allocated to healthcare. While I have previously suggested that a politically mandatory criterion for any kind of plan to be enacted in the United States would be that it be sufficiently generous to minimize the negative impact on those who currently have (for example) standard employer health insurance, there of course would be a limit or ceiling to the total funding (otherwise, there would be little to differentiate this kind of healthcare reform from the fiscally irresponsible approach we currently have).[86]

Any strategy to meeting healthcare needs must recognize the following practical challenges and facts "on the ground" about the United States: there are finite resources available for healthcare. The limitations are mostly financial, but there are also appreciable shortages of trained personnel (doctors, nurses, allied health, etc.) as well as the kinds of doctors (e.g., not enough primary care doctors) and where they are geographically situated (most in large population centers, fewer in rural and poor areas). The demands on personnel would be enormous if we moved to a universal healthcare system (see the projected demands for physicians—especially primary care doctors—under the Affordable Care Act (ACA) because of the enlargement of private insurance under the exchanges and subsidies, as well as Medicaid, in the states that expanded the program).[87] Due to existing inequities, some people are less well or less healthy or sicker than others and can reasonably be viewed as having greater healthcare needs (both in number and severity). For example, poor people tend to have less well-managed diabetes than those who are more well-off and thus have more complications such as hypertension, end-stage renal disease, and blindness.[88] Poor people also disproportionately have poor health habits such as cigarette-smoking, alcoholism, and obesity with their attendant healthcare problems (and hence, healthcare needs).[89]

It is unlikely that a wealthy country such as the United States, especially one that would transition from a hybrid, disjointed public–private healthcare system to a single-payer universal system, would be as cost-conscious and as underfunded (as some people view it) as the British National Health Service.[90] This has been the focus of Roger Crisp, who has rightfully proposed (in a Rawlsian sort of way) that the worst off have a greater claim on national resources to have their needs met in a healthcare distribution scheme.[91] This means that it would be doubtful that there would ever need to be a choice (at least initially) between meeting or satisfying the healthcare needs of those who are the sickest or least well-off (from a medical perspective) and meeting the needs of everyone else. This also implies that, although the needs of the worst off contribute substantially to the overall healthcare budget cost, they are not so overwhelming as to swamp the system and leave little for everyone else. That being said, however, it would behoove us to attempt to relieve or reduce some of the social and other causes of illness burden disparities by paying attention to the ultimate causes (albeit multifactorial as they are): this would be both fiscally prudent and morally responsible (see Chapter 6).

The implications are that the United States could (or should) afford to offer a reasonably generous package of healthcare benefits (and therefore satisfiers of medical/healthcare needs) without necessarily having to have a "tragic choice" prioritization scheme. Therefore, we must look for methods to distinguish and prioritize more important needs from others, presumably in some ordinal order of urgency and efficacy of the associated intervention. A number of approaches have been developed that attempt to accomplish this task, including cost-effectiveness analysis (see Chapter 2), clinical guideline construction, and assessments of clinical appropriateness. Before I discuss these, I must spend a short time considering the meaning of medical necessity because there are a number of different ways in which this term is used and how it might be transformed to a different meaning by my approach (to bring it in better accord with healthcare needs).

First, it should be emphasized that insurers generally use the term "medical necessity" in a manner fundamentally different from the way most of us (patients, physicians, nurses, etc.) would think under ordinary circumstances. The former employ this term in insurance contracts to indicate what is covered under a given policy. While the meaning was originally liberally interpreted in the 1950s and 1960s as whatever physicians thought was clinically indicated for a patient, the maturing of the industry (and the explosion in healthcare costs) has narrowed the definition considerably.[92] Nevertheless, the federal government characterizes it this way: "Health care services or supplies needed to prevent, diagnose or treat an illness, injury, condition, disease or its symptoms and that meet accepted standards of medicine."[93] This is obviously broad-based and open to wide interpretation. In practice, Medicare (and also virtually all private insurers) have applied this definition to cover almost everything that is approved by the FDA (both drugs and devices) so long as they are used in a manner that falls within either the approved use or one supported by "reasonable" evidence (and the clarification of reasonable can be a moving and flexible target as well as one open to contentious debate). Many have attributed at least some—if not a considerable percentage—of the escalating costs in healthcare to the relative largess and semi-scrutinized ease with which Medicare permits interventions to be reimbursed.[94] As I begin my examination of "medical necessity" and its relationship to healthcare needs, the means (and costs) to satisfy or address those needs, and how to decide where to draw lines of permissibility (and hence funding), I will start with a consideration of (clinical) appropriateness.

Appropriateness

Another way to look at what is reasonable to offer (at this point in the discussion, assume it is irrespective of the cost) is to employ a characteristic that has been labeled "[clinical] appropriateness." Essentially, this means that, for a given clinical indication—and there are literally thousands of them ranging from, say, a tension headache to chest pain/angina due to a severe blockage of the left anterior descending coronary artery—with a series of possible interventions, it is appropriate (or not inappropriate) to perform the intervention. Entangled in this consideration are characteristics of the condition as well as the diagnostic and therapeutic interventions available, how effective they may be, and the depth and quality of the evidence base supporting that judgment. In a collaboration between researchers from the Rand Corporation and the University of California (UCLA) in the 1980s, an attempt was made to elaborate what this might mean for practical use and how a convincing definition of appropriateness could be achieved. They devised a fairly simple statement saying that a given intervention was appropriate (be it diagnostic or therapeutic) if "the benefits sufficiently exceed the risks and that the procedure is worth doing."[95] The question remained as to how to determine both components of this assessment.

Ryan Abbott and Carl Stevens describe their adaptation of the *Rand appropriateness method* (RAM) as a way of fleshing out the meaning of medical necessity for specific clinical situations and available treatments.[96] This method is somewhat similar to the informed, expert multidisciplinary committees David Eddy has proposed that could evaluate the efficacy of interventions.[97] A committee of experts is convened to independently analyze the amount and quality of the evidence for a specified condition or clinical indication. It would be an iterative operation, one that continues until a consensus is reached. A major problem with this method is that it may be cumbersome and laborious. To adopt such an approach for all of clinical medicine would likely be a Herculean task when one considers the thousands of conditions and parameters that consist of the entirety of practiced medicine—even the "condition-treatment" pairs in the famous Oregon "list" would potentially pale in comparison since the potential budget for a national insurance plan would be presumably more generous.[98] Furthermore, with continuing progress in various fields of medicine, it would be an ongoing and evolving process.[99] Nevertheless, the healthcare enterprise has taken on similar challenges, such as the periodic revisions (and expansions) of the "bible" of psychiatry, the *Diagnostic and Statistical Manual*, and the recent roll-out and implementation of the 10th edition of the International Classification of Diseases (ICD-10). Nevertheless, while the reproducibility and reliability of the RAM has been questioned over the years, it is now reasonably accepted as a satisfactory and dependable approach to achieve this kind of agreement.[100] One of the major advantages of the "pure" RAM strategy is that it incorporates not only "hard" scientific evidence for and against an intervention (like a Cochrane review),[101] but it also utilizes clinical judgment, a much softer and subjective view which is undoubtedly influenced by the panel members' clinical experience, including anecdotal case experience.[102] But, by doing so, it can have a moderating effect on what could be actual (or perceived as) harsh, sterile, and possibly parsimonious decisions about clinical appropriateness. Considering judgments that may be more derived from the "art of medicine" as a corollary to the science may result in more interventions being approved for use—and hence inflating a budget. But this generosity could serve to mollify objections to what could be interpreted by some as a faceless, impersonal bureaucratic process.

What could be the "moral" force carried by appropriateness decisions made by an expert panel? Are they such that reasonable persons who were inclined to accept decisions of this kind would in fact accept them? Research has clearly demonstrated that careful attention must be paid to the makeup of the committees to avoid undue influence from overly zealous advocates one way or the other.[103] They might have more moral force if there were lay members and/or advocates for disease groups (breast cancer, for example) as participants. If the latter were included, the problem then would be that strident advocates for a disease (or groups representing other special interests such as device manufacturers, drug companies, etc.) could make the final decision for coverage or "appropriateness" look nothing like what the experts recommended. Nevertheless, I favor the approach of including interest group members (to a certain extent) up front. [104] There are a number of suggestions for including relevant patient representatives in the discussion, although the fact that many will lack the technical expertise to critically evaluate the scientific evidence may be a drawback.[105] However, I suspect that if the representatives were chosen wisely and came from large, well-recognized, and mainstream disease organizations (such as the American Heart Association or the American Cancer Society), they could be quite well-informed and could be expected to exercise their responsibilities conscientiously. Perhaps one of the roles of the moderator or leader of the group could be to clarify the participation role of the patient representatives and the degree of power their information should have on the outcome.[106] For example, Paul Shekelle offers some other suggestions to improve the RAM approach, especially the sources and currency of the information used to generate the appropriateness opinions.[107] It should also be noted that the original RAM method asked the panelists to not consider the costs of the intervention. Whether this should continue in my suggested approach is open to debate. However, I would venture that most very-high-cost interventions may fail the clinical appropriateness or necessity tests.

There have been numerous refinements and criticisms of the process and how it can be used (or abused) to create clinical guidelines.[108] Ideally, both the decisions and the process by which they were made and the reasons or justifications for them must be public. However, to avoid the system being bogged down in interminable objections from those who believe they may lose something because of the decision(s), there also must be a way to cut off debate or to winnow out reasonable appeals from frivolous ones.

Finally, the relationship between clinical appropriateness and medical necessity is worth discussing. A necessary intervention must be appropriate, but the converse is not true. What this means is that something could be appropriate—meaning reasonable to do under specified conditions—but the benefits outweighing the risks/harms are not so great to make it mandatory (or necessary) to do. Here are some approaches that have been taken to mark out these separate domains:

> Necessity is a more stringent criterion than appropriateness and refers to procedures that must be offered to patients fitting a particular clinical description. Necessity criteria have been developed for a number of procedures (coronary angiography, coronary revascularization) to measure underuse or "unmet need." Necessity is more difficult to measure than appropriateness, however, because it involves identifying a group of patients who might have benefited from the procedure, but did not receive it.[109]
>
> We define a procedure as necessary—or crucial—*if all four* of the following criteria are met:
>
> - The procedure must be appropriate, as just defined.
> - It would be improper care not to recommend this service.
> - There is a reasonable chance that the procedure will benefit the patient. Procedures with a low likelihood of benefit but few risks are not considered necessary.
> - The benefit to the patient is not small. Procedures that provide only minor benefits are not necessary.
>
> Note that necessity goes *beyond* the criterion of appropriateness, and it's more stringent. As the instructions emphasized to panelists, *appropriateness alone does not merit a high score on the necessity scale.* A high necessity rating means that it is improper clinical judgment not to recommend the procedure.... A low rating on necessity means that, whereas the procedure is appropriate, there are alternative procedures (possibly including no procedure) that are equally or almost equally appropriate.[110]

A number of questions are raised by this view. One of the most significant is whether only "necessary" interventions (assume for the sake of argument that this would be iteratively defined as earlier using a variation of the RAM approach) would (or should) be covered by a national health plan, or should we be more flexible and thus permit/pay for anything that is *not* deemed "unnecessary?" This would cover most interventions but eliminate inappropriate (and hence unnecessary) interventions that could include marginally beneficial or nonbeneficial care as well as unproved diagnostic tests and therapies. Special care would have to be devoted to giving due consideration to the claims of those individuals with rare diseases. For many of these illnesses, there may well be very effective (and hence appropriate) therapies, albeit very expensive ones. For example there is an enzyme replacement treatment for Pompe disease (type II glycogen storage disease) that is both beneficial and costly.[111] Since there are so few people affected by this disorder, one could argue that it may not make much economic sense to approve such treatments. On the other hand, I think it both reasonable and wise for the proposed RAM committees to rule on clinical appropriateness and avoid politically and socially contentious issues such as this.

Other challenges also arise. What is the relationship between appropriateness, necessity, and need as I have tried to define it earlier? Presumably, if something is necessary, it is also needed and appropriate to do; an example might be an appendectomy for acute appendicitis. An example might be knee replacement surgery for osteoarthritis. One could argue that this is necessary in the sense that it could reduce suffering and restore function, but it is not life-threatening, so it may depend on how stringent one's definition is of "necessary." That being said, in a wealthy country like the United States, it seems reasonable to support joint replacement surgery for these kinds of reasons. Finally, there is the set of circumstances when the proposed intervention is judged to be neither necessary nor appropriate, such as for platelet-rich plasma treatment for soft-tissue injuries,[112] continued ICU support for a patient with multiorgan system failure and advanced dementia or with advanced cancer, or renal dialysis in a patient with advanced dementia or in a permanent vegetative state.[113] Presumably, these sorts of conditions and interventions would fail the tests and not be supported. However, a current challenge to establishing reasonableness and clinical appropriateness that will undoubtedly continue to be a vexing issue will be the problem of interventions for which there exist little data for efficacy, but that are still desired by patients and their doctors.

In summary, medical necessity is currently a term of art utilized by the commercial health insurance industry (as well as by many publicly-funded payers) to designate that which will be covered (paid for) under the terms of a given policy. In this usage, it is contrasted with "unnecessary" and hence not eligible for payment. In more common lay parlance, it refers to something that is required to address a health-related condition without which a patient could suffer some harm that is potentially avoidable. It should not be construed that providing a necessary intervention (categorized in this manner) guarantees the avoidance of a harm or the provision of a benefit (I will discuss the uncertainty and probabilistic nature of this in the next chapter). The needs that would qualify to be considered for funding would be those on which a consensus panel agreed were both reasonable to address and that there were reasonably effective means to address them to provide a reasonable chance of a reasonable benefit, with the latter also judged by consensus. To flesh out this analysis further, I now turn to a discussion of demands that exist at the margins of needs; indeed, they skirt the cutoff lines.

It is unlikely that any healthcare reform will have any significant impact on demanding behavior of many patients. While improved education of what is clinically reasonable (and covered) under a comprehensive insurance scheme, as well as perhaps better training of physicians to listen to what their patients are expressing by their demands (which, of course, takes time, something that is sorely lacking in today's practice environment), may influence this activity, it is doubtful it will eliminate it. Nevertheless, the fact that it exists and will continue to do so must be taken into account. It is also likely that our commoditized healthcare system in which patients are increasingly referred to as "consumers" or even (on occasion) as customers, reinforces the mindset of medicine as a retail enterprise where patients may be empowered to demand services much as they would in a shop or store and hence expect to have their demands satisfied. The sole difference between a patient stating or requesting that she wants something and demanding it is one of demeanor; refusing to provide it may mollify the former but it is unrealistic to expect that it will pacify the latter. However, the differences between a genuine healthcare need matched with a clinically appropriate and valid intervention (satisfier) and demands that are expressions of wishes or preferences have become blurred with unsettling frequency. Not only does this lead to inappropriate care—as in the story of Sarah's unfortunate last weeks and days—but it is also a contributor to the massive amounts of money we spend in the delivery of fruitless attempts to prolong the lives of the dying. Establishing justifiable cutoffs that delineate reasonable expectations of what constitute reasonable needs and how they could be met is both necessary and plausibly possible.

I have illustrated this section with examples of what might be called unreasonable demands for interventions that are probably not clinically appropriate for the true needs of the patients. In each case, the interpretation of what these needs were and their relevant satisfiers differed between doctors and patients (or their families). However, if there had been agreement on the "need" for continued life support for Jahi McMath and Mr. Martinson, or further chemotherapy for my dying patient, Sarah, or Abigail Burroughs, then perhaps there would be little controversy.[114] But because there is, we must strive to create a fair, equitable, and acceptable mechanism for both setting cutoffs and limits of what kinds and amounts of care are reasonable to provide in a health system.

UNPROVED, EXPERIMENTAL, OR "INVESTIGATIONAL" INTERVENTIONS

A significant percentage of medical interventions are employed with minimal to no evidence supporting their use. Doctors are also well-known for seeing the value of anecdotal "evidence" or personal experience[115] or of notable cases they remember from their practices, thus falling prey to the "availability bias" or heuristic first proposed by Tversky and Kahneman (I will discuss this problem in greater detail in Chapter 5).[116] Most—if not all—practicing physicians (myself among them) constantly and consistently prescribe medications for non-FDA approved indications, the so-called "off-label use," of which only some are backed by significant scientific data.[117] Virtually all doctors who practice in this way (hence, almost all doctors in the United States) would claim that they are doing so for the benefit of their patients and that they either have strong beliefs that these interventions "work" or their patients are demanding that "something be done" and they are simply responding to their patients' "needs." Most of the time—but not always—third-party payers such as Medicare, commercial insurers, and, less frequently, Medicaid will reimburse physicians, hospitals, and patients for these practices.

It is not just therapeutic interventions that are the problem (although they comprise a significant percentage of unproved healthcare). Many diagnostic procedures, often using the most expensive and cutting-edge—read: truly, really, cool—technologies that are subject to what I call "clinical mission creep" (expanding applications without the benefit of evidence to support the use) also occupy front and center on this stage. Many of these types of imaging studies either have shown very little benefit or haven't been demonstrated to have any value at all, but still they enter the mainstream arena. And the more popular they become, the more patients want them and the more doctors use them (especially those doctors who get paid by a fee-for-service model and hospitals that make money from their use). Just because we think something should work, perhaps based on theory, intuition, individual prejudice, or personal experience, doesn't mean it actually does. Even if it is beneficial, it may only be marginally so and for very few people. Admittedly, some interventions have little downside and cause very little, if any, harm. Examples of these might include simple blood tests (although patients who have lots of blood drawn repeatedly may be subject to what we colloquially call "the anemia of chronic investigation") and ultrasound examinations. But all of these tests, studies, and even mild therapies cost money, and it adds up quickly.[118]

But there are two categories of these kinds of interventions: those that exist already and that have scant evidentiary backing, and those on the horizon or not even imagined yet. Unless the FDA and other agencies toughen up their criteria for entry into the market for devices and gizmos (and the even more relaxed standards for "new models" of already existing and approved devices), the uptake and implementation of technology run amok will continue unabated.[119] Of course, Americans have developed a mindset that "more is better," which discounts (or frankly ignores) the potential harms that can accompany many interventions (such as side effects, wasted time and money, etc.). There is little incentive for those who sell stuff to patients (including fee-for-service doctors) to attempt to challenge this view. And while Americans may believe that misuse and overuse of interventions are not good in the abstract, their views are often complex and probably differ when given specific examples if they or their loved ones are involved (e.g., antibiotics for a cold are a terrible idea but one wants them when one feels awful).[120] Unfortunately, this mindset also perversely leads to higher "patient satisfaction scores" that have become both a slogan and a goal of healthcare institutions throughout the country on the assumption that a satisfied patient is both a happy one who is also clinically better.[121] This is not surprising since people are generally happier when their desires or wants or preferences are satisfied, irrespective if it helps them (in a more general sense) or they are better off.[122] However, the "cost of satisfaction" (as Fenton et al. put it) can be considerable: increased spending on discretionary (i.e., nonappropriate, inappropriate and unnecessary) interventions.[123]

Ordinarily, when something is tried out with very little reasonable evidence to support its use (meaning evidence that could plausibly convince others that it would be appropriate), and whatever knowledge is gained from the attempt (such as patient response, lack of toxicity or side effects, etc.) might be employed in future patient care, we might be tempted to call this research or something resembling it. While we usually think of clinical research these days as an organized affair with lots of paperwork and oversight, it doesn't necessarily have to be so.[124] This state of affairs suggests that there may be a very fuzzy line (or occasionally no line at all) separating standard, evidence-based practice from what might be more properly identified as investigational or experimental interventions. This is important and germane to this discussion because health insurance companies (and Medicare) customarily may not pay for experimental therapies except under certain conditions (although the Affordable Care Act mandates that insurers cover ordinary health expenses for people enrolled in registered clinical trials).[125] However, how can we properly distinguish between the two, especially for those healthcare interventions that are not performed under the auspices of a standard clinical trial? Once again, I refer to the classification of needs, satisfiers, and appropriateness as I have described them. Unproven interventions are exactly that and can never be appropriate except under the controlled conditions of a regulated clinical trial that is attempting to determine the appropriateness of the experimental treatment (for example). The judgment of whether a medical intervention is or is not appropriate for a given healthcare-related need is by definition demonstrated by data derived by experiment (ideally in a clinical trial). All other data are less supportive by comparison.

In two very important papers, David Eddy summarized the conclusions of a workshop backed by the National Institute for Health Care Management that was charged with developing new language for insurance coverage benefit packages to attempt to eliminate the vague and ambiguous terms "medical necessity" and "medically appropriate" and try to delineate the difference between investigational and evidence-supported interventions.[126] Their workshop consensus language is superb. Even though it was developed for private insurance plans, all of which presumably differ somewhat in their products and packages, I think it quite useful as a starting point to create similar language. This is what they produced:

1. Health plans are required to cover health interventions within the specified benefit categories if they meet the following criteria:

1.1 the intervention is used for a medical condition.

1.2 there is sufficient evidence to draw conclusions about the intervention's effects on health outcomes.

1.3 the evidence demonstrates that the intervention can be expected to produce its intended effects on health outcomes.

1.4 the intervention's expected beneficial effects on health outcomes outweigh its expected harmful effects.

1.5 the intervention is the most cost-effective method available to address the medical condition.

2. Definitions

2.1 medical condition: a medical condition is a disease, an illness, or an injury. A biological or psychological condition that lies within the range of normal human variation is not considered a disease, illness, or injury.

2.2 health outcomes: health outcomes are outcomes of medical conditions that directly affect the length or quality of a person's life.

2.3 sufficient evidence: evidence is considered to be sufficient to draw conclusions if it is peer-reviewed, is well controlled, directly or indirectly relates the intervention to health outcomes, and is reproducible both with and an outside of research settings.

2.4 health intervention: a health intervention is an activity undertaken for the primary purpose of preventing, improving, or stabilizing a medical condition. Activities that are primarily custodial, or part of normal existence, or undertaken primarily for the convenience of the patient, family, or practitioner are not considered health interventions.

2.5 cost-effective: an intervention is considered cost-effective if there is no other available intervention that offers a clinically appropriate benefit at a lower cost.

3. Nothing in this language prohibits health plans, at their discretion, from covering health interventions that do not meet these criteria.[127]

One of the attractive features of this definition of a medical condition is that it allows for reconstructive surgery of the breast after breast cancer or the nose after an injury but not a nose job to "correct" a normal variation (unless it can be interpreted by consensus by dispassionate observers to be somehow so extreme that it may be a deformity and hence a "condition"). Another attraction is that it allows individual plans to include some things for "padded" benefits packages, such as dental and eye care.

That being said, there are some major issues with how the workshop chose to define clinical benefit in its quoted section 2.5 since it seems to be specified within the context of cost-effectiveness. Thus, an expensive intervention that benefits very few people or benefits very many only a small amount (or perhaps for only a short time) could be judged to be cost ineffective and thus not deemed officially "beneficial." Whether a nationalized healthcare plan that would restrict interventions to only those that provide modest to large benefits to large numbers of patients and ignore rare diseases for which there might be (or could be) a treatment that was very beneficial could be an open question (see earlier discussion). In a wealthy country such as the United States, I would hope that we would be able to continue to support both research and treatments for such patients. However, I find it truly admirable that there is a relationship between the clinical benefits of an intervention to a real (not simply measureable) health outcome that patients would be happy to have. What this means is that surrogate end-points that are so popular in many clinical trials are, with some exceptions, not adequate to assess the benefits of a treatment. One exception might be the effects of statins on cholesterol and HDL/LDL levels in the blood, although there is no current evidence that better control leads to the "real" improvement in clinical outcomes. Of course, the same could have been said about tight glycemic control of diabetes but now the data seem to be quite clear.[128] The problem is that for some of these kinds of outcomes, long-term trials and follow-up may be necessary. Therefore, surrogate markers *may* be acceptable if there is other evidence showing that they really do correlate well with relevant clinical outcomes.[129]

In his second paper on coverage language, Eddy discussed investigational (or unproven) treatments.[130] First, he needed to define what is meant by "investigational," and he decided that, for practical purposes, it would be best to relate it to "unproven" interventions, be they diagnostic or therapeutic. That doesn't mean that they are ineffective; it simply means that we don't know if they are beneficial or not and for whom. Perhaps a more apt term might have been "needs to be investigated" (although this is cumbersome). It is conceivable that some treatments might be proved effective for one indication and investigational for another. For example, using criteria for FDA approval of medicines, we can reasonably accept that they are "safe and effective" for their approved indication used in the approved manner (say, metoprolol for hypertension). However, when physicians then employ these drugs for different uses for which there exists little to no evidence (perhaps simply a theory the doctor has developed or their similarity to other drugs in a chemical class), under Eddy's classification we would label this as "unproven." The question is whether "unproven" or "remains to be investigated" healthcare interventions should be covered by some form of nationalized health insurance plan: would they be eligible for coverage, and how should we decide what falls into this category? Eddy views the evaluation of proposed treatments (for inclusion or exclusion in an insurance benefit plan on the basis of whether they are "proven" or "unproven/investigational") as a task that would be undertaken by a committee staffed by people with appropriate evaluative expertise:

Is the available evidence sufficient to enable appropriately trained, motivated, and impartial people to draw conclusions about the magnitudes of the effects of the treatment, compared with no treatment, and all the health outcomes they consider important? The reference to "appropriately trained" people recognizes that evaluating evidence requires some skills—knowledge of medicine and methods for analyzing evidence (e.g., statistics, experimental design) being the minimum. Given these needs, assessments of treatments are best done by multidisciplinary committees. (p. 180)[131]

Eddy proposes 10 steps of evaluation to decide whether an intervention is investigational (in his sense) or not. This is extraordinarily rigorous (and good) but perhaps an
ideal. Much debate would have to occur to see if such rigor would be broadly acceptable, especially in transition, because many drugs prescribed, procedures performed
for specific indications, and the like would be disallowed and not supported (i.e.,
funded).

These evaluation "committees" should be unbiased, without obvious (or even subtle) conflicts of interest. This has been a problem that has plagued clinical guideline
committees of national physician professional organizations such as the American
Heart Association, the American Society of Clinical Oncology, and the like. They
have discovered that many academic "experts" (i.e., the people who one would want
to sit on these boards to discuss the evidence and decide what is investigative, appropriate, etc.) often are also employed as drug and device company consultants, have
equity positions in companies that would be coming under their review, and more.
Simply declaring that they have such conflicts seems to be insufficient to minimize
or eradicate their damaging effects.[132] Methods would have to be devised to eliminate
or minimize these conflicts, perhaps by paying the committee members sufficient
amounts to reduce or remove the incentives to have profitable financial relationships
with the healthcare products industries. This can be problematic in a semi-priva-
tized system of health insurance since benefit determination committees are always
suspected of being one-sided, especially when in the service of a for-profit company.
This could be less of a problem with a national health system if physicians were sala-
ried and well-paid.

Initially, it would be wise to have practice runs to see how the rules play out within
the current clinical practice in a given area (say, cardiovascular disease or oncology):
how much of current practice would be eliminated, how much would be defined as
investigational or unproven? There also must be a more effective and time-sensitive
method to update the recommendations to reflect improvements in clinical understanding and scientific knowledge.[133] Nevertheless, committee recommendations of
"best practice" are the basis for clinical practice guidelines that have massively pro-
liferated in the past decade or so. While their ability to change practice is not as great
as would be hoped (meaning that practicing doctors don't change their habits so
quickly or are just unaware of changed recommendations), they have had a tremendous impact on healthcare.[134] Nevertheless, even though the Institute of Medicine
(IOM) issued comprehensive recommendations to protect the integrity of guidelines,
their impact has been less than optimal.[135]

It should be emphasized that this approach would be best if it were integrated into
a national health plan, not to any supplemental plans that people could be free to buy
on the open market and that would support stuff not available in the national plan
(e.g., nose jobs and stuff deemed investigational):

> The preceding steps are offered to help a committee approach the assessment
> of a treatment in an efficient and consistent fashion. . . . What they cannot do
> is make the actual determination. . . . This is equivalent to asking whether it is

possible to construct from the available evidence a defensible balance sheet for the essential outcomes. If the answer is yes, then the treatment is not investigational. If the answer is no, then the treatment is investigational . . . any patient at any time can receive the treatment if he or she can find a willing provider and is willing to pay for it. What a patient cannot do is expect other people to pay for it. And that is where the distinction between the investigational status of a treatment and his use becomes important. . . . If they were put through the proposed steps, many treatments that are considered standard and accepted would fail— not necessarily because they are worthless, but because the necessary research was never done. If coverage for them were withdrawn, public confidence would be shattered, wars would break out between practitioners and administrators, and medicine would be thrown into chaos. To avoid this, the proposed benefit language contained an escape clause that permits plans to cover treatments that do not meet the criteria. (p. 185)[136]

This being said, quite a large percentage of physician decisions (and hence costs of care) involve so-called discretionary decisions, meaning that there is an absence of substantive data to support them (such as contained in clinical guidelines, for example). Even though these kinds of interventions account for a significant amount of the difference in healthcare expenditures between high- and low-spending regions of the country,[137] there needs to be a mechanism to allow for bedside clinical judgment for physicians. They must have the flexibility to make these kinds of decisions (if for no other reason than to gain their assent or buy-in to a reformation of the system) to account for individual patient differences. Perhaps a way to do this is to have extensive RAM evaluations of appropriateness (or reasonableness as I rename it) and permit (almost) anything that is not inappropriate (or unreasonable), assuming that the clinical indicators are present.

Daniel Callahan approaches this problem with his customary insight: "If a consensus could be reached on medical necessity, the foundation could be laid for universal healthcare. If the same could be done for medical futility, we might then have a way to set some reasonable boundaries to such healthcare, useful for the purposes of individual patient welfare and for societal economic purposes."[138] However, I don't think this would have to be so rigid about medical futility, and we can draw the line earlier at inappropriate and/or marginally beneficial care. The advantage of using the label "inappropriate"—or unreasonable—is that one doesn't necessarily have to draw a fixed or inflexible line or cutoff point that is applicable to all interventions. For example, while we may say that anything with a less than 5% chance of "success" (however we wish to define this) in an 85-year-old with heart failure should not be used (meaning, the system won't pay for it, although there could be substantive reasons why it shouldn't be used no matter what), we might have different views (or feelings, more likely) about a 5-year-old and some last-ditch, low-probability chance to save her life.

In this same article, Callahan goes on to cite Tomlinson and Brody's essay in which they discuss the perversion of the social (and professional) ends of medicine when patient preferences rule what is and is not futile and thus off-limits.[139] However, they ignore the possibility that these kinds of decisions by doctors may not always be pure and that, for example, the concern and distrust of the medical system about undertreatment that many African Americans have and that is believed to underpin their higher use of intensive care resources at the end of life, may actually have a basis in factual experience.[140] In concluding he says:

> It long ago became obvious that a simple medical standard of necessity would not yield any minimally adequate level of healthcare. Such a standard cannot be developed independent of value and economic considerations. The final result, whatever it might best be, must be multilayered. At least five elements have emerged that must be part of that result: (1) medical need defined in some general way; (2) the efficacy of available treatments in meeting that need; (3) the comparative costs and benefits of those treatments; (4) the necessity of setting healthcare priorities; and (5) a political process capable of making the combined medical and moral judgments that will unavoidably be encountered along the way. To those elements I would add still another: (6) stimulation of public and professional debate on the substantive content of the moral judgments. It will not be enough just to consult the public through a decent participatory process. The public needs to be stimulated to think about what it ought to want, not just what it here and now unreflectively wants. The political process, that is, should do more than sum up existing preferences. It needs to help people think about what their preferences ought to be. (p. 34)

Therefore, it seems reasonable to claim that if a healthcare system must restrict access to certain kinds of interventions in the name of efficiency and cost-savings—even if the insurance or funding plan were generously financed—investigational or experimental or unproven therapies or diagnostic tools would appear to be prime candidates to target. This is not to say that clinical trials would (or should) not comprise a significant component of the healthcare system: indeed, more specifically separating out what is and is not investigational should help demarcate what could be central objectives for future clinical research. However, to continue to permit and pay for interventions that either have no benefit or are unknown to have any (and may actually harm patients) in an environment of cost-consciousness seems both reckless and foolish.

CONCLUSION

Inevitably, there is a tension between that which is judged to be clinically appropriate—even necessary—care and what is judged to be fiscally responsible or economically viable care. In a generous system that is well-funded, it can be presumed that this tension will be more relaxed than in our current hybrid and inefficient system and that the balance between the two sometimes competing goals (meeting patient needs and emphasizing patient welfare or well-being and staying within a defined healthcare budget and controlling costs) should be relatively nonintrusive. By this I mean that the requirements of fiscal restraint will not bear too heavily on what is deemed clinically imperative. However, at the borderlines (or the cutoff points), there undoubtedly will be controversial decisions that will deny some people what they think they need. Unfortunately, this is unavoidable. However, the generosity of funding should keep the disappointed population to a minimum and their complaints should mostly be about interventions that could arguably and plausibly be justified as inappropriate and certainly unnecessary in a *publicly funded system*.[141] Importantly, in a system that is predicated on meeting the reasonable medical health needs of (all) patients, it should be emphasized that the definition of what a reasonable need is (and what the justifiable—and fiscally supported—response to that need should be) should be made by a consensus of those individuals delegated to do so. Unlike other healthcare systems (such as the United Kingdom's National Health Service) where the authority to declare a need and provide the response to it is to a great extent left in the hands of primary care providers,[142] I have argued that a less arbitrary system would be more palatable socially and more defensible ethically. It could lead to fewer disparities and heterogeneity among similarly (clinically) situated patients in terms of what they receive based on medically and morally irrelevant characteristics such as socioeconomic class, ethnicity, gender, geographic location, and the like.

In this chapter, I attempted to tackle a very complex problem: namely, how to decide what is and is not clinically meaningful, beneficial care and that should be reasonable to provide to people enrolled in a comprehensive, national healthcare insurance plan in which all people living in the country would participate. In many ways, this is the most demanding challenge to the cutoff problem. It is important to remember that claiming that something is needed or that an individual has a need is not the same as the claim being valid within the framework of a system designed to meet needs of the sort we are considering here. This necessarily entails differentiating between what people may want (or demand) and what they could plausibly be thought to need. To do so, I have explored various methods that have been developed to distinguish wants from needs and then considered criteria that could be employed to separate out appropriate from inappropriate care. The two analyses dovetail nicely because both are based to a great extent on the evaluation of benefit and harms, balancing the two in favor of the former. Even though this makes a lot of sense and seems quite reasonable, there remains a tension and a number of unanswered questions.

The first is how we judge what counts as a benefit. It may appear straightforward to assert that saving someone's life from a ruptured appendix would without much doubt qualify as an unchallenged benefit. However, if this story were altered a bit to say that the patient was 90 years old and living in a nursing home with severe dementia, the calculus would probably be significantly altered. This raises the issue of the degree of benefit and the context in which that benefit is to be realized. I have already discussed that it seems sensible that we should restrict the evaluation of clinical benefit to those individuals who could appreciate the benefit (either in the present or in the future, as with young children) but allowing for a fairly broad interpretation of the ability to appreciate so that we can encompass those individuals with intellectual disability but who can purposefully interact with their environment. Next in this spectrum is to consider whether benefit should accrue to a population or to an individual, and here I endorsed somewhat of a compromise in an amalgam of the two, stating that, in many cases, they are inseparable. The heart of the doctor–patient relationship (and hence central to the goal of medicine) is the care and relief of suffering of individual patients. Of course, that can be accomplished at the bedside as well as in the public arena as, for instance, with mass vaccination programs, the provision of clean water and sanitation, and the like. Nevertheless, this concern becomes more germane when we ask whether it would be reasonable to pay for treatments that may offer clear benefit to a very few patients but be very expensive. A paradigmatic example of this situation is treatment for very rare genetic disorders such as infantile Pompe disease or Fabry disease, both of which affect only a handful of patients and for which the genetically engineered enzyme replacement therapy is extremely costly.[143] Fortunately, this is exactly the sort of challenge that could be discussed and decided by broadly representative evaluation committees such as I suggested in the section on appropriateness. This begins to address the related question of who gets to decide what counts as a healthcare need and what counts as a benefit for the purposes of funding.

Even if money were truly no object and we could afford to pay for all the healthcare interventions that people could conceivably want, they may not need all that they might desire and medicine should not feel itself obliged to provide interventions that don't work particularly well (or at all) or can actually harm significant numbers of people. If we focus on the central goal of medicine as the relief of suffering, as I have described it, then how we decide how to approach suffering and its alleviation becomes more tenable. The doctoring profession is one of expertise and knowledge, at once technical, intellectual, and social, which forms the core of the relationship between physician and patient. This is not to say that doctors have exclusive rights to this knowledge or that it is sacred or secret. Rather, they have been entrusted by society and by their training to use this knowledge wisely, well, and compassionately. Therefore, any group that is empowered with deciding what should be considered to be reasonable healthcare needs and appropriate responses to those needs (and their attendant suffering) should of course include physicians by dint of their special association to it and the people who seek them out. But since suffering is by its very nature an individual personal experience, patients ("real" people) must also be involved in this process because the information and understanding they have could only serve to assist in making the outcome of such deliberations more acceptable to those who would be affected by the conclusions.

Notwithstanding the apparent logic, rationality, and sensibility of this approach and these considerations, there is little question that "selling" this to the American public and the myriad of special interest groups and entrenched factions whose livelihoods are intimately connected with maintaining the status quo would be a very steep uphill climb. The public furor over recent recommendations of the US Preventive Services Taskforce on the utility (and disutility) of early annual mammogram screening and prostate-specific antigen (PSA) screening gives caution to any one-sided declarations of inappropriateness. Of course, the fact that physicians who had major financial interests in performing these tests (radiologists and urologists) argued against the Taskforce's conclusions did little to calm the general hubbub.[144] Paul Starr's summation of the American healthcare predicament at the end of his book on the history of healthcare reform in the United States is beautifully written and concisely encapsulates both the problem and the difficulty of the task of reform, so it is worthwhile quoting him at length:

> But though the health insurers, drug companies, and other interests profit from the health system, they are not alone responsible for maintaining it. The bias against change also comes from members of the protected public. No other major democracy created a financing system that provides the biggest tax breaks to the people with the best private insurance; no other major democracy established a separate program for the elderly. A variety of other programs protect particular groups. These partial measures have become major obstacles to efforts to control costs and to extend protection to the uninsured. The resistance to reform didn't arise because Americans were such determined individualists that they rejected all government help; much of the resistance has come from members of an entitled majority with a privileged position in the public-subsidy system. The potency of these entitlements lies in the psychology of self-exemption they instill; the beneficiaries do not understand themselves as benefiting from government assistance or sharing a common condition with the excluded. The tax subsidies are nearly invisible to those who receive them; Medicare invites the elderly to believe that they have earned its benefits, whereas other claimants have not. Morally armed, they can reject helping others in need as a matter of high principle; after all, Americans shouldn't look to the government for help.
>
> What is also peculiar about the American struggle over healthcare is that the problems do not just afflict the least powerful in the society. Many middle-class people who have to the bad luck to get sick also get stuck without protection. Most of the uninsured are not the poorest of the poor, but working people in low-wage jobs—the kind of people who Bill Clinton used to say, "play by the rules." It's just that the rules of health insurance in America have been stacked against them. Americans are supposed to value work but apparently do not value it strongly enough to give workers a right to protection in ill health.[145]

In this regard, there is also this quote from a participant in the CalPERS conference on designing a health benefit plan using clinical guidelines. The speaker was a representative of the California public employees union:

> The statement was made that the way to do it is by saving enough money on the insured to pay for the poor. I wanted to be clear that I can't support my members giving up health benefits so that pork can be insured and still allow a few rich people to go out and buy anything they want. And there is a reality there that needs to be faced as well. I don't think you're going to find working people ready

to give up their health benefits for anything that is life-sustaining or important to them as a trade-off to having the poor insured.[146]

However, if we focused on true healthcare needs and defined them as clinically appropriate interventions with appropriateness judged by an inclusive process similar to the RAM method, we would automatically eliminate the most grievous abuses of the system whereby inappropriate care is rendered. This would go far to decreasing the massive amount of waste that seems to be embedded within the current system in the United States. Combined with the drastic reductions in administrative overhead that would naturally follow the creation of a nationalized healthcare insurance plan and system, we should be able to realize both significant savings and fiscal restraint for future cost control while maintaining high quality. Furthermore, we would set an ambitious and broad-based research agenda for the future because comprising those interventions that are deemed inappropriate would be those that could never be appropriate as well as those for which evidences of efficacy is lacking and therefore would be reasonable targets for clinical research. Nevertheless, a modified RAM approach has been found useful in clinical guideline development, so there certainly is potential for this methodology and it seems suited to the strategy for which I would recommend its adoption.[147] Building consensus among a group of experts and dedicated laypersons, all of whom would be predisposed to reaching agreement on what would qualify as valid medical or healthcare needs and clinically appropriate and reasonable means to address those needs, could be the solution to the cutoff problem. Nevertheless, there are many potential roadblocks along the way that must be considered, and I will devote the remaining chapters to considering the most significant of them.

It is not unreasonable to hold that everyone has healthcare needs, as I have described them. Some have more than others, and, throughout an individual's life, there will be times when one has more or less of these sorts of needs. Analogous to the variety of quantity and timing of needs are the ability to meet those needs by the resources one has at one's disposal. In today's healthcare environment, those people who are fortunate enough to have good jobs with excellent insurance and also possess the financial wherewithal to easily afford co-insurance costs have a multitude of options available to them. For everyone else, such as those with no insurance, bare-bones insurance with high co-pays and deductibles, minimal or no prescription drug coverage, and the like, the ability to have healthcare needs met is precarious. Delays in diagnosis and treatment initiation, subtherapeutic medication use due to high costs, poor access to primary or specialty care, all can lead to inequitable results and undoubtedly contribute to the overall poor outcomes that are a hallmark of American healthcare. In his monograph on inequality, Harry Frankfurt maintains that it is not necessarily that the rich have too much; rather, it is that the poor have too little.[148] A similar conclusion can be drawn about the distribution of healthcare resources in this country. I would not begrudge the well-off their excellent doctors, facilities, ease of access, and ability to purchase and hence take effective treatments for their diseases and conditions. Of course, one could argue that a significant amount of what the affluent purchase may be ineffective or superfluous to their health, but the fact remains that they can choose (or not) to obtain what they and their doctors think they need. I would suggest that we aim to raise up the poor as opposed to lowering the rich. Instead of taking away the excellent healthcare from those who have it, the goal should be to offer similar benefits to those who currently lack it. Certainly, we should also trim the fat, the bloated administrative costs, and other excess in the system, as well as carefully determining what healthcare interventions are effective within the context of a comprehensive understanding of health needs (and their satisfiers) as I have described in this chapter. This approach will serve the demands of both compassion and social justice without a wholesale redistributive scheme that is often believed to be so alien to the American ethos. By focusing on addressing and satisfying the requirements of healthcare needs and recognizing that all people have them to some extent and that we all can suffer from them, we then must meet the demands of social justice. Suffering is suffering: while it may come in grades of severity, it does not come in degrees of worthiness, some of which should be relieved by the powers of medicine more than others. By centering attention to needs and defining them broadly and contingently, we can eliminate—to the extent this is possible—those morally irrelevant differences between people that can detract from the overall objective of fair distribution of healthcare resources to those who need them and thus deserve them.

Approaching the cutoff problem not as a matter of defining hard metrics dependent on physical or other characteristics about people that bear only a weak (or no) relationship to clinically relevant factors that should matter in access and receipt of healthcare resources, but instead as a deeply personalized challenge that demands care and caring to solve is one that has eluded most scholars who have attempted to grapple with it. I have assumed from the outset that the goal is to be fair in the allocation of healthcare resources, thus making this primarily a moral enterprise. To do so, I have deemed it essential that the focus of efforts to decide what sorts of states of affairs should be eligible for what should depend on both clinical need and the appropriateness of what is available to meet that need. By attending to needs and distinguishing them from mere desires or wants that people may have, I have eliminated any obligation to become distracted by proposals to utilize both clinically irrelevant and morally objectionable features such as age or immigration status.

The challenge of the blurry borders is the same definitional one present in attempts to outline distinct boundaries of categories such as "rich," "smart," "bald," and the like. "Marginally effective treatment" is another of these. Just as we can say with confidence that life support for a dead person is absolutely nonbeneficial, we could probably agree that a man with absolutely no hair on his head is bald. But then we face the sorites situation of a patient who is not dead but has no functioning cerebral cortex (say, because of prolonged anoxia or an anencephalic infant): would prolonged life support be beneficial to them? And so on. I would suggest that we focus on the word "agreement." I suspect that consensus could be reached on resolving many of these tough borderline questions by utilizing a version of what John Rawls called "reflective equilibrium" (as employed by the RAM committees, for example), in which well-meaning people who were disposed to reaching agreement would, by rational moral argument, reach a compromise accord to which all could concur that could be justified to themselves and others.[149] By this mechanism, boundaries or cut-offs could then be seen as legitimate by large groups of people who would be affected by the decisions, and, from this state of affairs, it would achieve its moral authority.

Sick people who are suffering are all the same in a fundamentally important sense. Their needs may vary somewhat, as will the means to address them, but it is their need for help and their very human experience of suffering that helps define the nature and solution to the cutoff problem. By considering *all* people who suffer on the basis of their healthcare or medical needs and by judging the approaches to satisfy those needs on the grounds of efficacy, we can meet the demands of both social and medical justice. Finally, in developing a solution to the cutoff problem by proposing that representative groups of experts and lay people, free (to the extent possible) from overt conflicts of interest and well-meaning, be empowered to analyze medical data to decide what are reasonable needs and reasonable satisfiers, I believe I have advanced a feasible strategy to resolve contentious issues at the blurred boundaries. What remains is to consider other problems raised by this approach.

4

PREDICTION, PROGNOSIS, AND UNCERTAINTY

INTRODUCTION

One of the greatest challenges faced by physicians and their patients—and for the latter, a source of immense aggravation and occasional anger—is the fact that the ability to predict the exact outcome of a treatment for an illness in a specific patient is uncertain. Moreover, for many people who are clearly suffering from symptoms they are undoubtedly experiencing, they must face an often implacable medical bureaucracy that seems resistant to calling what ails them a "disease" and thus worthy of the kinds of responses we ordinarily have to sick people. It is this uncertainty, coupled with incomplete and imperfect knowledge of the world and how it interacts with the monumental complexity of biological systems, that leads to enormous difficulties in translating the vague and fuzzy to the concrete answers we crave. These various forms of uncertainty—inconclusiveness, ambiguity, and indeterminacy—about what the future could or will bring, or even what to call the constellation of complaints a patient has, plagues the practice of medicine. It is intrinsic to our attempts to conquer human illness, and this lack of clarity when precision and confident exactitude are desired can be immensely frustrating. It is a prime contributor to the cutoff problem. I will begin my discussion of this topic with two clinical cases to illustrate the direct challenge faced by patients and physicians that then directly influences the decisions that policymakers have to face in this realm.

The first symptoms that Jessica's parents noted were her weak cries that were unresponsive to their attempts to soothe her.[1] She wasn't interested in eating and was almost inconsolable even while rocking in their arms, an activity that had never failed to comfort her before, even in the throes of what her pediatrician had called "colic attacks." But Jessica was now 11 months old—her parents' first child—and they were terrified that something was seriously wrong with her. They measured her temperature as they had been taught, with a rectal thermometer, and were even more alarmed to discover that she had a fever of 39.5°C (103.1°F). They called their pediatrician, and the doctor on call told them to give her some ibuprofen and call back if she wasn't better in an hour or so; he guessed that maybe she had an ear infection. Jessica did not improve, so they called the doctor again and he told them to go to the hospital emergency room. There, the resident examined Jessica and quickly got a worried look on her face. She noticed that Jessica's liver and spleen were enlarged, she was very pale, she had big lymph nodes in her neck and groin, and she had tiny red dots all over her skin. Some blood tests were done, and the news got worse: Jessica had a very high white blood cell count, her platelets (cells that help the blood clot) were very low, and she was profoundly anemic, accounting for her pallor and the red dots on her skin (petechiae). There was little question that she was very ill, but with what? After a few more tests, including a bone marrow aspirate to look at her blood-forming tissue, flow cytometry to better characterize the white blood cells circulating in her veins, and tests to determine if any of these cells had genetic abnormalities of the chromosomes, it was clear that she had acute myeloid leukemia. Since she was under the age of 1 year, she would be classified as having infantile leukemia, a particularly severe and difficult-to-treat form. This was when I met her and her family. We had effective treatment for this disease, although not as successful as we would like: only about 50% of children could be cured. Bone marrow transplantation had somewhat better outcomes, but one needed a brother or sister who was a complete tissue match for this procedure and Jessica was an only child. Her parents of course asked me what her chances were. When I cited the statistics, they were confused and implored me to tell them what was Jessica's possibility of a cure, not anyone (or everyone) else's. And I was stumped, because there was no way to tell: I was reduced to repeating the mantra of the probability numbers, which was not what they wanted—or needed—to hear.

Mr. M. was a 55-year-old man who had previously been in excellent health. He was rarely sick, watched his diet carefully, got plenty of vigorous exercise and was proud of the fact that he could wear the same size clothes he had when he was a 20-year-old college student. He didn't smoke, and he drank wine and hard liquor socially and not to excess. He was married and had two grown children. He regularly had an annual check-up as recommended by his health insurance plan and occasionally boasted about how impressed his doctor was with his excellent blood lipid profile. So he initially ignored the slight feeling of discomfort in his upper abdomen, assuming it was something he ate that was disagreeing with him. However, over a period of several weeks, it got progressively worse until he became scared. He also noticed that his stools occasionally had flecks of blood in them. He then decided to consult his physician who thought she felt a fullness or mass in his mid-abdomen. She confirmed that he was bleeding from his bowels. She immediately ordered a CT scan of his belly and arranged for a gastroenterologist to perform a colonoscopy. The CT revealed that he had a mass in the middle part of his large intestine (colon). The endoscopy with a biopsy showed that he had an aggressive and large adenocarcinoma of the bowel. He was referred to a surgical oncologist. After surgery to remove the tumor(s), he was gratified to hear that the surgeon was absolutely certain that he "got it all" so there was "nothing to worry about." What gave him the confidence to be so certain?

Health systems and the governments or other public and private entities that run them have always been interested in the health and welfare of *populations*: how well are the American people doing? What are the latest infant mortality statistics for the United States as a whole? Or for individual subpopulations such as African

Americans or Latinos? Doctors, on the other hand, while acknowledging their incal-
culable debt to the scientists who conduct clinical trials and the epidemiologists who
collate, analyze, and interpret data collected from around the country and the world,
are quite rightly concerned and devoted to the health of individual patients. This is
not to say that doctors do not rely on their personal experience with patients with
similar clinical conditions or their diagnostic and therapeutic trials with an "n-of-1"
or anecdotes; indeed, some might say they rely on this mode of reasoning much too
often.[2] But it is a continuous and often frustrating challenge to abstract information
derived from the lumped many and apply it to the bedside of the individual patient.[3]
And even though most modern physicians acknowledge the facts of group data even
when it conflicts with their own direct practical "knowledge," they nevertheless may
have difficulty reconciling the two, especially when the drive to heal the suffering
person in front of them is so strong.[4] They are not always incorrect in this assessment
because some trials lack what is termed "external validity" or the ability to be applied
to a large segment of "similar enough" patients. However, it is most often up to the
judgment of doctors whether their patients fit the profile from which the data generated in a trial could be relevant. Whether from bias, ignorance, inertia, or some combination, doctors' not infrequent resistance to adopting new information (especially
that promulgated by clinical guidelines derived from studies of populations) can
often be detrimental to patients. In any event, no matter how confident she may be
in her prognosis for the outcome of a treatment, a doctor can never really be certain.

Roughly beginning with Louis Pasteur's mid-19th century disproof of the previously dominant scientific theory of spontaneous generation, to Fleming's discovery
of penicillin and its widespread introduction after World War II, to the decoding
of the human genome in the late 1990s, the explosion in medical knowledge and
the rapid expansion of scientific medicine has led to the optimistic assumption that
cures for all human ills are either here or on the horizon. Never mind the fact that
millions of babies worldwide die before their first birthdays or that many thousands
of women die giving birth to them; those of us fortunate enough to live in wealthy,
industrialized nations such as the United States have been raised to believe and have
faith in the overwhelming power of modern medicine to fix everything. We want
and expect definitive answers and are gravely disappointed when faced with either
pessimism or doubt.

There is little question that advances in the scientific understanding of how
the world works since Newton and Galileo (among many others) has reduced the
total amount of uncertainty over what the future may hold. Increasingly, we are
able to predict with seemingly amazing precision both what will happen and when.
Thousands of years before they occur, we can tell the exact dates and times of lunar
eclipses. Astrophysicists and cosmologists have even been able to tell us when our
universe "began." Even meteorologists have become progressively more accurate in
their predictions of the weather. While quantum mechanics may be based on unpredictability, the macro-world in which we live would seem to obey simple laws of cause
and effect that, although correct for the motions of the planets, are much less so for
the biological world. There remains a startlingly large number of areas affecting our

lives in which we might be said to be almost clueless about what the future holds. While it is true that cigarette smoking causes lung cancer, it is still only *probable*—not certain—that many years of smoking will lead to the development of malignancy in a given individual smoker; indeed, the evidence underlying this assertion is mostly epidemiological in origin and hence a statistical association or correlation. There are still some people who smoke two packs of cigarettes a day for 50 years who will never get cancer, and we do not yet know how to pick them out from the cohort that starts their exposure as young people. This is only one example of an intrinsic and most likely irreducible feature of medicine and human biology.[5]

In the previous chapter, I introduced the concepts of medical need and its differences from patient demands and desires. I also discussed clinical appropriateness and its distinction from medically inappropriate interventions. I concluded that, in a generous and well-funded universal healthcare system, fiscal restraint could be realized by offering reasonable answers to patients' reasonable needs while at the same time reining in both excessive administrative costs and healthcare wastage by minimizing the support for unproven interventions. I argued that the most practical approach to deciding what would be reasonable needs and the most appropriate interventions to address them would be a variation on the Rand Appropriateness Method (RAM) approach in which expert medical opinions integrated both the most up-to-date scientific understanding of diagnostics and therapeutics with those of the lay public. By this procedure, consensus judgments on how to draw boundaries at inherently fuzzy borders would be the most satisfying option to solving the cutoff problem. This could be a strategy to determining what might be reasonable to include in a comprehensive and generous healthcare benefits package in which caring and sensible restraint on the use of resources (i.e., rational rationing) was a central component. Moreover, by utilizing this form of decision-making by group agreement and focusing on clinically relevant information on which to base determinations and recommendations, we avoid resorting to using ethically unjustifiable personal characteristics that are morally (and medically) irrelevant and highly arbitrary.

However, expert and lay thinking is based on settled facts to which all can agree and beliefs that may or may not be supported by uncontested data. Indeed, the bedrock of clinical information is population statistics derived from both epidemiological studies and scientifically rigorous controlled clinical trials (some more so than others), which then must be abstracted and applied to individual patients. This, it turns out, is both a challenge to accomplish and even more of a challenge to understand (for patients as well as doctors). Many of the decisions by my proposed RAM committees would be overtly obvious. For example, they undoubtedly would offer standard surgical and/or antibiotic treatment for acute appendicitis. However, many others would be considerably less certain because the evidence base on which they would be determined is also less certain. They not only would have to contend with the possibility of making a mistake or error, they also would need to decide in some cases that providing or rejecting an intervention could be akin to a moral judgment. The sort of rationing envisioned to be necessary for a healthcare system as a whole is population-based in its conception but individual patient-based in its application, and transforming this knowledge from numerical calculations to singular implementation can be problematic. This is where any kind of methodology that would be adopted would have to incorporate and cope with uncertainty.

In her seminal 1957 essay on the central role of unpredictability in medicine, "Training for Uncertainty," sociologist Renée C. Fox defined the pivotal function that this lack of confidence in hoped-for outcomes and the future played in the education of young physicians.[6] She rightly pointed out that this feature is a characteristic and inherent component of medicine itself, and learning to understand it, cope with it, and help patients come to terms with it was a cardinal attribute of doctoring. She described the problem succinctly:

> In Western society, where disease is presumed to yield to application of the scientific method, the doctor is regarded as an expert, a man professionally trained in matters pertaining to sickness and health and able by his medical competence to cure our ills and keep us well. It would be good to think that he has only to make a diagnosis and to apply appropriate treatment for alleviation of ills to follow. But such a Utopian view of the physician is at variance with facts. His knowledge and skill are not always adequate, and there are many times when his most vigorous efforts to understand illness and to rectify its consequences may be of no avail. Despite unprecedented scientific advances, the life of the modern physician is still full of uncertainty. (p. 208)

Remember that these words were written almost 60 years ago, and things have not changed much despite the enormous expansion in basic medical knowledge and the growth in our diagnostic and therapeutic armamentarium that Fox's physicians could not imagine existing even in their wildest dreams. In the succeeding years since Fox made her observations (echoed to a great extent by Fred Davis),[7] they have stood the test of time and the radical alterations in medical practice heralded by the relative demise of physician paternalism and the rise of respected patient autonomy in clinical decision-making. Today's doctors still face what Kathryn Montgomery has called "radical uncertainty" every day of their clinical lives, whether they admit it to themselves or not.[8] And that is because uncertainty may be due to two mutually exclusive causes, one of which is epistemic owing to lack or gaps in our knowledge of human physiology and pathophysiology and hence amenable to improvement with research. The other, and perhaps most troubling because of its immunity from minimizing or eradication, is the inherent unpredictability of natural systems in the world.

The dilemma facing doctors, patients, and policy-makers is how to accept the fact of uncertainty and incorporate it into planning for a rationed healthcare system. Decisions at the bedside or in the clinic, as well as in the boardroom and floor of the legislature (or wherever system allocation and funding strategies are formulated, debated, and then finalized), all must acknowledge that there is an unavoidable amount of guesswork involved in clinical medicine. In the same way that we cannot be completely confident in our projections about the future course of the economy (even those who act like they "know" are not sure), we are more or less able to predict what will happen to individual patients. While that may not—and perhaps should not—have significant influence over macro-policy decisions about what is reasonable to include in a comprehensive benefit package, it does have enormous effects on the quotidian concerns of patients and doctors. For most medical interventions, there may very well be someone, somewhere who could benefit from some intervention, even if the overwhelming majority would not. Those charged with developing policy must not lose sight of the concerns of suffering individuals even though their choices will hinge on population (and hence anonymized group) data.

Thus far, I have argued that a sensible, universal rationing plan that was generously funded would seek to limit access to those interventions that lacked excellent to reasonably good evidence for efficacy. Recognizing that the state of medical information is far from complete and that many treatments and diagnostic tests in common use have not been studied or have data supporting their use, the groups charged with developing a list of offered interventions would have to manage the entire range of illnesses and these gaps in knowledge. Simply because there is little proof that some accepted therapies work for a given disease does not mean that we can afford to ignore the fact that it causes suffering in afflicted patients and that we should try and offer something for their relief. This state of affairs could stimulate at least two responses: first, it would behoove us to establish a system that will use such cases to set a research agenda (in both basic and clinical science); second, simply because there is no effective treatment for a disease (say, glioblastoma multiforme, an almost uniformly fatal type of brain cancer) does not imply that we have nothing to offer such patients because suffering can almost always be relieved. Nevertheless, the task of these committees (such as the RAM-like panels I have already suggested) would be difficult. One significant aspect of their challenge will be to render the population data on which their decisions will depend into a language that can be readily translated and transmitted to physicians and their patients. In so doing, they inevitably will retain the essence of the uncertainty inherent in medicine and, indeed, biology itself. I will spend the remainder of this chapter discussing a variety of difficulties to establishing reasonable cutoffs presented by uncertainty in clinical (and scientific) medicine and then suggest some strategies for effectively coping with them. I will first discuss uncertainty in a bit more detail.

UNCERTAINTY

At its best such a trial shows what can be accomplished with a medicine under careful observation and certain restricted conditions. The same results will not invariably or necessarily be observed when the medicine passes into general use; but the trial has at the least provided background knowledge which the physician can adapt to the individual patient.[9]

This brief description of the fundamental and perhaps unsolvable problem of individual patient prediction summarizes the predicament facing physicians, patients, and health policy creators. In the system I am arguing for, there will be at least three levels of overlapping uncertainty enveloping healthcare delivery: first will be that which the RAM committees will need to confront when recommending which among the vast array of services are reasonable to (and clinically appropriate) offer. To a great extent, they must do so by considering anonymous populations rather than individuals. Second, physicians (as they do already) will need to translate what they observe and measure at the bedside and provide advice to patients that is based on abstracting from population data to the single person in front of them. And third, patients must grapple with the blurriness of prognosis that is also based on group cohorts.

Biology entails diversity, even at a molecular level. Although it is assuredly true (if not redundant) that all people are humans and we share that community, each of us is biologically unique in many ways, whether it be from the massive individuality in the slight differences in our genomes, to acquired alterations to our genes by epigenetic processes, to the normal "wear and tear" of everyday life. These differences contribute to the varying ways in which we express physiological dysfunction, react to our environment, and respond to medical interventions designed to ameliorate or mitigate symptoms or even cure us of pathology. The ability to predict how these interactions will work and whether the result will be as expected (or hoped for) exists somewhere between prophecy and inferences based on probability estimates. This state of affairs results in an inevitable and assured friction between the demands of population-based health policy and those of individual patient-based healthcare.[10] Applying the former in a manner that makes the latter comfortable and willing to accept the decisions made at the policy level is a major challenge. There is ample reason to believe that the explanations and rationale provided to the public will be inadequate to convince them to abide by what could be interpreted as arbitrary verdicts or judgments coming from anonymous experts hiding behind an Oz-like curtain. People will quite justifiably want to know how these decisions affect them and their families at a personal level. Attempts to avoid the managed care debacle of the 1990s—wherein multitudes of patients (and their doctors) were furious at the overt efforts to save money by apparently skimping on what many were convinced was necessary care—should be a priority.

In terms of designing a healthcare system in which some interventions would be covered and others not, the dual problems of clinical and scientific uncertainty will pervade the design and decision-making process (it is worth noting that this general state is identical in many ways to what currently exists). This will occur at both the systemic, policy-making level as well as in the patient–physician interaction. Both must be recognized and dealt with as successfully as feasible. Whatever the mechanism chosen to create a list of conditions and associated interventions to be covered by a comprehensive health plan (I have suggested a strategy to do this in Chapter 3), the people entrusted with this authority will need to understand and manage this variability. Therefore, a central challenge will be how to incorporate the inherent necessity of outcome uncertainty—of applying population data to individual patients—into both the evaluation of needs and interventions and then their practical application to clinical practice. In particular, I do not wish to discuss some abstract notion of uncertainty as a philosophical or even psychological construct that saturates healthcare (especially medicine). Rather, I want to explore the particular kind of uncertainty that is a fundamental allied component of prediction based on probability estimates. Let us consider a seemingly simple but illustrative example.

If someone goes to the doctor with a sore throat and an examination reveals a red, inflamed posterior oropharynx with what appears to be a pus-like exudate over the tonsils, the physician might very well estimate—based on her experience, training, and knowledge of this constellation of physical signs (the appearance of the throat) and symptoms (pain, perhaps fever, etc.)—that there is a good *chance* that the patient has a strep throat (infection with *Streptococcus pyogenes*). To improve the *probability* that she is correct, she might obtain a throat culture to attempt to grow and identify the causative organism.[11] Or, alternatively, she might just *bet the odds* and prescribe an antibiotic (say, amoxicillin or cephalexin) because she is reasonably sure (not certain) that this is what the patient has. If she's right, then the patient should get better within 48 hours. But this is not guaranteed because one might actually have a viral infection masquerading as a bacterial infection, or one might have been infected with a strain of strep that is resistant to the antibiotic the doctor chose. Or, she might also wait and see: a small but real percentage of patients with true strep throat will get better on their own without treatment. Indeed, it may be higher than we suspect because it is conceivable that many patients with mild strep throat never see a physician. Nevertheless, we treat true or highly suspicious infections due to the relatively small but severe risk of not treating them (such as complications like rheumatic fever, poststreptococcal glomerulonephritis, retropharyngeal abscess, etc.).[12]

All these decisions embrace uncertainty: diagnostic, therapeutic, and outcome. Of course, this is a simple case where we can say with a fair amount of confidence that the odds are very high (but not 100%) that the doctor will be correct and the risk of being incorrect and overtreating is relatively small compared to the risk of undertreating. These sorts of assessments and decisions occur routinely in the practice of medicine. In ideal circumstances, doctors take what they hear, see, touch, feel, and detect by the history, physical examination, and laboratory and imaging findings and integrate these data with their knowledge of what all this might mean for this *particular* patient in this *specific* situation and what might be reasonable to recommend. All of these numerous steps are fallible and riddled with uncertainty. Furthermore, the physician (and the patient) may be influenced by other factors that introduce even more unpredictability about the efficacy of an intervention. Individual patients are rarely the prototypes envisioned even in the most well-designed clinical trials, and applying what is learned and true for the study population to everyone else can be very difficult.

Even in clinical situations in which a condition and its appropriate and reasonable diagnosis and treatment were covered by my hypothetical reformed healthcare system, there are variables about whether the therapy may be the most sensible approach for a specific patient.[13] There are a multitude of factors that influence the suitability of an intervention. These can include such considerations as the patient's social situation (encompassing her family and friends available to support her and help her both physically and psychologically), her financial situation (can she afford to take off work while recuperating?), her will and wish to undergo whatever is reasonable to prescribe (does she really want intensive chemotherapy and radiation for her breast cancer?), her age and degree of debility (will the treatment actually improve her quality of life?), to name just a few.

For example, suppose in some future imagined version of a universal healthcare system, hemodialysis for end-stage renal failure would be considered appropriate to fund for people who have diabetes and are still ambulatory, have controlled hypertension, and have stable coronary artery disease. Let us say that the hypothetical patient is a 70-year-old obese man who lives alone and must rely on a van to take him to and from the dialysis center. He is a widower with no children and few friends. He (along with his physician) may make the reasonable decision to either give dialysis a try for a while to see if he finds it an acceptable way of life or forgo it altogether, knowing full well that he would die within a relatively short period of time. Such flexibility for personal decision-making—not mandating that an intervention be used, simply that it is available if wanted—would be a true good of such a system.[14] To permit this kind of freedom of choice for clinicians and patients represents a strong moral argument in favor of generosity of funding and granting of benefits. The fact that it would be a priori decided that such expensive therapy would be funded for elderly (however that might be defined; see Chapter 2), friendless, socially isolated people helps minimize the chances and opportunities to force tragic choices and even more tragic results.

Even for very unlikely outcomes, there are some people—perhaps only a very few—who will respond as hoped for. The question is whether the system should support treatment for either marginally beneficial effects or for "rare" cures? What I mean by the former is that the benefit obtained is minimal compared to baseline, and the latter is where the benefit could be great, but only a few patients receive the big payoff. Not infrequently, the two are related. We are far from a state of affairs where we can predict up front who will respond and who won't. For instance, if I take 100 people with a serious condition, say, advanced cancer, and wish to treat them with a drug that we know has only a 2% chance of working, what could this mean? Well, it depends on the clinical data on which this prediction is based. It could mean that 2% of patients (2 out of 100) respond by being cured and 98% do not respond at all (98 out of 100 got worse). Unfortunately, all the patients initially look more or less the same, so we can't pick out the two lucky ones. Moreover, most treatments, especially for serious diseases, are not benign and there are always side effects, sometimes quite severe. So, the 98% who didn't respond in this hypothetical scenario both didn't receive any benefit (their tumors were still there and growing), and they experienced many of the side effects. Regrettably, this is quite common.[15] Nevertheless, decisions must be made, hopefully with the prime Hippocratic directive *primum non nocere* (first, do no harm) in mind. Alternatively, a larger percentage of patients could respond—say 30%—but no one would be cured and the effect would be temporary.[16] Finally, it is important to note that, for a given individual patient, the chances of success or failure are either 0% or 100%, depending on how one defines each outcome; as

I discussed in the previous chapter, almost everyone is interested in one thing: feeling and getting better, if not immediately, then eventually—or certainly not feeling worse. Even though the probability of a hoped-for result is derived from population data, patients (i.e., sick people) only want to know one thing: will it work for me?

Another way to look at this is the personal story made famous by Stephen Jay Gould in an essay he published in 1985 several years after receiving an unexplained (and perhaps inexplicable) diagnosis of abdominal mesothelioma.[17] This rare and almost invariably fatal form of cancer is most often caused by asbestos exposure and presents with either (or both) lung and belly masses. Rarely, patients do not have a known history of exposure, but they seem to have the same sort of terrible prognosis as the majority. Gould fell in the former camp. After abdominal surgery, he was informed of the diagnosis and its grim future by his physician who explained that the "median mortality" was about 8 months. Once he recovered from the shock (and the pain of surgery), he resumed his level-headed scientific worldview and his knowledge of statistics to more properly investigate and interpret what these words actually meant. Indeed, when he examined the extant medical literature on this disease and its clinical course, he discovered that people such as himself—young and with presumably idiosyncratic disease—fell on the right half of the 8-month median. Moreover, the distribution of patients on the graph was not Gaussian or "normal," and the right-hand longer survival group was quite skewed. He convinced himself that this was where his case lay. He was fortunately correct in his bet because he lived another 20 years, eventually dying from a different, unassociated malignancy.[18] Nevertheless, he could never be certain, only perhaps less uncertain about his prospects, so his spirits rose not because of absolute conviction (he was too good a scientist for that) but because of the odds being in his favor.

Benjamin Djulbegovic and his colleagues recently wrote an excellent and comprehensive review of many of these challenges.[19] They highlighted one of the most vexing conundrums of clinical uncertainty, one that persists even in an environment in which scientific evidence for and against various interventions is both improving and increasing and is inherent in a probabilistic world: "the application of probabilistic statements based on group averages to individual patients at the bedside . . . is permissible as long as we espouse the idea of exchangeability of the past and future events. . . . [T]he characteristics and circumstances of the patients are not demonstrably so different that one is easily able to dismiss the relevance of the group data" (pp. 325, 326).

While it may be somewhat more straightforward for the experts to understand and manipulate these often confusing probability estimates, the necessity of conveying decisions based on them to the lay public who will be affected makes developing approaches that can readily communicate salient and salutary information a vital concern. The fact that clinical data about harms and benefits are almost always available as uncertain predictions about the future based on past events entails three levels of uncertainty that Paul Han and colleagues have described: probability (e.g., there is a 40% chance of cure), ambiguity (e.g., there is a 30–50% chance of an effect), and complexity (e.g., there is a 50% chance of cure, but only if the patient has certain specific features; if she doesn't, then there is a 40% chance, etc.).[20] As Han describes the problem in a more recent paper:

> The most fundamental uncertainty in clinical evidence is probability, and the conceptual problem it entails arises from the endeavor to apply objective probability estimates to the domain of single events experienced by individual patients.... The problem, however, is that objective probability estimates are logically incoherent when applied to the prospect of a future event experienced by a single individual with only one life to live.[21]

Perhaps most disconcerting to patients (if they were informed about this unsettling fact) is that uncertainty entails the possibility of error.[22] The chance of mistakes pervades the entire medical enterprise from interpreting signs and symptoms and their (perhaps) associated complaints to deciding what laboratory or diagnostic tests to order to understanding what they all mean, giving the patient a diagnostic label, and then deciding on appropriate therapeutic recommendations (including doing nothing at all). The risk of misinterpretation, lack of pertinent knowledge, missing a vital piece of information because the doctor forgot or didn't think to ask about it when obtaining a history, all contribute to the potential for blunders, miscalculations, or omissions or commissions that could harm the patient unintentionally. And some doctors are simply better diagnosticians and "therapeuticians" than others. Sir William Osler, the "father" of American academic medicine, was renowned for his clinical acumen and skills, and most physicians can recall master clinicians from their days in medical school or residency training, physicians who were almost always right. But even they were sometimes wrong. And if they really were good, they would also tell you of the occasions when they weren't correct and warn you of the dangers of hubris in diagnosis and prognosis.

Some errors might be more excusable than others, but how to know the difference is very difficult. In the classic report from the US Institute of Medicine *To Err Is Human,* issued in 2000, it was estimated that perhaps as many as 100,000 people per year die in this country as a result of medical error, with untold thousands (perhaps millions) more injured for similar causes.[23] Of course, modern healthcare is a very complex system with innumerable components and actors, so some errors and mistakes are unavoidable, but many are not. Merging into the arena of blunder, miscalculation, and error is the wide variation in training, skill, and intelligence of physicians, nurses, technicians, and the rest of the panoply of human actors involved in the modern medical enterprise. Doctors differ widely in their abilities to take histories and perform physical examinations. This can lead to underdiagnosis, overdiagnosis, and huge disparities in the kinds, quality, and amount of interventions patients receive.[24] There are also wide discrepancies in doctors' knowledge base and their willingness to follow evidence-based clinical guidelines.[25] Whether one's physician decides to send a test, investigate further, ignore or pay attention to something one said (or didn't say), has kept up with the medical literature in her field, or, for that matter, remembers that the spleen is on the left and the liver on the right is almost a matter of luck.[26] The bottom line is that there is huge variability in educational attainment and maintenance of skills. Generally speaking, the criteria for becoming a practicing physician (and remaining one) are relatively low, all things considered.[27] Not surprisingly, this can lead to large differences in practice style, intervention usage, and patient outcomes. Therefore, the underlying uncertainty in medical practice can be amplified almost immeasurably by these other poorly controlled factors.

Exactly how to convey probability estimates to a public whose numeracy and other academic skills (such as general and specific health literacy) are sketchy at best remains a significant challenge both for providing intellectually understandable and digestible information and its effect on health behaviors and adherence to treatment regimens.[28] Americans may have worse performance in these areas than people from other countries.[29] Even physicians may be taxed to understand the sorts of data they are presented with from guidelines committees and the primary scientific medical literature, especially when compared with their own clinical experience, which they may judge to clash with what the "experts" say.[30] In addition, there is good reason to believe that not only the uneducated or unsophisticated public is in the dark about biomedical statistics and what they mean; physicians are probably no better.[31] If a cardinal focus of "accountability for reasonableness," an adaptation of the Daniels and Sabin method that I used to explain how rationing can be accomplished with public support, is the necessity of transparently disclosing and discussing the reasons underlying decisions for what is and is not included for insurance coverage, then the difficulty of doing so with a population who lack the ability to understand the rationale may be one of the more onerous and vexing problems in this process.[32] We should also not discount the inherent distrust that Americans often have for "expert authorities" representative of government or some other relatively faceless bureaucratic organization versus the trust they frequently place in their doctors; patients who trust their physicians are more likely to try to follow their advice (notwithstanding if they have difficulty remembering to take which pill when), even if they cannot understand the details of why the advice is being given.[33] Finally, techniques may need to be devised to avoid the well-known psychological mechanisms people have for viewing negative news positively; this kind of thinking is commonly observed in intensive care units when families are told of poor prognoses.[34] When this form of analysis is used in response to decisions to not offer coverage of an intervention because of its low likelihood of benefit, it could prove to be an obstacle for acceptance, although there may be ways to counter this effect.[35] On the other hand, in a possibly positive note, there is considerable evidence that alternative strategies of presenting statistical information (especially using visual aids) can improve the ability of both patients and doctors to comprehend the data and constructively incorporate them into their decision-making.[36]

Due to the irreducible and unavoidable uncertainty inherent in clinical medicine, even well-performed research that also asks the correct and relevant questions will not go far to eliminate or even minimize the probabilistic nature of illness, interventions, and outcomes. As Djulbegovic and Paul point out, physicians seem to prefer to make errors of excess or false-positive mistakes as they attempt to lessen uncertainty as well as respond to the increasing demands of their patients to "do something."[37] This ineluctably leads to what they call "indication creep." The widespread use of drugs for off-label indications with little regulatory oversight contributes to this excess.[38] Similarly, the attraction of technology (and the seemingly indiscriminate way that Medicare will pay for things) also leads to "gizmo creep," as noted by Daniel Callahan.[39] As medicine becomes ever more powerful, doctors have grown more uncomfortable with powerlessness, and as patients become more empowered and more knowledgeable (even if the knowledge they possess may be wrong), their requests for interventions—diagnostic and therapeutic—become more urgent (often stimulated or egged on by increasingly seductive and psychologically manipulative advertisements on television, in print, and on the Internet placed by the drug and device companies); thus, the chances of a clinical encounter resulting in watch-and-wait becomes rare. However, physicians skilled in clinical medicine also learn to adapt to changing and unpredictable circumstances, often by doing what has been called "improvising," but which is actually considerably more structured (and less free-wheeling) than the term seems to imply.[40] As Peter Bernstein has written:

> Under conditions of uncertainty, the choice is not between rejecting a hypothesis and accepting it, but between reject and not-reject. You can decide that the probability that you are wrong is so small that you should not reject the hypothesis. You can decide that the probability that you are wrong is so large that you *should* reject the hypothesis. But with any probability short of zero that you are wrong—certainty rather than uncertainty—you cannot *accept* a hypothesis. (emphasis in the original)[41]

There is little doubt that the methods by which the chances of success (or failure) of an intervention are presented or framed to patients (and doctors) can heavily influence their willingness to do something or accept the results of a decision; this is true in everyday life as well as in healthcare situations.[42]

Due to both the undeniable scientific and therapeutic successes of Western medicine over the past 100 years and the curiously strong role played by consumerism, commercialism, and hucksterism in American medicine, the public not only expect new cures and "breakthroughs" to be announced on a regular basis, but also that "miracles" will occur every day, especially to them and their loved ones.[43] Healthcare providers—doctors, nurses, drug companies and their advertising agencies, medical researchers, etc.—do nothing to dispel this illusion of all-powerful potency over the ravages of disease and even age. No one trumpets their failures; only triumphs make the front page and the display ads in magazines, newspapers, and TV.[44] Moreover, old tried-and-true technologies or even "watchful waiting" or the admonition "it will get better with time" are considered old-fashioned, behind the times, and ineffective even if there is little reason to believe that the latest device or drug is any better than what it purports to replace (or, for that matter, no intervention at all). This obsession with the new increases demand for the most current thing, which can only inflate costs related to technology usage.[45] Even if the newly introduced device, test, or procedure is found to be ineffective or no better than what preceded it, once people have become accustomed to it, no amount of data will change their minds. The only exception might be if insurers refuse to pay for it any longer, although even this brave act may be subject to both "consumer" (i.e., patient) protest and even legal challenges.[46] These unrealistic expectations that are partly based on misplaced certainty, partly on hope, and the remainder on misinformation will represent a significant obstacle to committees trying to decide what is reasonable to offer as elements of a comprehensive health benefits plan.

John Steiner explained some of this predicament in 1999 when he characterized the difficulties in translating data from randomized clinical trials whose results seem to be statistically sound and consistent with previous data. In one succinct paragraph, he demonstrates the almost Sisyphean task of attempting to discern the most appropriate way of discussing whether a patient should or should not take a given medication (for example). He utilizes the "number needed to treat" (also a favorite of H. Gilbert Welch in his book),[47] which describes how many patients meeting the study inclusion criteria (which he emphasizes may be dissimilar to the clinical condition of the patient at hand) would need to be treated with the study drug (the experimental conditions) to realize the benefit in one patient. This also can be translated as the number of people who receive the medicine and potentially suffer all of its side effects and receive none of the benefit:

> If the number needed to treat were 1, we could guarantee benefit to an individual patient and would not need to choose between measures of treatment effectiveness. However, the formula used to calculate the number needed to treat is $1/(P_C - P_T)$. In this formula, the number needed to treat would equal 1 only when all untreated persons developed the adverse outcome ($P_C = 1$) and all treated persons avoided it ($P_T = 0$). In other words, the treatment would need to be invariably effective for a condition with uniformly bad outcomes. Few diseases are that bad, and no treatments are that good. Thus, the number needed to treat never provides assurance of individual benefit.[48]

Similar kinds of challenges will face those charged with explaining the rationale for covering certain interventions with low likelihoods of benefit for very few people.[49] Likewise, the manner in which the results of clinical trials are "framed" can easily lead to a framing bias and misperceptions of both the benefits and the risks of a proposed intervention. Interestingly (but perhaps not surprisingly), both physicians and patients are equally susceptible to this form of distortion and in the same manner.[50] Moreover, doctors continually edit the content of the information they provide to patients as well as the "menu" of reasonable options they believe are (or should be) available in a particular clinical situation. While this is often done consciously, it also has an unconscious component, the latter of which may contribute to hidden bias and prejudice and may go some way to explain why ethnic minorities receive fewer indicated interventions than white patients (even from doctors who share their ethnicity).[51] Finally, patient satisfaction as it is currently determined may be heavily influenced by the manner in which physicians convey uncertainty. In one interesting investigation, middle-aged women facing cancer therapeutic or prevention decisions were studied to determine their satisfaction with how their doctors presented information about their options in which there was no obvious advantageous choice; more highly educated patients and those who were less involved in the discussion and resulting discussion were less pleased with the encounter and the role of uncertainty, suggesting that there may be strategies to mitigate this problem.[52] Another study has demonstrated (at least in Great Britain) that patients have less satisfaction when a female physician conveys uncertainty, especially when the patient is male.[53]

Throughout this discussion, I have emphasized the importance of data-driven healthcare decision-making, both at the organizational and individual physician (or other provider) levels. Ideally, these data would come from randomized and controlled clinical trials. However, there are significant areas of medicine that have yet to be studied in this manner for any one of a number of reasons, one of the most salient being too few patients (as for a rare disease, for example) for a statistically relevant conclusion to be drawn. In pediatrics, there are huge gaps in knowledge, especially with respect to the safety and efficacy of drugs in different age groups, due to some of the challenges associated with performing clinical research in children and the poor "market potential" of this population for many kinds of serious illnesses. With this in mind, what kinds of evidence do doctors commonly rely on when there is either little reliable data, no expert-generated guidelines, or the physician simply hasn't kept up? A very common tool used by doctors is their "personal experience" or that communicated by colleagues about their similar observations. This sort of reasoning has been called "anecdotal experience" and has been both criticized (justifiably, in my view) and lauded.[54] There has also been the relatively recent promotion of a new kind of evidence generator, the so-called "N-of-1" trial. These are more formalized methods of deriving usable and potentially generalizable information from anecdotal data obtained from clinical experimentation with an intervention using one patient.[55] This technique, while seemingly attractive because it can utilize relatively easily available data, may have other problems because the unreliability of anecdotal recalled experience data injects further uncertainty into prognostication.[56]

While it is often said that the only undeniable truths are death and taxes, Americans are increasingly loath to accept the former as something that happens to them, and their doctors do little to dissuade them of this fallacy. Organized medicine and the healthcare industries in the United States have done a stellar job of convincing people that not only is there a cure or a fix for everything that may ail them, but that there are more things that ail them than they could have possibly imagined. The medicalization of symptoms and "conditions" is a relatively recent phenomenon, but it has been a financial bonanza for companies meeting the created demand for their products.[57] Not surprisingly, the creation of disease labels for constellations of "symptoms" leads ineluctably to increased spending to diagnose and treat these newly discovered or identified illnesses.[58] It does not take very long for recent basic science discoveries to invade the healthcare market and be medicalized, as the modern fields of genomics, microbiomics, and proteomics readily demonstrate.[59] Not only is there the generation of novel markets, but there is a concomitant demand for insurance companies to pay for a product whose utility is hardly proved.[60] Short of a massive reorganization in the regulation of direct-to-consumer advertising (DTCA) of healthcare-related products, the pressure on those empowered to decide what should and should not be paid for will be intense, and it will stem from both the affected industries as well as patients/consumers/customers.[61] If the inappropriate use of healthcare resources (such as expensive prescription drugs) can be influenced by publicity, regulation of DTCA activity—a multibillion-dollar business—might be a reasonable place to begin.[62] Unfortunately, the very goal of DTCA—irrespective of the publicly noble sentiments expressed by the companies responsible for the content that they simply wish to educate the public—is to sell more drugs or, in the case of diagnostic testing firms (such as genetic testing), to sell more test kits. Since the linkage between one's actual need for a drug (stimulated by drug advertising) may be tenuous to nonexistent, but the desire to have the drug (or think one needs it) can be very strong, effective ads promote the potential needless overuse of a variety of healthcare interventions (not to mention the associated visits to the doctor often required to generate the prescription for the medication) can be profound.[63] Not surprisingly, DTCA content does not emphasize either the potential downsides, such as side effects or adverse reactions to drugs (to the extent the Food and Drug Administration [FDA] permits them to evade this issue) or the unpredictability of the (hoped for) responses. Yet the ads must be effective since the industry keeps on churning out more of them every year. Even if one accepts the argument that some of this activity can be helpful, such as encouraging or galvanizing a reluctant public to seek help for a problem they may have been ignoring or alerting some others to a potentially remediable health risk that is reasonable to address, it is likely that the market expansion sought by manufacturers is not confined to this relatively small group but also to the more juicy target of those who are at low to no risk of a specific condition.[64] Nonetheless, the goal of these ventures is to improve sales of drugs, devices, and the like and to "educate" consumers (i.e., patients) about their symptoms or ills; in effect, these ads aim to reduce uncertainty by introducing simplicity and clarity into the true vagueness of clinical medicine. And obviously they do it quite well. I will discuss this in more detail a bit further on.

DISEASE, ILLNESS, AND SUFFERING

It is not just the uncertainty of prognosis or clinical outcomes that decision-making bodies (and individual practitioners as well as patients) must contend with. They also must address the issue(s) of what qualifies as a disease or illness as a category of human suffering sufficient to be addressed in a comprehensive health plan. To do so must involve recognizing or acknowledging a constellation of signs and symptoms (not always obviously physical, such as a rash or a fractured bone) and possibly laboratory surrogates (such as a blood cholesterol level or blood pressure measurement) as both real and worthy of being identified as a bona fide medical pathology. Essentially, this process must address two fundamental questions: first, what is the difference between normal and abnormal (alternatively, the distinction between health and illness); and, second, how much of a departure from what is judged normal or healthy is worthy of recognition by a national healthcare system in which not all medical issues will be met (financially)? Obviously, these issues are of fundamental importance both ethically and because of their core significance in maintaining the fiscal soundness of a system. I addressed one aspect of this problem in Chapter 3, when I examined what might be plausible differences between reasonable healthcare needs and desires or wants. Both needs and what counts as illness that we recognize as such are contingent, subjective, and, in a very real sense, probabilistic in their nature. All have a cutoff problem that must be solved due to their inherent blurred and indistinct boundaries.

Ordinarily, such a measure would not depend on the existence of a treatment (or treatments) because that would negate the millennia of observations and naming by generations of physicians about disorders for which they had neither effective therapies nor coherent understandings of their cause(s). Simply because we do not have a directed, curative, or beneficial treatment does not mean that someone does not have a true disease. However, the converse is also true: simply because we have a pill that does *x* does not imply that there is or must be a disease that can be treated by it (see later discussion). Nevertheless, as perhaps exemplified by the explosive increase in identified diagnoses in the various editions of the *Diagnostic and Statistical Manual of Mental Disorders* (DSM) as well as in the International Classification of Diseases (ICD; published by the World Health Organization), we are constantly discovering new ways to classify both old ailments and finding new ones. Some are uncontested true disorders typified by infectious diseases, as the stories of severe acute respiratory syndrome (SARS), HIV-AIDS, and, most recently, Middle East respiratory syndrome (MERS) can readily attest.[65] Others may be more ambiguous to diagnose and treat, and, indeed, may even be equivocal as to their actual existence as a true disease. Those conditions on the borderline between what some might call the vicissitudes of normal life—especially the losses of function associated with advancing age, but also those encountered during everyday living—will prove especially challenging and vexing for both the experts and the lay public.

This is not to say that there are not physical (and perhaps psychological) problems that people routinely encounter that can be bothersome—even somewhat debilitating, albeit often temporarily, such as a bad cold—that can be readily ameliorated symptomatically with pills and nostrums (including the much-ridiculed chicken soup), most of which are manufactured by drug companies. But no one would suggest that a health insurance plan should offer to pay for aspirin or other over-the-counter medications. It is the invasive procedures, the prescription drugs, and expensive diagnostic tests for questionable or dubious clinical indications that are the problem. To be even more specific, it is those conditions for which there does not exist a clear boundary between the normal and abnormal—when does sadness become depression? when does a certain blood pressure measurement become hypertension? when does hyperglycemia become diabetes? when does a cholesterol level become hypercholesterolemia? etc., etc.—and hence are amenable to discussion, disagreement, and amendment that will pose the greatest challenge. Not surprisingly, the stakeholders in these debates will be very powerful: both people who think they have something wrong with them and demand acknowledgment of their suffering by a disease label, and the pharmaceutical and medical devices industries that stand to gain (or lose) enormously from what is and is not labeled as disease and thus is or is not covered.[66] Those with financial interests at risk must be resisted, coddled, mollified, and negotiated with in order to develop and implement a comprehensive and practicable healthcare plan for all. Patients and the groups representing them are particularly vulnerable and working with them requires recognizing that not all claims are legitimate, and while the pain and anguish of those who suffer may indeed be genuine, the validity of their misfortune dose not depend on the bestowal of a disease name.

Of course, another distinction drawn by this classification scheme is one of both personal and societal identification of those who may be called well and those who may be labeled as sick or ill. While most us desire the former, the latter designation bestows a number of ancillary benefits, not the least of which is the sympathy that naturally is elicited by the unwell. In addition, sick people are entitled to certain other perks, including access to paid time off from work (if needed), potentially workman's compensation if one can prove that one's condition is work-related, and even disability payments if one's illness results in a debilitating state that compromises one's ability to earn a living. Thus, expanding the ranks of the sick by increasing both the breadth and number of discernable and "approved" diseases seems to work to the advantage of all: people suffering from symptoms who now have an official name to apply to their distress, drug companies that can now sell more pills for this now-official disease, and even doctors who potentially can cash in on treating these new patients. But there is something lost as well as we overdiagnose and contract the range of what is considered normal.

Nevertheless, there is little question that people who have these various symptoms are suffering; the question is whether they are suffering from what we usually think of as a disease, amenable to 21st-century medical and surgical interventions. It is now widely accepted that human diseases per se are organic biological entities with discoverable pathological causes. This reductive, materialistic approach has proved time and again to be correct and has led to unveiling the causes of many heretofore mysterious ailments, especially in the realm of single-agent causative disorders.[67] Where it becomes much more complex is in multifactorial disease (e.g., atherosclerotic heart disease) or in disorders that are often without symptoms (e.g., hypertension) or are hallmarked by more vague and poorly measured (or immeasurable, subjective) symptoms (e.g., chronic fatigue syndrome, anxiousness vs. anxiety, chronic pain, etc.). It is in the latter that the difference between the normal and the abnormal is blurred and often quite variable between people; what bothers one person and leads him to suffer may be different for someone else. The threshold effect is thus highly mutable, as is the cutoff between what we term normal and abnormal, ill and well. Upon whom should we rely to label someone sick or not? If a diagnosis largely depends on the physician evaluations of patient-reported complaints, the challenge is easily seen.[68]

The medical-industrial complex, notably the drug industry, has taken advantage of this uncertainty with often alarming consequences. For example, it is interesting to note that there are only two countries (the United States and New Zealand) that have expressly permitted pharmaceutical marketing to the lay public. While this activity is regulated in both nations, it is completely banned most everywhere else for the reason of its proven ability to distort the demand and need for prescription medications.[69] Nevertheless, although specific advertising of named products or drugs is prohibited in European Union member countries, drug companies have managed to find ways to market their pharmaceuticals. For example, a company that makes a drug for fungal infections of the nails initiated an "information campaign" to alert the public in the Netherlands of the signs, symptoms, and dangers of this disorder and not-so-subtly suggest that sufferers see their doctor. Even without advocating a specific remedy, prescriptions for the drug produced by the company (Novartis) increased significantly.[70] It turns out that such "disease awareness" approaches are not uncommon in those countries that prohibit DTCA of drugs but may have similar effects.[71] Ray Moynihan and Alan Cassels refer to this as "*astroturfing*: the creation of fake grassroots campaigns by public relations professionals in the pay of large corporations."[72]

It is an unfortunate reality of medicine that many diseases are defined or categorized as distinct entities on the basis of where the scientific facts or features that are believed to be their cardinal characteristics fall on a population distribution curve.[73] And the demarcation point between someone who has a "disease" or a "condition" is often a somewhat arbitrary line (i.e., a cutoff point) on a relatively smooth continuum. An excellent example is how we decide that a patient is hypertensive—a pathological condition—versus someone who simply has high blood pressure,[74] or an individual with a blood cholesterol level that falls somewhere on a continuous plot of population cholesterol measurements but is stamped as hypercholesterolemic or perhaps borderline hypercholesterolemic or simply has high cholesterol. Both are exemplars of the shifting nature of disease categorization as we learn more about the natural history in populations of untreated groups of patients (or treated ones) over time with given blood pressure or cholesterol measurements. Of course, the definition of a pathological condition is relative to what we specify as normal (or more usually, a normal range). This is often conveniently +/−2 standard deviations from the arithmetic mean in the population, signifying that 5% of the population is inescapably abnormal (2.5% too low and 2.5% too high). In addition, such is the nature of physiological measurement that those individuals at the borders could fluctuate a bit and be normal on one day and abnormal on the next.[75]

One of the many problems associated with the attempts to transform physical conditions associated with normal aging (e.g., male pattern baldness) or even birthright (e.g., a big nose or small breasts or short stature) into medical conditions is that there could then be a plausible argument made that there is (or should be) an affiliated medical need to ameliorate them, especially if there also exists some form of "treatment." If we accept this open-ended argument, then it is possible that there could be no limit to what could qualify as a medical need. This could make many plastic surgeons, dermatologists, and drug companies very happy, but it also could corrupt and erode—as well as undermine—attempts to check spending. This concern does not intend to deny or denigrate the suffering of people who are dissatisfied with their baldness, breast or nose size, or height; far from it. But there may be more fruitful—as well as less dangerous and expensive ways—of helping people cope with these sorts of issues than to say that they have a medical condition or illness and hence may be owed payment for "therapy." Nor does this view relegate those individuals born with other disabling conditions to the ranks of those whom we would characterize as "not medical" or not sufficiently serious or disfiguring or painful enough to warrant not only our sympathy but our (society's) financial support to mitigate.

Perhaps, we could agree that short stature caused by growth hormone deficiency would be acceptable as a medical condition, and a reasonable and generous health insurance plan should pay for growth hormone treatment. Likewise, failure for a girl to undergo puberty due to estrogen deficiency would also qualify as a medical condition for which a health plan should pay for treatment. But what are the distinguishing features that differentiate these conditions from short stature not due to (relative) growth hormone deficiency (perhaps due to constitutional or genetic reasons such as short parents)? Is this simply a matter of quantitative differentiation or are there qualitative differences that can be demarcated? For some conditions, there may be a measureable answer to this. Alopecia not due to male pattern baldness may be reasonable to consider a bona fide medical condition. What about breast or nose size or shape? Or deafness? Most of us think it is reasonable to address the latter as a medical condition (if the deaf person desires it to be so addressed) but not the former. Of course, we have also come to the conclusion that breast reconstruction surgery after a breast cancer operation—including using the same sort of implants employed for elective cosmetic surgery—is a reasonable *medical* condition to pay for. It seems to me that the solution to these thorny, more questionable problems might be an open and impartial discussion by representatives empowered to come to a final resolution. It would be unseemly—in addition to politically suicidal and immorally disrespectful—for physicians to completely commandeer and control the apparatus and procedure to decide what is and is not a medical need, what should and shouldn't count as a medical intervention, and the like. However, to not give physicians who possess clinical and scientific expertise and are free of financial (and other) conflicts of interest a major voice in these debates would be unwise.

We can argue about whether medicalization is all bad or all good or some mixture, but, for my purposes, the most relevant aspect is how to distinguish medicalized conditions worthy of being covered (if any) and what features make them so and differentiate them from those that are not/should not be covered (an obvious normative issue). The multinational drug companies are intimately and heavily invested in devising new ways of transforming what had heretofore been considered normal parts of life (menopause, male pattern baldness, low testosterone levels) or sad, but not unexpected failures of body functions (impotence), into true diseases deserving of treatment by pharmacologic means. By marketing these symptoms as illnesses and enlisting celebrities to exploit their fame by appending it to the condition, many people (and their doctors) could become convinced that they needed therapy and that there was a pill (or pills) designed just for their needs.[76]

There are several significant issues my proposed RAM-like committees would need to confront that deal with definitions and their social and ethical ramifications:

- There could be a decision to not cover something because it is not deemed enough of a disease (say, male pattern baldness or male impotence) even if it may produce suffering (not to be deemed medical suffering); this could lead to the creation of a market for medications for these conditions that would only be available to those able to afford them privately (outside of the universal coverage system). One could then argue that this would exacerbate existing inequalities: poor men would have to live with impotence and baldness and the attendant suffering due to them, while more well-off men would not. This could also apply to unorthodox or unproven interventions for well-established and accepted illnesses. One could imagine that drug companies would reorient their drug development and marketing to aim at these customers (assuming that the target population was deemed sufficiently large) and develop drugs of special interest to higher socioeconomic groups (while at the same time aggressively lobbying to expand the market by convincing the RAM committees that these conditions are truly diseases and hence deserve to be covered).
- Given that treatments (drugs, for example) are rarely—if ever—totally benign, the medicalization of common issues that may or may not be diseases is by no means risk-free. Perhaps significant numbers of people being treated for a discomfiting but benign condition (such as impotence or baldness or restless leg syndrome) would experience deleterious side effects that may be considerably more dangerous and harmful than the conditions they are purportedly treating. Some have called this "disease mongering."[77] The question would then arise as to whether the system (a universal healthcare plan) should cover complications or adverse side effects arising from interventions that were not covered. For example, assume that elective cosmetic surgery would not be part of a standard benefit plan. If an individual decided to purchase such surgery (say, a nose job or a tummy tuck) on his or her own, who should be liable for paying for a postoperative wound infection requiring hospitalization?[78] It would seem unreasonable for the taxpayer-supported insurance plan to pay for this. If the surgery were covered by a private health plan, then it makes sense that a regulated private insurance market would require that these plans would also cover unexpected (but possible) additional costs. The quandary would be for people who paid for the surgery privately (as most do now).
- Another approach that drug and device companies commonly use to improve market share and increase sales is to support or sponsor disease interest groups whose members are or could be users of the products of these manufacturers. Indeed, their semi- or completely blinded backing of these groups may enhance the palatability of the message as the veneer of commercialism is removed or diminished.[79] For example, in their effort to promote a drug they made that was

approved for another indication, GlaxoSmithKline initiated a campaign to increase public consciousness of what they called "restless leg syndrome."[80] They also covertly sponsored the Restless Leg Syndrome Foundation that was created to publicize this condition and intensify advocacy.[81] Industry support for disease and patient advocacy groups is both common and extensive and not restricted to the United States.[82] Indeed, as mentioned previously, these groups offer an effective venue for advertising products in those countries that ban direct marketing. Of course, it is not just drug companies that wish to increase their market share; medical centers, hospitals, and individual doctors and practices are doing the same thing with similarly questionable misleading and biased copy.[83] These groups also bring enormous influence to policy-making groups, and it could be anticipated that the RAM-like committees would be similarly affected. Martin Gilens has shown that special interest groups do have a significant influence on the outcomes of public policy debates and laws passed or not passed at the federal level. This influence appears to be additive or subtractive and separate from the influence of general public opinion.[84] However, in an often-ignored aspect of federal policymaking, one of the most significant areas open to influence is rulemaking after a law is passed and promulgated to the agencies responsible for implementing it. At that point, the agencies create the rules that govern how that policy actually works, and, perhaps not surprisingly, special interest groups can have their greatest influence at this level.[85]

This is not to say that a market-driven healthcare products industry may not be an efficient or even the most suitable mechanism in a modern economy to develop the pharmaceuticals, diagnostic and therapeutic devices, and the like that will demonstrate both innovation *and* benefit for the general public. However, because of the arguably unique role that illness and health play in human society, and the comparable role that *effective* medicine can perform, the tools provided by these industries are vital constituents in this moral enterprise. As such, they deserve careful scrutiny, oversight, and suitable incentives (e.g., to develop medicines that will help large numbers of people, such as treatments for malaria, drug-resistant tuberculosis, etc.) so that they (and their practitioners, owners, etc.) cannot take undue advantage of vulnerable people. This is especially germane in the United States, where a significant percentage of new products originated in academic research funded by the federal government (the National Institutes of Health and National Science Foundation) and hence by the American public. However, this view should not be interpreted as denying the contributory significance of profit to the inspiration of innovative products; it is simply to state that the degree of financial gain should not be excessive and should be managed in the same way that we tend to limit the effects of price gouging when vital commodities are in short supply.

THE CHALLENGE OF PERSONALIZED OR "PRECISION MEDICINE"

The year 2004 heralded the arrival of a new scientific journal, *Personalized Medicine*. It announced its aims and scope: "*Personalized Medicine* translates recent genomic, genetic and proteomic advances into the clinical context. The journal provides an integrated forum for all players involved—academic and clinical researchers, pharmaceutical companies, regulatory authorities, healthcare management organizations, patient organizations and others in the healthcare community. *Personalized Medicine* assists these parties to shape the future of medicine by providing a platform for expert commentary and analysis.... Topics addressed include:... Cost-benefit issues for personalized medicine, Ethics in personalized medicine ... Integration of diagnosis with therapy," among others.[86] This path-breaking periodical was followed by others: *Journal of Pharmacogenomics and Personalized Medicine* (2008), *The Journal of Personalized Medicine* (2011), *Personalized Medicine Universe* (2012), and *The EPMA Journal* (official organ of the European Association for Predictive, Preventive, and Personalized Medicine; 2010). This must be a very hot area to spawn so much research and venues in which to publish the results. What is personalized medicine, what are its hopes and promises, and what are its challenges for healthcare delivery and especially for establishing cutoffs?[87] Presumably, the goals are to reduce uncertainty and unpredictability, enhance prognostic accuracy, and improve our discriminatory abilities in diagnosis and treatment. This sounds unobjectionable and laudable in theory; what could be wrong with it? Let me begin with some historical examples that first show the benefits.

Isoniazid was one of the earliest effective drugs developed for the treatment of tuberculosis (and it continues to be a mainstay to this day, even with the emergence of multiply-drug-resistant organisms). Soon after it entered into widespread clinical usage, it was noted that some people metabolize the drug much more rapidly than others, resulting in its rapid disappearance from the blood.[88] It appeared this was due to how swiftly enzymes in the liver detoxified the primary drug by chemically modifying its structure by acetylating it to render it inactive. Some patients were deemed "fast-acetylators" and others "slow-acetylators," and their dosing was adjusted accordingly. This was an initial excellent example of "personalized medicine" and how such information could be used to improve patient care. There were (and are) millions of people worldwide who are infected with *Mycobacterium tuberculosis*, and the ratio of fast to slow acetylators varies in different genetic populations.[89] Deleterious side effects are more often observed in slow metabolizers.[90] One could easily conclude that the sort of information revealed by this form of personalized medicine is a definite benefit to all involved.

Clopidogrel is a direct inhibitor of the function of platelets, the cells that circulate in the blood that helps it clot at the sites of injury and/or inflammation.[91] It has been widely used clinically when patients are at high risk for arterial clots, such as after myocardial infarction (a heart attack) and insertion of coronary artery stents.[92] Like isoniazid, this drug is also metabolized in the liver, and the principal enzyme responsible for its chemical alteration (and change in activity) comes in a variety of alleles or molecular types dictated by one's genotype. Therefore, some current recommendations suggest that therapy with the drug should be adjusted based on the findings from genotype testing (although there is some controversy over this).[93] This is another potentially excellent, clinically useful example of personalized medicine in action, and one that also affects large numbers of people and that may be judged cost-effective.[94]

These are but two illustrations of how advances in genetic and other biomedical sciences may have improved how we deliver treatments to people based not on how similar they are but by recognizing how different we are from each other and how those differences not only may dictate what diseases we may be more or less susceptible to catching or developing, but also how we respond to the treatments we have created to combat them. However, the future may lie elsewhere. For example, in 2012, Vertex Pharmaceuticals based in Cambridge, Massachusetts, announced the FDA approval of their new drug for cystic fibrosis (CF), ivacaftor (Kalydeco).[95] This highly specialized drug was designed to target the G551D mutation in the CF gene with exquisite sensitivity and specificity. Unfortunately for the vast majority of the 30,000 or so Americans with this disease, the drug will only work in the 4–5% or so who possess this particular mutation. Furthermore, this life-altering medication costs almost $300,000 per year.[96] Who can pay for this form of highly personalized medicine? Is it worth it?[97] If ivacaftor were a "one-off" medication, unique in not only its method of action but also in its existence, that would be one thing. But the promise and allure of personalized medicine is that this will not be the exception, but the rule.

If the dreams and predictions of proselytizers for personalized—now rebranded as "precision"—medicine (both genomic-based and not) ever become true, how might this affect our ability to limit the availability of medical treatments and control costs? Currently, if we decide to restrict access to treatments that have very little chance of success, we make that assessment based on population data. For example, if a patient has metastatic, progressive cancer of some type and it is stated that there might a 5% chance of response (the tumors and/or symptoms improving) after a treatment of one form or another, this means that in a sample of 100 patients or so, 5 would respond well and the other 95 would not. We would not be able to predict ahead of time to which group an individual patient would belong. We would make the judgment that this treatment would not be "worth" offering under a rationed (even if generous) medical insurance system due to the small chance that it presented to a population of reasonably similar patients. However, if there were a "perfect" or idealized system of personalized medicine, we could imagine that we would be able to predetermine who the 5% of responders would be and separate them out of the pack. We would then be left with the perhaps more troublesome and difficult question of whether it would be worthwhile to offer the treatment to those patients, knowing that it would probably be effective. Would effective (and perhaps expensive treatment) for very rare diseases or conditions affecting very few patients be reasonable to pay for? This is a different way to look at treatments that work a little bit for the few. Perhaps we might take the approach used for some "orphan" diseases, where expensive treatment may be life-saving (such as some genetically engineered enzyme replacements for metabolic diseases)[98] but where relatively few patients are affected. It may well be reasonable to save someone's life with an expensive drug but not if it was solely palliative or offered only a marginal benefit, even if one could be virtually guaranteed that the patient would experience the benefit (i.e., "marginal" benefit could be defined on an individual as well as a population basis).

If a cardinal rule of morality is that similar situations should be treated similarly if one wishes to be fair, then the prospect of individualized, personalized, and particularized medicine poses a challenge. By the very nature of drawing distinctions between people by their inherent and acquired specific characteristics, one diminishes the degree of similarity between people that fairness demands. Of course, the proponents of personalized medicine would say that the goal is to individualize treatment from the "one size fits all" that we currently use most frequently. But the minute we are able to say that my prostate cancer is uniquely different from yours and should thus be treated differently, we have the potential for physicians (or the "system") to state that perhaps my cancer is too uncommon or too rare to merit treatment or that the treatment is too expensive for a publicly funded system to afford (for example), or some other arbitrary—but perhaps not entirely unreasonable—approach.

Alternatively, we would have to address demands for consideration from those people who now would have a "rare" subtype of a perhaps common disease. For example, today we classify lung cancer into four or five different disorders using the tools of microscopic appearance, some genetic "signatures," and the like. A truly personalized medicine might distinguish many more, say, 30 to 40, accompanied by a number of different host "genotypes" that could contribute to the metabolism of the drug(s) selected and hence their efficacy (as in the stories of isoniazid and clopidogrel).[99] While such a reductive approach could, in theory, improve therapeutic accuracy and potency by narrowing the number of patients receiving a treatment to only those who could benefit from it, it could also contribute enormously to cost. It is no doubt less expensive to treat many people with one drug than lots of different people (with now newly distinct different diseases) with lots of different drugs. Finally, if the financial incentives were set in such a way to stimulate new drug discovery or design for disorder subtypes that affect even smaller populations of patients, the size of the customer base over which to amortize the costs of research and development also becomes smaller, thus increasing prices.

In many ways, the utopian goals of personalized medicine are to minimize or even eliminate the problems of uncertainty that I have discussed throughout this chapter. It aims to accomplish this by adapting diagnosis and treatment options, as specifically as scientifically possible, to each patient's unique biomedical characteristics. However, it is unclear whether to do so will require such enormous amounts of information about everyone matched with the call for such huge varieties of individualized medicines that there may be insufficient funds as well as demand to make the program fiscally viable. As Donna Dickenson vividly explains, "me medicine" gives short shrift to the perhaps unglamorous but hugely effective public health and population-based interventions that have led to such prodigious gains in the overall health of generations of people.[100] Personalized medicine's dependence on a concept of reasonably strict genetic (or metabolomics or proteomic) determinism may be misplaced, overly confident, and fail to take into consideration the complexity of the interactions between what might be labeled our native biomedical endowment and the myriad different environments in which we live and which affect our futures.[101] At least theoretically, the form of uncertainty due to a lack of knowledge is amenable to the sort of information that could conceivably be provided by the forms of analyses favored in personalized medicine, as described as a new branch of healthcare (as, say, distinct from public or population health). Hence, a complete knowledge of how the human body works and how it interacts with its environment (assuming that such knowledge is even possible) should reduce this form of uncertainty to near zero. Of course, this sort of terminal reductionism may be inherently fallacious as a way to describe, know, and finally manipulate nature, but personalized medicine's adherents seem to hew to this view. However, even if such knowing were possible, it would do nothing to attack the other contributor to uncertainty: the irreducible nature of complex systems.[102]

In many ways, the ultimate end-point in personalized medicine (the *reductio ad absurdum*, if you will) creates what might be called "boutique" services, in which each individual patient is "uniquely unique", requiring highly specialized and exclusively particular services that can only benefit her (and no one else). While this ideally removes uncertainty, it also requires some very heavy lifting on the part of those who would supply the boutique services or answers to the unique problems presented by each individual patient. This would include the enormously complex knowledge base that would need to be understood by physicians; rather than learning about disease X, the physician of personalized medicine would have to know about disease X in patient Y and what drug or intervention is required for this particular situation from the now potentially huge number available to meet the multitude of different clinical situations. It would be as if a surgeon was surprised each time she opened a patient's abdomen and discovered that the organs and their interconnections were different in each patient. Another challenge would be for those charged with coming up with answers. In a world where one size doesn't fit all, the number needed to treat would be just one, but the array of treatments from which one would need to choose for a given patient could be vast. No company would embark on the expensive venture of developing drugs or machines that could only be used effectively in a select few individuals; if they did, they would have to price them like Kalydeco, but probably charge much more. Such a system is not only unsustainable, but unimaginable.

One final complication of personalized medicine that has yet to truly enter the clinical sphere (but is poised to do so in the near future) is the challenge posed by the rapidly expanding knowledge of epigenetics. This field of study concentrates on the semi-reversible chemical modification of genomic DNA that can radically alter the activity of genes.[103] This is a highly regulated system and has served as the target of novel sorts of therapies aiming to unmask the activity of genes that have been silenced in certain kinds of cancer, for instance. While epigenetic changes are usually acquired during one's lifetime after exposure to a variety of environmental agents, most notably various toxins, of great significance is that some of these alterations can be passed onto one's children in a sort of odd vindication of a form of Lamarckism.[104] What is relevant for my discussion is that the patterns of epigenetic modification can be radically different between patients and thus can influence not only the expression of disease but also its response to therapy. Hence, this adds another complication of uncertainty into the personalization of medicine.

Onyebuchi Arah insightfully emphasizes that health or disease of the individual cannot be separated from the context in which that individual lives, both physically and socially.[105] He notes that personal health is inextricably intertwined not only with one's present circumstances but also with those that preceded in time and place:

> Health is not entirely individual; it is relative to the individual's context, which in turn is fashioned out of the interactions that exist between members of any defined collective whose health (read: population health) is defined by the health and context of its members. The circularity of this concept and argument is not lost on us. Many diseases such as allergic, cardiovascular, and even genetic disorders seem to have contextual antecedents. And these contextual causes, determinants or facilitators tend to accumulate from, probably, before conception and birth through adult life.[106]

Thus, the success of the person cannot be untangled from that of the population in which she is situated and lives. We are much more dependent on others than many would care to accept, as Donne's lines describe: "No man is an island, Entire of itself, Every man is a piece of the continent, A part of the main."[107] Nevertheless, when going to the doctor, people don't do so in groups: they go as individuals, and they want to believe they are being considered and treated as such. No one would find being blended into a crowd very satisfying or comforting. We are reassured that our doctor is looking out for our best interests and not others'. The "market" for personalized healthcare services, ranging from genetic and other forms of laboratory testing services (now including commercial microbiome services)[108] is still developing and evolving, and it remains to be seen what will emerge when it matures. However, it has the possibility to profoundly affect the sorts of probability information available to the public and which segments of the public have access to it.[109]

Of course, we wish to continue to treat patients as individuals with their unique needs, hopes, desires, and goals. However, this does not mean that medicine itself must develop individualized treatment in the particular, such as is the hope and goal of personalized or precision genomic medicine, because to do so would create both incredible obstacles and overwhelming costs. Furthermore, it is unlikely to benefit the vast majority of patients. Just like custom-made clothing costs significantly more than off-the-rack goods that can be adjusted to fit almost everyone, "made-to-measure" drugs and genetic treatments also promise to lead to skyrocketing costs without proportionate benefit. One might object and point out that patients already get custom-made prostheses, for example. True. But they come from a standard model (and they are also *very* expensive).

CONCLUSION

The task of nosological classification is not one that constantly deals with ontological truths, of black and white, of the presence or absence of self-evident and obvious disease states with which few—if any—would quibble. Even the less ambiguous illnesses, such as streptococcal pharyngitis, must co-exist with chronic nondisease "conditions" such as stable colonization with the strep bacterium. Who is to say categorically that a deviation from statistical norms qualifies as a state of disease that we recognize and regard as sufficiently abnormal that we can behave as if the person suffering from it is afflicted with a true illness and hence has a need (for something)? Trying to decide who is sick—or could be in the future if a preventive action were introduced—is an essential corollary to defining medical needs and therefore also to establishing what would be reasonable interventions to permit.

If we had a universal healthcare system that had to cope with such fiscal constraints that it could only afford to support interventions for the most grievous of illnesses or injuries—perhaps akin to a parsimonious Oregon Health Plan-like system—the choosing between what to include and not could be much simpler (although perhaps tragically heart-wrenching). But, as I have maintained, we live in a wealthy country and even if the powers that be had a tendency or philosophy to be niggardly in their generosity to those less well off than themselves, generosity would mark the system simply out of political expediency.[110] And therein lies the conundrum, for the very generosity of healthcare coverage benefits entails that conditions that are more debatable in their reality will be considered as worthy or not for inclusion. Again, we have the problem of where and how to draw a justifiable cutoff between what is and is not a health condition, a kind of suffering that generates a healthcare need that should prompt both concern and compassion and, if the means are made available, interventions to respond appropriately. In actual practical application, we should run out of diseases (hopefully) for which we have reasonable treatments well before we run out of money (assuming we also make the other systemic changes that would be required in a complete overhaul of the healthcare system, such as a vast decrease in administrative costs, minimizing wasted or ineffectual interventions, etc.).

How do we (society) cope with the flexible and fuzzy borders that are entailed by guaranteed uncertainty and the penchant for classifying collections of symptoms, complaints, and occasionally physical signs into disease categories that are often difficult to distinguish from the normal trials and tribulations of life? Jeremy Greene offers a particularly trenchant and insightful observation about the blurry lines that surround diagnosis and also treatment (even though he doesn't specifically address this):

> If the threshold is a thin dividing line, a precise curtain marking the break between normal and abnormal, the category of the borderline as commonly used in medicine refers not to the line itself but to a space or territory made up of individuals or populations who sit, problematically, within a reasonable margin of error from the line. As a space around a threshold, the borderline soon develops

its own boundaries, with new thresholds on either side. The space of the border-line simultaneously acts as as a buffer zone between the territories of pathology and normality, while at the same time offering itself as a colonizable land, a fertile area for future disease expansion. The experimental treatment of a borderline state makes the treatment of non-borderline states seem less experimental and thus less controversial as a form of therapeutics. Additionally, the presence of the border tempers the potential for conflict between individually minded practicing physicians and the standardizing intent of guideline-producing bodies by offering a sanctioned area in which idiosyncratic patterns of practice are still permitted. Although failure to treat a clearly pathological individual is grounds for malpractice litigation, failure to treat a borderline case is no failure at all; in these gray realms, some individualization of medical practice remains possible. Thus the borderline functions as a pressure valve for those who might dissent from therapeutic guidelines by maintaining a sanctioned space for therapeutic libertarianism.[111]

Greene's thesis is centered on what some think is an unholy alliance between drug (and medical device and, increasingly, molecular diagnostic) companies to expand the categories of abnormal conditions and diseases for their self-interested profit (or perhaps more accurately, pre-conditions and pre-diseases since so many of these are detectable only by a blood test or other technical investigation and go unnoticed by those who "suffer" from them).[112] On the other hand, there is little question that the expansion of people who are treated with cholesterol- and lipid-lowering statin drugs will likely lead to lower cardiovascular morbidity and mortality (at least that fraction due to hyperlipidemia). However, the widespread and universal use of mammograms, prostate-specific antigen tests, and the like may lead to both overdiagnosis and overtreatment.[113] This is not to say that these increasingly sophisticated and sensitive devices and blood (and now genetic) tests are not picking up things that appear to depart from the normal (depending on how this is defined). But simply because something is "abnormal" does not necessarily mean that it is something to worry about. If an 85-year-old man with prostatic hypertrophy (an enlarged prostate gland)—i.e., almost every man who is this age—were discovered to have a mildly elevated PSA and a biopsy showed noninvasive prostate cancer, should he undergo surgery to have it removed, or even radiation treatment? Does he have a disease? I suppose that technically he does, but chances are very good that he will die of something else well before his prostate cancer has a possibility of making him sick.[114]

Even more puzzling is the proclivity to increase the number of entities we are willing to label as "real" diseases, often at the not-so-subtle behest of organizations and individuals who stand to gain materially (and otherwise) by these designations. This pursuit is most frequently observed with conditions that are hallmarked by distress of one sort or another that is causally ascribed to some underlying sometimes-speculative pathology. Many observers have questioned the reality of these disorders, ranging from Georges Canguilhem to Thomas Szasz to Ivan Illich to Greene and Welch, to name but a few.[115] Despite their critical analyses and commentary, there seems to be little evidence of a slow-down in the proliferation of new official illnesses, all of which command attention, diagnostics, therapeutics, and hence money.[116]

In an essay entitled "The Meaning of Normal," John Ryle warned of the confusion brought about by the introduction of any new diagnostic or investigatory technology that is more sensitive than its predecessor, hence opening up new and heretofore unseen measurements and variations that can be viewed as abnormal:

> Many a new diagnostic instrument or technique capable of adding a greater precision to medicine has at first been abused in the same way and has added to the tale of clinical error. The stethoscope, through misinterpretations of natural sounds or of innocent murmurs, at one time created its thousands of cardiac invalids. With the introduction of the chest radiography, the diagnosis of "hilar tuberculosis"—based on misinterpretations of the normal root shadows—was once dangerously fashionable. The barium meal led to diagnoses of "dropped stomach" and "dropped bowel" and the prescription of expensive abdominal supports and unsound surgical procedures.... Blood-pressure readings within the normal range have been accounted as evidence or signals of arterial disease. In each instance there was an initial failure to appreciate the importance of examining a large series of sound and symptomless individuals before extending the clinical uses of the method. Other findings due to laboratory methods have been similarly liable to misconstruction.... There can be no sharp demarcation between the inborn variations of health and the induced variations of disease where bodily function is concerned.[117]

Even though he was writing more than 50 years ago with a much less technologically sophisticated medicine, his insights are just as pertinent today. Radiologists and clinicians, while delighting in the exquisite sensitivity of the latest spiral CT scanners in their ability to detect tumors and other abnormalities only millimeters in cross-sectional diameter, bemoan the constant intrusion of "incidentalomas" and, like their forebears misinterpreting chest radiographs to show TB, have no idea what to make of them.[118] Are the people with these "abnormalities" sick?

In essence, we must distinguish between the normal and the abnormal in the present tense or the proto-abnormal in the future tense. The former would refer to people who are obviously sick in the here and now; they have an infection, a bone fracture, cancer, or some other readily identifiable and acknowledged illness that warrants our intention and empathy. The latter alludes to those individuals who are not noticeably sick. Indeed, they may feel perfectly well and be alarmed to be told that there is something wrong with them. They are the ones who have occult illnesses—the patients with small tumors discoverable by sensitive blood testing (say, PSA) or precancerous colonic lesions only detectable by colonoscopy. But they also include the people who have other forms of abnormal measurements—such as what we label an elevated blood cholesterol level or high blood pressure—which, even though asymptomatic, are causally associated (many believe) to the later development of disease in some—though not all—patients so afflicted. Since we cannot predict who will develop heart or kidney disease, we err on the side of caution and recommend treatment for all, knowing full well that many who we treat actually don't need it and hence may risk the harms associated with therapy without realizing any benefits. Because our primitive abilities to foresee the future for individual patients is so poor, we condemn all as if all were doomed, even though only a few may be. As we learn more about the risks inherent in modern life and continue to develop interventions that may prove beneficial for a handful, we will be forced to confront the ongoing questions of whether it is worth it—worth the expense and the dangers associated with widespread population therapy. As we lower the bar for what is an acceptable or tolerable "normal" (e.g., by decreasing the cholesterol and HDL levels that should be treated with statin drugs), an ever-greater number of clinically well people will be declared "sick" and warrant interventions. We should question this trend for at least three reasons: first, by reducing the criteria for treatment, the "number needed to treat" to avoid clinically important events also decreases; second, with the quantity needed to treat getting progressively smaller, the number of patients unnecessarily exposed to the harms of treatment proportionally increases; and third, the costs associated with treatment will also continue to increase with diminishing returns in benefits. Indeed, this same problem affects decisions about what we call "marginally beneficial" treatments, although the term is often reserved for very invasive, high-risk care such as that offered in intensive care units or for advanced cancer patients. Nevertheless, the similarity holds: if an intervention is thought to work in 1% of patients with a given condition, on average 100 people will need to be treated in order to benefit the one.[119]

Aside from the political advantages of endowing a health system with generosity is also the distinct cushion or insurance it provides to hedge against the undoubted likelihood of making mistakes. What this means is that, due to our incomplete knowledge of disease and health, and the inherent large amount of uncertainty in applying the knowledge that we do have (based on populations) to individuals, it is almost certain that we will make mistakes both as individual physicians and as a society. For example, we could decide not to provide a given intervention because we had erroneously concluded, based on limited evidence, that it is not sufficiently beneficial to be included in a healthcare plan. Of course, this means that some patients will do without an intervention that could conceivably help them if we had more evidence to that effect. However, when evidence like that becomes available, the people who missed out might be considered victims of an error. Hence, it could be better to be generous and potentially make mistakes of commission than to make mistakes of omission. On the other hand, as Welch and others have abundantly demonstrated, doing things for people can have negative consequences as well.[120] Nevertheless, it is also conceivable that physicians (and patients) faced with fewer options in the universe of covered interventions may find their choice(s) not only simpler but also more beneficial in the balance.[121]

Indeed, while the effect was small, one randomized study of physician decision-making found that the use of specific clinical guidelines (created via the RAM approach) demonstrated a significant effect on specifying suitable recommendations rather than leaving the standards more nebulous or open-ended.[122] Moreover, over the past 25 years or so, the methods of developing and updating the guidelines have improved a great deal and have been adopted not only by specialty societies, but also by national entities such as the National Institute for Health and Clinical Excellence (NICE) in the United Kingdom.[123] However, two of the biggest challenges to having existing guidelines are having them used by practitioners and accepted by patients. I suspect that tying guideline clinical practice penetration and agreement by patients (the latter undoubtedly highly influenced by their doctors) to financial incentives, such as penalties/rewards for physicians and possibly some financial risk for patients, would go a long way toward successful implementation.[124] Nevertheless, one of the biggest advantages that could result from having a uniform system of coverage— albeit one that does leave some discretion of applicability to physicians at the bedside or in the clinic—is that it should reduce the large discrepancies in the use (or disuse) of various medical interventions that have been documented for a number of years. Stark variations in practice mean not only that what is available is often determined by where a patient lives and thus the local "custom" standard(s) of care, but also that the attendant costs (as well as injuries or harms) vary in the same manner.[125]

Ezekiel Emanuel's view of population-based healthcare delivery offers a stark contrast to what I have discussed in this chapter.[126] In his argument for the necessity to move from the Hippocratic ideal of individualized and person-centered healthcare, as idealized in mythology and the common media, to that in which population-based measures of communal health are optimized, he offers guiding principles that would govern both how this could be accomplished and what sorts of interventions would be covered. Unfortunately, he tends to overlook the singular significance to sick people of having an individual physician (and nurse) care for and about them (or even having people worried that they are sick, not to mention having their families worried about them). I believe that patients need to know that someone in authority is looking out for their welfare and cares about their suffering enough to do what needs to be done to relieve it. Emanuel's prescription to create cutoff points at 15% efficacy are as harsh as they are arbitrary, especially when applied to a country with the abundance of resources and wealth as the United States and that could afford to be generous. While he presents a formula for merging individualized care with population care, it seems to me clear that his emphasis is plainly on the latter. Perhaps I may be reasonably charged with the opposite by stressing the former, but that is only because I am attempting to cope with the reality of the true concerns of patients as well as the overall social medical needs of all Americans. We cannot blithely dismiss the importance of the doctor–patient relationship and encounter. No one—especially those who are sick—wants to rely on a one-off liaison with a "doc-in-a-box" in an urgent care center or an emergency department physician; as helpful as they may be in a critical situation, they don't develop long-term relationships of trust and reliability with the patients they see.

In a recent review of communications to (individual) patients, Haroon Ahmed et al. wrote:

People perceive risk differently depending on their awareness and understanding of the risk in question and also depending on the way the risk information is presented to them. Therefore, effective risk communication should involve the sharing of information that improves risk perception and understanding and that allows shared decision making. *Sometimes this may be at odds with apparent "public health" messages that may, for example, promote uptake of screening tests to achieve programme [sic] effectiveness at population levels.*[127] (emphasis added)

This is an extraordinarily important point that distinguishes between the ordinary, quotidian concerns of physicians and their patients and those that must be reckoned with by the committees determining what will and will not be included (or should and should not be) in a comprehensive healthcare plan. Undoubtedly, there will be patients who individually could benefit from coverage and application of a particular intervention that, because of its lack of benefit for the vast majority of similarly situated patients, was not considered sufficiently beneficial to include. While these relatively rare patients and their doctors may believe that they "need" this intervention, it will be unavailable unless the patient wishes to pay for it herself (and, for some types of treatments or diagnostic tests, it may very well be that the private market is so small that it will be unavailable at all).[128] However, the remainder of the population would be saved the potential harm from receiving something of no benefit. Another problem with widespread screening programs in large populations is that the harms and benefits are experienced by two (mostly) mutually exclusive groups. While the people with breast cancer who have positive mammograms may have risks and harms associated with their treatment, they do so as informed patients. But they are different from the larger group of women who may undergo unnecessary surgery, worries, and the like since one doesn't know pretest in which group one will be, all while accepting the testing as important or vital and assuming that they will belong to the former group.

This is a specialized scientific medical problem, as well as one of human psychology and healthcare economics. Diagnostic and therapeutic guidelines-writing committees (or modified RAM groups as I have suggested) will be charged with devising reasonable recommendations that would, in my suggestions for radical overhaul of the healthcare system, be available for participants (i.e., everyone except those who might have the means and the desire to purchase their own insurance in place of or in addition to the nationalized program). But, as I have also argued, fairness and transparency dictates that these decisions be open and justifiable to those affected by the decisions, meaning the people.[129] Indeed, I have proposed that informed citizens be members of the committees to give them a "seat at the table" (literally; see Chapter 3). However, I also noted the tremendous hullaballoo that accompanied the public announcements of the US Preventive Health Services Task Force recommendations on decreasing the widespread use of PSA testing and routine screening mammography to more selective and higher risk populations: getting people to accept these changes will not be easy. These events took place in an ongoing toxic political environment polluted with misrepresentations by the various factions that had a stake in the outcome (and I am not simply talking about men and women scared about possibly missing a detectable cancer that might kill them). Rather, I refer to radiologists who would lose income from performing fewer tests, the manufacturers of mammography machines who would potentially sell fewer machines, surgeons who would perform fewer breast biopsies and further surgeries, the PSA-testing labs that would stand to have decreased business, the urologists who would certainly do fewer prostatectomies (and hence earn less), the makers of the latest robotic surgery machines (a particular favorite of urologists), and hospitals who make money on radiology and surgery procedures—the list can go on and on. The truth is that there is an unholy alliance among all the actors in contemporary American healthcare; they all have a personal conflict-producing stake in the outcome of any decisions that are made.[130]

Without question, one of the largest challenges facing the implementation of generalized coverage guidelines will be selling the idea (and the decisions that are made) to both physicians and patients. The currency of language used to communicate the value in each decision will need to employ a number of different approaches. First and foremost must be the knowledge of how the decision-making process was carried out: what the rules were (are), who does the deciding, what information was considered relevant. This information must of course be widely available and accessible before the deliberations start and must be open to some degree of amendment, but not so much so that the very process is undermined and corrupted by those who stand the most to gain or lose from the outcomes. Second, it will be vital to make all stakeholders understand what sorts of data "count" as both relevant and reasonable. For example, anecdotal case series and beliefs not supported by reliable facts (that more than one person or group can accept) should not be considered if there are more reliable data available. An ancillary task to discussions of this kind will be to agree on a common statistical language that avoids the use of obfuscatory terms and euphemisms and uses such terminology as natural frequencies, absolute risks, risk reduction, and the like that have been demonstrated to be much easier to understand and assimilate by both the lay public and professionals.[131] Finally, doctors, healthcare industry representatives, patients, and disease advocacy societies or groups will need to know that the process is not immutable or perfect and can be amenable to change, but only under certain conditions (but not including such influences as political donations, sophisticated and divisive publicity campaigns, etc.).

Canguilhem (and others) argues persuasively that our decisions about what is normal (or normal enough or not sufficiently abnormal) can be heavily influenced by the prevailing social mores and customs of differing eras. Recall that it was only a few decades ago that homosexuality was declared a mental disorder and now no longer is; indeed, it is increasingly accepted as simply a normal variation in the panoply of human sexuality. However, it may be true that conditions that are more subjective or "lifestyle-affecting" without detectable anatomical and/or chemical pathology are more susceptible to shifts in culture. One of the greatest challenges faced by physicians and patients is the degree to which we view clusters of "symptoms" with opprobrium or sympathy or indifference and how this is so highly influenced by the prevailing tenor of the times (think of alcoholism as being a vice or a disease). Canguilhem goes on to write "the borderline between the normal and the pathological is imprecise for several individuals considered simultaneously but it is perfectly precise for one and the same individual considered successively. In order to be normative in the given conditions, what is normal can become pathological in another situation if it continues identical to itself. It is the individual who is the judge of this transformation because it is he who suffers from it from the very moment he feels inferior to the tasks which the new situation imposes on him" (p. 182). Unlike mechanical structures in which the setting of norms must adhere to strict and narrow conformities or tolerances in order to achieve the specified results (e.g., a machine that performs as desired), what we consider to be normal in biological systems often has wide ranges and encompasses a fairly lenient forbearance for differences from the mean or what is arithmetically the most frequent. Nevertheless, both common intuition and gut feeling can readily detect deviations from the normal that can be influenced by prevailing cultural liberalities and some evaluation of functional performance. While his observation is very astute and no doubt true, one can easily see the impossible situation this would present to those who would design a healthcare system where one must impose cutoffs. Translating his rules of internal normativity to a population would be virtually impossible. It would be both impractical and implausible, if not ridiculous, to evaluate whether the system should cover conditions based entirely on a decision made by each patient about whether he or she was sick.

5

RULES, RESCUES, AND MIRACLES

In the previous chapter, I discussed the challenges posed to the creation and implementation of a comprehensive healthcare system by diagnostic, prognostic, and therapeutic uncertainty. In particular, the ambiguity and often disturbing unpredictability inherent in biology and medicine guarantees that the task of developing reasonable cutoffs to determine what are sensible health conditions to include in a comprehensive insurance coverage scheme (and, of course, what to exclude), as well as acceptable interventions to prevent or treat them, will be fraught with difficulties. I have suggested that committees composed of informed experts and lay representatives could be charged with formulating consensus and binding recommendations for coverage decisions as a mechanism for coping with blurred, continuous, and indistinct borders. Consensus recommendations by experts and other representatives charged with this responsibility may serve as the most morally sensitive and justifiable solution to resolving the cutoff problem. In this chapter, I wish to continue analyzing potential obstacles to my argument that could either complicate or even possibly derail my prescription unless adequately acknowledged and managed. I will focus on three such issues: the Rule of Rescue, the power of anecdotes in medical decision-making, and a unique form of patient demand for care while they pray for a miraculous intervention.

THE RULE OF RESCUE PROBLEM

Jessica McClure (popularly known simply as "Baby Jessica") fell down a well in Midland Texas when she was only 18 months old. One might think that there was not much going on in either the country or the world by the enormous amount of publicity that attended the protracted rescue attempt over the next few days. Peter Applebome, a reporter for the *New York Times*, explains what happened:

> The drama, in which hundreds of workers from the surrounding oil fields worked day and night to rescue the child, Jessica McClure, peaked in the final, emotional hour as workers reached her and gingerly hoisted her to the surface amid wild applause of onlookers and quiet tears of the burly workers. "All across the world people were watching this thing in Midland, Texas, and if they didn't get a tear in their eye, they're not human," said James Shaw, who helped operate the drilling rig used to free Jessica. "I know there were tears

in my eye, and I'm not afraid to tell you that." ... She was admitted to the intensive care unit and was being fed intravenously. Her first solid food since falling in the shaft Wednesday morning was a Popsicle, Dr. Rubin said. Jessica's rescue ended a maddeningly slow process in which workers drilled a 26-foot-long shaft parallel to the one where the girl was caught, and then a 63-inch horizontal tunnel through solid bedrock to join the two shafts.... The girl's plight has captured worldwide attention. The switchboard at the police station here has been jammed with callers offering suggestions on how to rescue her and neighbors have been receiving calls from news organizations as far away as Australia. After two days of digging and drilling, workers were able to touch Jessica for the first time today. Their efforts were slowed after they found that one of her legs was caught in a crevice. At times she cried for her mother. But rescue workers, using a speaker lowered into the shaft, soothed her with nursery rhymes and words of encouragement. At one point, workers said, she sang along with a Humpty-Dumpty rhyme. Fans blew warm air into the well to ward off the chill. Relatives and friends described the girl as an aggressive, inquisitive child. Officials believe she tumbled into the well after children removed a rock or flower pot covering the opening. The shaft is in the backyard of the child care center operated by the girl's aunt.[1]

The story riveted the attention of the world, no less so than that of the 33 Chilean miners trapped after an explosion in a mine and their heroic rescue.[2] Both were examples of the so-called "Rule of Rescue," a deep psychological impulse that almost all of us have to empathize with the plight of an identified individual in difficulty or who is suffering. They differ from the anonymous thousands—indeed, millions—of children who we constantly hear about and whose circumstances are no less desperate than Jessica's, and who "statistical" lives, lumped together into an impersonal, characterless mass, easy to erase from our minds. But put a face and a name to a sufferer with a personal, heart-rending story and that's all it takes to evoke massive outpourings of emotion and the desire to help in whatever way we can. The Rule of Rescue represents the ultimate in distinguishing the specific and particular from the general.

While the modernist version of the Rule is often attributed to Albert Jonsen's explication,[3] it actually owes its first iterations to Thomas Schelling (who conceived of the term "statistical lives") and Charles Fried.[4] They described our propensity to direct our concerns to the "real" people whose identities are revealed to us and hence plucked out from the masses of everyone else. As Fried pointed out, the Rule emphasizes the here-and-now and the known at the expense of the future and the unknown others (as well as our unknown selves).[5]

When in the emotional grip of the Rule, we no longer view its subjects as anonymized members of a mass of humanity; rather, they are living, breathing, suffering souls who could easily and understandably be our daughter, son, sister, brother, or even ourselves. No wonder charities looking for donations put photographs of the obviously desperate in their advertisements, often with a name attached, pleading for you, the reader of the ad, to help this innocent child (and the millions like her).

Filling the same space with a dull recitation of the unspecified numbers of people who suffer from whatever calamity for which the organization wishes to claim your attention (and money) would only bore us by numbing the senses, no different than the hoary, boring supplication of parents trying to get their children to eat their vegetables by invoking the "starving children in Africa."[6]

In addition to these generalized, publicized identified lives, there can be no greater identified life than the one that physicians have in their examining room at any point in time because the essence of the duty that physicians have to their patients is devoted to bettering the latter's interests—obviously a highly individualistic endeavor.[7] Indeed, multiple experiments and observations have demonstrated that doctors make different kinds of decisions for individuals and for groups.[8] But strict adherence to the Rule entails ignoring or minimizing (or perhaps putting on the back burner) the plight of the nameless many for the immediacy of the dire straits of the proximate and known individual. And this is exactly what patients quite understandably want; indeed, one of the main causes of the failure of the managed care fiasco of the early 1990s was the perception—and not entirely unwarranted—that managed care organizations created incentives for their employed or contracted physicians to diminish their primary duty to their patients' welfare in order to cut costs.[9]

The assumed diversion of significant resources and potential risks (to rescuers) in asserting the Rule is frequently used as an argument against employing heroic efforts (and money) to save the few at the presumed expense of the many. This view has been expressed by those arguing for various versions of nonsystematic bedside rationing (for example) as well as others who realize how concern for the present crisis heavily discounts future concerns (and needed expenditures).[10] Aside from psychological arguments explaining why the pull of the Rule is so powerful for most people—and, indeed, why it may be ultimately beneficial to have such easily evoked emotions—there may be good instrumental reasons to not reject application of the Rule as part of everyday life, and especially in the domain of healthcare, for several reasons. Knowledge that one's physician cares uniquely about you as her patient and will go to great lengths to secure and advance your interests is both ennobling and serves to strengthen the sometimes frayed fabric of the modern doctor–patient relationship.[11] Second, utilization of the Rule to publicize what would ordinarily be obscure or even unknown rare medical conditions can lead to both productive research that is beneficial for those afflicted with the disorder as well as unanticipated scientific findings that could help many more people who have much more common illnesses.[12] Third, the knowledge that the Rule was electively ignorable or, perhaps more corrosively, was illegitimate in the practice of medicine could very well undermine essential trust in the role and authority of physicians.[13] Finally, it must surely be of some benefit and comfort to people (and their loved ones) to know that someone cares about them as particular persons and not as nondescript or anonymous "patients" lumped together with others in some indistinguishable mass.[14]

On the other hand, there are numerous reasons to reject incorporating the Rule into a planned, centralized healthcare system, as in the United Kingdom and as explored by Tony Hope.[15] Interestingly, since his paper was published, the main authority of the UK's National Health Service (NHS) responsible for evaluating new (and frequently extremely expensive) technologies (the National Institute for Health and Care Excellence [NICE]) and deciding whether to have the NHS cover them has explicitly incorporated considerations of equity that are at least sometimes addressed by the Rule.[16] Hope suggests that his analysis could also apply to managed care organizations in the United States (or to large insurance pools covered by the same policy, etc.). Unfortunately, he fails to note the significant differences that exist in the breadth and depth of coverage of private and even public insurance policies in the United States. Thus, there are large variations in the need to appeal to the Rule to gain a service or intervention that may be wholly dependent on the kind of insurance coverage one has. For example, in the well-known case of Coby Howard in Oregon from the 1990s, the then newish Oregon Health Plan did not cover the sort of bone marrow transplant that his mother and his doctors stated was the only chance he had for a cure of his leukemia.[17] His case was publicized, and the relevant authorities reversed their decision (unfortunately, too late for Coby who had died). Nevertheless, it is highly likely that if Coby had been covered by private health insurance, he would have had little difficulty getting the expensive transplant procedure approved. The point is that, in the United Kingdom, while local and regional health jurisdictions have a fair amount of leeway in allocating resources, big decisions for the NHS are made nationally and apply everywhere.

In his (limited) defense of the Rule, Mark Sheehan discusses an extremely important point that is only becoming more obvious as social media penetrates ever further into our world of mass communication.[18] Even though he, too, is writing from (and about) the UK, he notes that one argument against the Rule is that it can be exploited by those people savvy enough to use the media to publicize their situation. Indeed, it is the publicity that makes the victim identified to a wider audience and generates the visceral emotional reaction that is at the core of the Rule. While he notes that this is a problem, he does not regard it as a deal-breaker and goes on to offer other reasons why the Rule should not be reasonably rejected (in a national health system). However, the facility with which people can engage social media to immediately and widely announce their tragic circumstances to the world is an ever-increasing component of daily life in the digitally connected globe. And it is not simply the generation of a "private" campaign of publicity that contributes to this state of affairs, but also the attractiveness of these terrible cases as a vehicle for standard media outlets such as local TV news, commercial websites, and the like that plays a major part in amplifying the message and the audience. In many ways, the Rule is a product of modern means of communication and the rapidity with which news tidbits go viral. Whereas 25 years ago one might only hear about a child being denied an organ transplant or a very expensive drug if the wire services picked up the story or the national news networks (in the United States) thought it an interesting enough human interest item on which to expend a few precious minutes of airtime, social media make these older sources antiquated, even quaint.

Another excellent example where the Rule comes into play (and into conflict) with the just allocation of scarce resources is in the arena of solid organ transplantation. As

I (and others) have noted, the organ transplant system in the United States is devoted to the equitable allocation of organs (although walking a fine line in balancing the inherent tension between equity and efficiency) and has embarked on a number of efforts to improve both transparency and fairness in how organs are distributed.[19] An unfortunate, but not rare, problem is the need for a second transplant after the initial one has failed. This can occur either in the immediate postoperative period as, for instance, when a major blood vessel in the allograft has clotted off or there is hyperacute rejection that cannot be successfully treated and that results in organ failure, or much later (even years later) when the organ (most commonly of cadaveric origin) simply slowly "wears out." Should people who have had their chance at an organ be given a second one—emergency or not—before others on the waiting list have had even a first opportunity? This is a situation where the Rule can come into play.[20] Physicians quite naturally wish to save the life of the desperately ill person in front of them, especially if they had previously made the commitment to venture into the perilous realm of transplant.[21] They may feel they "owe" something more to the identifiable patient who has been through so much and sacrificed greatly as opposed to an unidentified patient from someplace else (or even in the same hospital) waiting for a first transplant. The issues are both clear and tragic.[22] Even though retransplantation continues to be controversial and the outcome for patients receiving their second (and even third) organ(s) is significantly worse than for those undergoing primary transplantation, it continues to be a practice that is accepted and acceptable within the organ transplant community. Indeed, while being a repeat recipient is entered into the calculations of prioritization and counted somewhat against one's chances, the negative weight accorded this status does not appear to be all that great and is superseded by the gravity of the patient's medical condition.[23]

Consider the story of Sarah Murnaghan:

(6/12/2013) Sarah Murnaghan, the 10-year-old Pennsylvania girl with cystic fibrosis who has been at the center of national controversy over transplant policy, was receiving an adult lung transplant on Wednesday. Family spokeswoman Maureen Garrity said the child is getting lungs from one adult donor, ending a campaign by the family in the highly publicized case, which involved pressure from lawmakers and more recently intervention by a federal judge, to allow their child to receive adult lungs. Garrity said the family got a call about the donor Tuesday night and found out the organs were a match Wednesday morning.... Sarah Murnaghan went into the operating room shortly before noon Wednesday. "Sarah got THE CALL. She will be taken back to the OR in 30min. Please pray for Sarah's donor, her HERO, who has given her the gift of life," her mother, Janet Murnaghan, wrote on Facebook on Wednesday morning.... Right now patients under 12 are effectively ineligible for adult lung donation; they wait for a pediatric donors instead. But those donors are much rarer. A national organ transplant policy committee is reviewing the policy and is allowing an independent expert panel to review the cases of individual children in the meantime. In a highly unusual move that sent a shockwave through the transplant community, a federal judge last week ordered Sarah Murnaghan and Javier Acosta, 11, onto the adult waiting list. Both children are dying of cystic fibrosis and need lung transplants to survive. Acosta is still awaiting a transplant.[24]

(6/24/2014) A year ago, Sarah Murnaghan, an 11-year-old Pennsylvania girl, was fighting for her life while her family waged a campaign to change a national policy on lung transplants for child recipients. Their battle has now led to permanent policy change. On Monday, the Organ Procurement and Transplant Network (OPTN) and United Network for Organ Sharing (UNOS) announced their decision to allow some children ages 11 or younger to receive additional priority for lung transplants, including lungs from older donors, according to a statement from UNOS. The previous policy required lung transplant candidates to be at least 12 to receive lungs from an adult donor. Following an appeal by the Murnaghans, in June 2013 a federal judge issued a restraining order to prevent the age-restriction policy from being imposed in Sarah's case. Sarah received lungs donated by an adult. The first transplants didn't take, requiring a second transplant, again from an adult donor. "Sarah receiving adult lungs means she is now breathing on her own," her family said last year, "after three years of being tethered to machines." On Monday, the family called her new lungs "beautiful" and said Sarah will be returning to school in the fall.[25]

Sarah (and then others) received her lung transplants solely because of her parents' persistence in publicizing her case via social media and the commercial press. They were obviously successful both for her and other older children in that they got her what she arguably needed (from a personal, medical perspective) as well as going further by changing the national policy on lung allocation by UNOS. Undoubtedly, none of this would have happened if they had remained silent and accepted the decision of her doctors with equanimity (even if it was wrong). Of course, they were savvy and educated enough to take advantage of an existing system to widely advertise their plight. We don't ever hear about the many other patients (indeed, we have no idea how many there may be) who do not make use of social media, TV news, and the like to make their situation known and thereby activate the Rule. They are either shy or ill-advised ("it won't work") or ill-informed or submissive or some combination. Even patients who are clinically similar to those who speak out and protest would be left behind, especially in situations where public policy is not altered (as it was in the case of Sarah).

This observation points to one of the significant moral problems of the Rule as it is "practiced" in the United States; the reason why I specify this country is because we lack a coherent, consistent, and unified single healthcare system in which future planning for healthcare needs and costs is coordinated. For the most part, this means that publicizing the case of a single individual will often not generalize to others like him or her (although there have been exceptions).[26] Thus, those who can manipulate the media and insurance companies and the like will gain an advantage over those who cannot for whatever reason (poverty, poor education, etc.). The upshot is that this tends to further disadvantage the already disadvantaged. And, of course, there is no reliable way to determine—once an individual or class of individuals is identified as needy in the special manner required to activate the Rule of Rescue response—if the needs of these people are actually legitimate or if they truly can be helped in a meaningful way by whatever intervention(s) they are requesting. The unique power of the Rule is that the publicity required to identify an individual patient beyond her small circle of intimate acquaintants and family can have a transformative effect on what qualifies as a healthcare need under normal circumstances. Certainly, in some cases, it can serve to broadcast a previously unknown inequity to a wide audience; in these circumstances, a true need may have been unfairly ignored for unjustifiable reasons. But, in many other situations, the Rule may be employed to shame an organization into providing an intervention that was legitimately denied solely to avoid the negative consequences of bad publicity.[27] The reasoned scrutiny of evidence-based medicine is relegated to a minor role (or none at all) once a case becomes public in this distinct way.

Another interesting aspect of the Rule is that it seemingly must focus on people who are in grave and probably imminent danger—either of severe and permanent injury or death—and who are in such a state acutely. People who are merely bad off either because of unfortunate social circumstances, such as the homeless, impoverished, and unemployed, may kindle our sympathy but not the systematic outpouring of overwhelming emotion that customarily accompanies the Rule. While one may feel sorry for the homeless veteran standing at the streetlight corner with a sign asking for money to buy food, and one may occasionally even donate some small amount to his cause, it is not the same as if he were prominently featured on the nightly television news as a "unique" case deserving of our special concern. The exception to this generalization may be those patients with chronic diseases for whom there is an existing treatment, albeit not a cure, and on whose behalf sponsors are beseeching donations for research or supportive care.[28] Therefore, one should not be lulled into thinking that the Rule only applies to those in immediate life-threatening circumstances. Indeed, as is made clear by Largent and Pearson in their careful analysis of so-called "orphan" diseases in the United States (operationally and legally defined as a prevalence of fewer than 200,000 cases), there could be many thousands of patients covered under this definition.[29] While these individuals may not meet the strict definition of having their lives at imminent risk, there would be little doubt that they could be sick—some gravely so—and may therefore generate some sympathy for their plight when suitably portrayed to the public in a manner designed to activate the Rule.

On the other hand, the Rule by no means guarantees that the cause that is publicized is just or warranted as one deserving both our empathy *and* our resources. Consider this case. Amelia Rivera is a child who was born with Wolf-Hirschhorn syndrome, "a complex genetic disorder caused by deletions in the short arm of chromosome 4 (4p) and occurring in 1 in 50,000 to 1 in 20,000 births. The phenotype of WHS consists of a broad range of clinical findings. The core features include a typical craniofacial appearance, growth deficiency, developmental delays, intellectual disability of variable degree and seizures (or EEG anomalies) in most patients. Variable clinical findings include feeding difficulties, congenital malformations including orofacial cleft, cardiac, renal and urogenital malformations, skeletal and dental anomalies, hearing loss, recurrent infections and other complications."[30] By all accounts published in the press, Amelia had numerous manifestations of this disorder, including a severe and global intellectual (cognitive) disability; she could neither walk nor talk but was able to interact in a restricted way with her surroundings and the family who clearly loved her. By the age of 3 years, her kidneys began to fail. The institution where she received her care, Children's Hospital of Philadelphia, considered her as a candidate for kidney transplantation (dialysis would have been an option because cognitive dysfunction is not a contraindication). However, she was denied a spot on the list for a cadaveric transplant. According to news reports "Mrs. Rivera told ABC News she initially 'thought we were just finding out how a transplant works and how we could be a donor. But then, I was told we couldn't because she was mentally retarded,' she said. 'Those were the exact words on a piece of paper.' Medical staff also expressed concerns about Mia's ability to cope with taking medication for the rest of her life, and especially when her family were [sic] no longer around to look after her, Mrs. Rivera claims."[31] Amelia's family went public, and a firestorm of mostly negative publicity (for the hospital) ensued. They relented and attempted to save face; eventually, Amelia received a living related donor kidney (from her mother) at the age of 5. Irrespective of the merits of this kidney transplant in this particular patient, it is unlikely that Amelia would have received a kidney if her parents had not alerted the news media and had her plight not been publicized. The story line was that she was denied due to "mental retardation" and not to any other factors that may have been involved but that might have been lost in the public kerfuffle that ensued. The very fact that her family resorted to engaging the public transformed her story to one of rescue rather than individual patient care, hence losing all semblance of reason (and reasons).[32] It is also worth noting that insurance, in this case Medicare, would pay for all or most of her transplant-related care because she would qualify for the End-Stage Renal Disease Program benefit (indeed, Medicare would have picked up the tab for dialysis as well). Finally, since Amelia received a kidney from her mother and thus was not entered into the much larger—and considerably more competitive—pool for a deceased donor organ, it is likely that considerations of the judicious use of scarce resources did not enter into the initial evaluation.

There are clearly definite downsides to permitting the Rule to play a major role in the allocation of healthcare resources, even in such a messy system as exists in the United States. In a centrally controlled and regulated health system, one of the most consequential arguments against the Rule is that it unjustifiably allocates resources to the few (albeit the identifiable few) in the present at the expense of the future anonymous many. When the future comes around, would our later selves (or our descendants) be grateful to us for jeopardizing their endowment—even, perhaps, their entitlement—to save or treat a few known individuals in the past? Is the investment in the present worth the possibility of endangering the resources of the future?

Forbidding or preventing the Rule from being used in healthcare may indeed save some money, but, in the United States, it is not money that would be reallocated to pay for other, needed healthcare because of the disjointedness and uncoordinated manner in which we deliver healthcare.[33] Thus, when an insurance company fails to approve an intervention that a beneficiary (and her doctor) claims is needed, the money that is not spent is not *necessarily* used to benefit other patients; indeed, in a for-profit environment, it could easily be used for executive bonuses or shareholder dividends. Similarly, one does not necessarily know beforehand the chances of success of a rescue effort (such as the attempt to save the life of the little girl who fell down the well) and if the money and effort expended would be considered to be worthwhile. However, there are times when the large expense and the minimal percentage of a favorable outcome can be predicted, but if the pathos of the situation is portrayed in manner sufficient to evoke our sympathies and stimulate the Rule, then expense and small chances may be irrelevant.[34]

Of course, virtually everyone is identifiable or identified by one or more individuals, usually relatives, friends, and the like. But the Rule does not seem to play a major role in generating anything more than the group-restricted sort of empathy and outpouring of a desire to help that is usual when people who are loved and cared for by others are suffering or are in other desperate straits. It seems that it is only when others who do not know the "victim(s)"—those who are otherwise strangers—become aware of his/her/their identity that the almost universal emotion that grounds the Rule is activated. And, as I have mentioned, savvy people can take advantage of this proclivity even if they have never heard of the Rule. But does the Rule merely publicly capitalize on singling out those patients (or miners, little girls trapped in a well, etc.) who, all things being equal, should deserve our empathy and our help simply because we extend this kind of compassion to all those of whom we are aware need our help? Occasionally, as in the case of Sarah Murnaghan, the publicity created by her parents served to notify a wider audience not only of her plight but that of many similar older children who, because of a vagary of the lung transplant allocation system then extant, were shut out of a larger pool of potentially available organs. In this case, the Rule exposed an inequity and arguably led to an improvement in the fairness of the system. In other cases—perhaps the majority— that may not be true.

But we must consider how to place the demands of the Rule within the context of a healthcare system that is standardized to employ rationing of the type that I have suggested could be both workable and fair in the United States.[35] I think to ignore the Rule could jeopardize the legitimacy of an entire system that would depend on an endorsement by the majority of the populace. One could employ an explicit recognition of the powerful psychological and emotional grip the Rule has on people and their willingness to embrace a healthcare system that exhibits the sort of compassion that is believed to be exemplified by the Rule. Such is the case in Australia, where the national Pharmaceutical Benefits Advisory Committee (PBAC) unequivocally recognizes the Rule and has issued guidelines for approving appeals for noncovered medications. However, they do not give carte blanche automatic support to anyone who applies. There are four prerequisite conditions that must met before consideration for payment approval may be given:

- No alternative exists in Australia to treat patients with the specific circumstances of the medical condition meeting the criteria of the restriction. This means that there are no nonpharmacological or pharmacological interventions for these patients.
- The medical condition defined by the requested restriction is severe, progressive, and expected to lead to premature death. The more severe the condition, or the younger the age at which a person with the condition might die, or the closer a person with the condition is to death, the more influential the Rule of Rescue might be in the consideration by PBAC.
- The medical condition defined by the requested restriction applies to only a very small number of patients. Again, the fewer the patients, the more influential the Rule of Rescue might be in the consideration by PBAC. However, PBAC is also mindful that the PBS is a community-based scheme and cannot cater for individual circumstances.
- The proposed medicine provides a worthwhile clinical improvement sufficient to qualify as a rescue from the medical condition. The greater the rescue, the more influential the Rule of Rescue might be in the consideration by PBAC.[36]

They additionally qualify these four conditions with the following contingent statement: "As with other relevant factors, the Rule of Rescue supplements, rather than substitutes for, the evidence-based consideration of comparative cost-effectiveness. A decision on whether the Rule of Rescue is relevant is only necessary if PBAC would be inclined to reject a submission because of its consideration of comparative cost-effectiveness (and any other relevant factors). In such a circumstance, if PBAC concludes that the Rule of Rescue is relevant, it would then consider whether this is sufficiently influential in favour of a recommendation to list that PBAC would reverse a decision not to recommend listing if the Rule of rescue is not relevant."[37]

Importantly, the open acknowledgment that the Rule exists and that it can (or will) be intentionally manipulated by individuals on behalf of themselves or others whom they believe to be in dire straits and whose predicaments would otherwise be ignored concedes that these situations predictably arise and that a mechanism for coping with them is wise. One could certainly argue that PBAC's strategy is vague or concentrates on the harmful aspects of the Rule,[38] but the fact is that their methodology represents a not unreasonable strategy, especially if it were endorsed by those to whom it might logically apply.

In 2006, the United Kingdom's NICE and its Citizen's Council—a broadly representative advisory group—examined how (or even whether) the Rule should be considered in the NHS. Their report first suggested that the term be abandoned completely and reference should rather be made to "exceptional cases," which they believed was a more accurate description of the sorts of situations that would be encountered by NICE for outside-the-planned-budget funding.[39] The document is interesting to read because arguments both for and against incorporating special urgent clinical situations and the social, budgetary, and larger systemic implications and effects were presented. Nevertheless, and not surprisingly (and perhaps necessarily), it is reasonably vague in a way strikingly similar to the position taken by PBAC. Some might view it as balanced, even nuanced, in this respect, while others might consider it to be so indeterminate to be almost vacuous.[40] However, both documents and the processes they represent signify good-faith attempts to substantively admit the reality of the Rule and that healthcare systems must contend with its effects.

But both PBAC and NICE work within coordinated, centrally structured, and regulated healthcare systems very different from the distorted market-oriented, profit-driven system in the United States. I have already given a number of examples of how the Rule has been used by patients and their advocates to obtain what they would not have received had they not appealed to the Rule. While the courts remain a stable space in which to argue for the merits of one's situation, they can be slow and cumbersome and lack the sort of technical expertise that might be necessary to fairly adjudicate claims that rest on clinical and scientific evidence. Far better to utilize the power of modern social media, the Internet, and the like to attract the sympathies of the widest public possible. Since the Internet is (mostly) free and easy to access, all it would take is a smartphone to make one's situation known to millions and marshal their heartfelt opinions against the monolithic, faceless, and for-profit insurance companies (or government, in the case of Medicaid or Medicare) who would deny some life-saving drug or operation to some desperate patient. In a system that seems always willing (and to the extent possible to date) to pass on increased expenses to others—customers/policy-holders, employers, federal and state funders, and the like—the penalties for caving in to the demands of Rule of Rescue exploiters is only temporarily painful. And the lessons of hard-fought and won battles of this sort will only serve to encourage others.

How could a reformed and reformulated US healthcare system that incorporated generous and rational rationing such as I have suggested accommodate the Rule? If rationing were implemented according to substantive medical need (Chapter 3), most patients would get what they needed (and presumably, wanted). Of course, those who have been denied something that they believe is important and needed will be frustrated and angry. Assuming that the life-saving intervention that would trigger the Rule has more than a minimal chance of being successful, it seems both reasonable and morally right in a wealthy, munificent nation to pay for this. However, when clinical trials demonstrate that a very expensive drug is minimally life-extending in an incurable situation (such as many new anti-cancer drugs that have been approved for advanced disease), then it seems just as reasonable to limit or even bar publicly funded payment. This is not to say that drug companies developing such treatments could not offer them for sale on the open market; simply that the public, national insurance plan would not pay for them.[41] Currently, people are able to trigger the Rule by engaging the almost universally held antipathy to "heartless" and faceless insurance companies that are viewed as making decisions in an opaque manner and with the express purpose of refusing to approve "needed" interventions solely to save or make money. But if the deliberations and decisions that produced these conclusions were made openly and with public input and comment, and if there was also a mechanism to appeal adverse decisions that was credible, they could be considered legitimate.[42] Of course, nothing would be able to stop unhappy, disappointed, and disgruntled people who regarded themselves as losers in this process from "going public" to drum up sympathy and support, but the strength of their case would be considerably weakened if this happened after they were turned down by a valid and sanctioned process.

As a matter of policy, it may be that society has more sympathy for some of its citizens than others (or conversely, less). For example, stories of children suffering from the ravages of incurable cancer tend to elicit more emotion than the similar suffering of older adults. Aside from the fact that there are vastly more adults who die from cancer than children, this seems only natural, and so we may wish to make allowances for appeals from the parents of these children and give them a "credit" that we might not extend to their grandparents. However, there is an invidious side to this consideration. Just as invocations of the Rule bring to the fore newly minted and probably temporary VIPs, it could also publicize the cases of people who I have previously labeled Very Unimportant People, or VUPs.[43] The undocumented immigrant or incarcerated felon who receives an organ transplant are good examples.[44] Without arguing the fairness or morality of policies that restrict or permit access to scarce resources for various groups (I have done this elsewhere), one would have to guard against the corrosive effects this could have on the system as a whole.

I think it is both fair and reasonable to suggest that most of us would feel better living in a society in which the Rule was ready and waiting to be activated rather than discouraged or even prohibited. There is little question that a wealthy society such as the United States could easily afford to engage in periodic rescues of one kind or another, both in its healthcare system and outside of it. The problem comes when rescues, rather than being one-off or relatively uncommon, unique events, become unexceptional. Or they become engrained into policy, such as believing that we should always try to cure the sickest first no matter what, even if they may have less of a chance of survival (lest one think this is fantasy, the rules governing the allocation of transplantable organs more or less follow this strategy). A wise, compassionate, and judicious use of resources would argue to keep rescues to a minimum and not make them the standard of care.[45] While widespread use of the Rule could serve to make such rescues commonplace and hence less dramatic (if everyone were "special" then no one would be), the restriction of its application to truly exceptional cases (whatever they might be) can certainly have a socially salutary effect. For run-of-the-mill, quotidian allocations of resources to anonymous others, however, fairness in share distribution still prevails as the norm.[46]

One way to avoid this conundrum or tension with our psychological and compassionate desire to help those in immediate and obvious (i.e., identifiable) need is to pair this with a commitment to minimize the future requirement to practice rescue medicine. Of course, there will always be little girls who fall down wells (unless we eliminate wells or demand that there be steel mesh covers on all of them) or even

Chilean miners who get trapped (assuming we have maximized the ability to make mines safe). And, similarly, even in the cars of the future with minimum human control (maybe a fantasy, maybe not), parts will break unexpectedly and accidents will happen and people will be injured, just like those who will trip on curbs or fall down stairs or get struck by lightning: we cannot eliminate risk and unanticipated catastrophic illness. We would always wish to have a "rainy day fund" or the financial and medical wherewithal to care for people in sudden unfortunate circumstances. Similarly, there undoubtedly will always be people who believed that their cases were treated unfairly and that the denial of a service was unjust, irrespective of whether it was or not. The problem arises if the definition of rescue becomes blurry and/or there become too many people who need or want rescue help such that we sacrifice the needs of many others—both current and future others—for the few. Quigley and Harris describe this as benefitting the few at the expense of the many and discounting the future within the realm of public (preventative) health and private health.[47]

One of the benefits of living in a wealthy nation is that it affords us the opportunity to make more decisions of choice as opposed to necessity and sacrifice. It is highly unlikely, if not implausible, that the United States in the present or foreseeable future would find itself in such dire financial straits that it would have to choose between "rescuing" the current needy because of concerns about being able to afford general healthcare provision for the population in the future. Nevertheless, our affluence should not blind us to the potentially corrosive effects of being too empathetic to every plaintive plea for help that arises. As more people take advantage of simple, rapid, and pervasive means of communicating their desperate situations—including perhaps misrepresenting the gravity of their predicament to better tear at the heartstrings of a gullible and easily swayed public—this could get out of hand and lead to erosion of the system of fair allocation on which rationing would be based. With increasing numbers of people portraying themselves as deserving of special treatment or consideration, including jumping ahead of others in line or requesting exceptions to the rules, this can only serve to lead others to believe that they may do the same. For every successful well-publicized case on the Internet pleading for special dispensation, more will be spawned. This is not to say that we should abandon the Rule of Rescue and the genuinely good emotions and moral intuitions it awakens in us. Rather, we should be more selective in its applications. Rescues cannot be permitted to become commonplace; they must remain exceptional.[48]

As a final note to this subject, I should mention that the Rule has a corollary opposite or antithesis that we might call the "Rule of Abandonment." In much the same way that we blithely go about our business, blissfully unaware of the constant tragedies that might engage our sympathies until the Rule is activated by publicity, we also remain ignorant of those individuals and situations that could arouse our ire. For example, while it may be well-known in some segments of the legal (and perhaps even the bioethics) community that in 1976 the US Supreme Court decided that incarcerated individuals were entitled to receive the prevailing standard of medical care, most are probably unaware of this (and succeeding cases).[49] This decision was based on the reasoning that the removal of prisoners' physical liberty prevents them from freely availing themselves of the opportunity to access healthcare (this is irrespective of whether they would have done so). Hence, to deny them healthcare while imprisoned would be a double penalty and would violate their Constitutional right against cruel and unusual punishment, in much the same way that denying them adequate food, water, and shelter would be wrong. While many people might not mind that prisoners would receive routine care, they could become quite upset if they learned that the standard of care for many disorders in America is quite a bit beyond simple antibiotics, high blood pressure pills, insulin for diabetes, and the like. They are also entitled to interventions like expensive chemotherapy (this is not to say that they always receive it) and, perhaps most provocatively, organ transplants. Indeed, there is nothing like a headline such as "Prisoner gets $1M heart Transplant" to get the blood boiling for any number of people.[50] Or consider the furor over the 2003 case of Jessica Santillan, a teenager who suffered a grievous medical error while receiving a heart-lung transplant at Duke University Medical Center; she received a second set of organs, only to die of complications. While the mistake was bad enough, the enduring story was the public furor over the fact that she and her family were undocumented immigrants who traveled to North Carolina expressly for medical care and transplantation.[51]

These are cases that arouse the opposite sentiments and moral feelings as those stimulated by the Rule of Rescue. While the circumstances and the needs of these individuals and patients may be "out of sight, out of mind" most of the time, the power of modern publicity technologies to hit the right emotional buttons, both positive and negative, can be extremely powerful and can be just as easily manipulated for both good and bad reasons. We are justifiably proud of the instantaneous outpouring of good will when we hear of the desperate plight of someone we consider "deserving." At the same time, darker emotions are triggered by those viewed as social outcasts, the less than equal, and those undeserving of our sympathies and generosity. However, since the definition of who is categorized in this way can be varied and shifting with time (which immigrant group is ostracized this decade? Are prisoners in jail for robbing a convenience store to feed their families more deserving of a kidney transplant than convicted murderers or rapists?), we should be very wary of this negative side of what might be termed "rule psychology" or "rule morality."

ANECDOTES

Physicians love their anecdotes. While the rise of the evidence-based medicine movement over the past 30 years has attempted to relegate the significance of anecdotal reasoning and recall to the dustbin of history, it continues to exert a powerful influence on the way doctors think and act. The Oxford English Dictionary defines an anecdote as "The narrative of a detached incident, or of a single event, told as being in itself interesting or striking."[52] Drawing conclusions based on these sorts of noticeable and personally memorable and impactful events informs a common logical fallacy called *inferential reasoning* by which one attempts to make a generalizable declaration or assertion about the state of the world based on an inappropriate or an inadequate evidence base (i.e., the anecdote). Anecdotes draw their strength both from their power to influence and dominate memory and the grip they frequently have on our emotions and hence our ability to express those sentiments to others. In as much as we wish our doctors to care about us as individuals and not as anonymized members of a population (see Chapter 4 and earlier discussion in this chapter), the emotive force of our physician telling an anecdotal story about another patient she cared for "just like us" can readily trounce the dry, colorless data from any number of clinical trials. Consider this common scene:

> Dr. Smith's patient, Mr. Jones, was recently diagnosed with Stage 4 metastatic lung cancer. By the time it was discovered the cancer had already spread to his bones and he also had a suspicious lesion detected on a brain CT scan. Mr. Jones and his wife had already researched the disease on the Internet before their first consultation with Dr. Smith, a noted oncologist at a major National Cancer Institute-designated Comprehensive Cancer Center located at a nearby academic medical center. They knew that the prognosis was dismal, and there were essentially no curative options. They were therefore surprised by Dr. Smith's somewhat upbeat demeanor. When they asked him why he seemed to be more optimistic than appeared to be warranted by the literature they had reviewed, he mentioned that while he was well aware of what the clinical trial data showed, he had had several patients over his 25 years of practice who had done extremely well with advanced disease just like that of Mr. Jones. Indeed, he remembered them quite well. Mr. Jones and his wife were extremely gratified to hear this uplifting news and were able to tell their children that there was hope after all. They agreed to the intensive chemotherapy and radiation therapy regimen recommended by Dr. Smith.

There is little doubt that Dr. Smith meant well and that he was attempting to instill some level of hopeful thinking in an otherwise horrific and undoubtedly terminal clinical situation. Indeed, he may have even believed that Mr. Jones was similar to those few patients who seemingly beat the odds (out of the thousands whom he had seen who had not). The few stood out because of their uniqueness. If the chances of success are 0.5%, then 1 out of 200 will do well, and we certainly remember rare, unusual, and idiosyncratic events. They are impressed on our memory, and we can recall them instantly using the "availability heuristic" first described by Amos Tversky and Daniel Kahneman in 1973.[53] And there is little doubt that a personal story (and memory) can influence not only the kinds of recommendations made by physicians but also the decisions patients make in response to the narrative anecdote.[54]

Physicians also use their anecdotal experience in the all-too-common practice of off-label use prescribing (OLU). An exception to the Food and Drug Administration (FDA) rules governing prescriptions for medications permits doctors to order drugs for anything they believe will be in the best clinical interest of the patient, irrespective of the evidence base or indication. Thus, if I am convinced that a specific drug will work for a patient with a given disorder because drugs of a similar class (for example) may be effective for similar kinds of conditions, I am free to write a prescription.[55] I may be held to account if an untoward (although perhaps not an unexpected) adverse event occurs with harm to the patient that is caused by the drug and that could have been avoided if I had not prescribed that medication (or perhaps prescribed a more appropriate one), but I am well within the bounds of legal and clinical practice to take this action. Most physicians do. This is not to say that there are many clinical conditions that are treated with drugs for which FDA approval is lacking (for that specific indication) and for which there exists ample clinical data, including from well-controlled clinical trials. However, much OLU occurs in situations with little or no supportable evidence of this type. Indeed, many doctors refer to their expert judgment and clinical experience with a given treatment in deciding whether to employ it again. A singular positive experience (which may be correlative rather than causally related to the drug) may be sufficient to induce a doctor to try it again under similar circumstances. As I have stated, anecdotes of this kind exert a powerful effect on future behavior. Doriane Coleman and I have suggested that this practice be curtailed and controlled to limit the ability of doctors to prescribe in the absence of evidence other than anecdotal experience.[56] We outlined a number of reasons to do so, but for the purposes of my argument here, one of the most salient would be that, within the confines of a universal health insurance plan in which coverage was determined both by medical need and the appropriateness of interventions, the role and strength of physician experience based on anecdotes would be both limited and subject to outside scrutiny by peers. With these constraints, the power of anecdotes to influence clinical practice would be diminished in one respect—physicians would not be completely free to prescribe whatever they wanted for whatever indication—but they could make their case (with their patients) utilizing an appeals process.

The powerful appeal to both physicians and their patients of the sort of customized, personalized attention and care epitomized by the application of anecdotal reasoning and "n-of-1" experience could serve to hamper any attempt to limit its use. We already see the tremendous backlash that can occur when faceless bureaucrats (i.e., insurance company employees, including physicians employed by these firms) deny access to treatments that doctors think will help their patients, irrespective of the amount and quality of data that support what they think is best.[57] It is likely that at least some of the animosity toward those issuing denials stems from the source: for-profit insurers and other opaque decision-makers. It is not unreasonable to suggest that a more transparent system that was open and free of (most) overt conflicts of interest (such as my proposed RAM committees) could issue decisions and the reasons for them in a manner that could both appear to be more fair and actually would be and hence be more tolerable. Nevertheless, we should not underestimate the long—and often noble and well-intentioned—tradition of doctors incorporating personal experiences and beliefs (what is sometimes referred to as coming under the umbrella of the "art of medicine") into patient care and the compelling role this convention plays in clinical practice.

MIRACLES

Finally, I wish to discuss what I will call "illegitimate requests (or demands)" and the obstacles they may represent for establishing cutoffs and having them respected. By this I intend to convey a very specific and context-dependent meaning. Illegitimate requests are not simply those that, within the framework of a publicly funded, universal healthcare system, do not meet the previously agreed-upon criteria for need that is inclusively worthy of being supported by the healthcare system. Rather, they are demands to continue or initiate care that on its face has little to no relationship with what medicine can or should have as its reasonable or justifiable goals. This could incorporate demands for both physiologically and prognostically nonbeneficial (or futile) interventions or those that have been declared as not meeting true medical needs (see Chapter 3) as defined by the cutoff system(s) that comprise the benefits package. This section will introduce a topic that is a more specific examination of the application issue introduced in the prior chapter. In the United States, many people have become accustomed to the healthcare system acceding to their demands for certain types of interventions, even if there is little clinical justification for doing so (indeed, much of the futility debate at the bedside is related to this problem).[58] There is a genuine disagreement among an ethnically and religiously diverse population of patients and families about the goals of medicine and what legitimate and illegitimate requests can be made of doctors (such as keeping people alive indefinitely with intensive care while the family prays for a miracle to occur). This section will discuss some of these challenges because there is little doubt that any kind of reasonable rationing system that limits care based on efficacy will necessarily have to develop ways to cope with these demands.

For example, the system could refuse to meet patient requests that are determined to arise from irrational thoughts (not simply unusual ones) such as delusions, hallucinations, or other expressions of psychiatric conditions like body dysmorphic disorder (a rare illness in which patients focus on one or more parts of their anatomy as unconditionally ugly and/or intolerable and wish it/them altered or even removed).[59] The system could also make the a priori decision, similar to what presently exists with most standard commercial insurance policies, to not pay for non-reconstructive cosmetic surgery (nose jobs as opposed to breast reconstruction after mastectomy for cancer); or when the family of a patient declared to be dead using neurologic criteria ("brain death") insists that life support continue because members of their faith do not accept this category of death;[60] or when parents insist that full life support be maintained in a child with complete anencephaly.[61] All these would be cases of what I am labeling "illegitimate" because they are *prima facie* invalid, and refusals to provide the sought-for interventions are appropriate and cannot be violations of either individual rights or fairness.

It is now well-established in Western medicine that the autonomy of patients with decision-making capacity must be respected almost absolutely. That means that patients have an unfettered right to make (rational) decisions about what happens to their bodies and themselves in a medical encounter. They can refuse any intervention proposed by a physician unless it can be proved that this decision is the product of irrational, diseased, or disordered thinking such as that produced as a consequence of a sufficiently incapacitating mental illness or ingestion of a substance that has a similar effect on cognition. Merely unwise or even what others might consider stupid or ill-founded decisions are accepted as valid (even if they might be controversial). Of course, as with other domains (such as those discussed throughout this book), there can be blurry boundaries, especially when it concerns systems of belief that are outside the mainstream (meaning that they are held by a small minority of people). For example, when does a set of religious beliefs transform from the suspect, spooky, weird convictions of the few (and hence unacceptable) to beliefs that may still be considered by many to be odd, but not so odd that they are thought to be crazy? The borderline—or cutoff—is difficult to establish.

But there are other demands that patients or their families make that are more complex and troubling, especially those that derive from beliefs based on religious faith that may be more mainstream. I will concentrate on miracles as paradigmatic of this sort of request. What follows should not be construed as an assault on the depth of faith that people possess who believe in the reality of miracles. Nor is this a debate intended as an argument against the existence of God or deism in any of its iterations. I simply wish to frame a discussion of what a generous, publicly funded healthcare system that aims to be fair as well as control costs would reasonably offer to beneficiaries, as well as reasonably deny them. I hope to discuss a fairly common demand by patients (and especially their families) in America when faced with dire medical straits such as a diagnosis with a very dismal prognosis or a less than optimal or expected response to therapy: namely, to "do everything while we pray for a miracle." My goal here is not to argue against the existence of miracles (although I will do that to some extent) but rather to explore how an evidence-based, reasonably rational healthcare system that must place some limits on what is provided can respond to such requests. Indeed, what is perhaps most important is not the metaphysical truth of whether supernatural causation and the production of miracles (i.e., events that contravene the known laws of nature) occur. Rather, it is that many people believe that they do exist and occur and that this belief needs to be respected in a special, action-compelling way by others, particularly members of the medical system (irrespective if they hold similar beliefs). No one is asking me to believe in miracles, but many are demanding that I respect their belief in such a way that my actions concerning my decisions on treatment interventions and the like will be guided by their beliefs and not my professional expertise and judgment.

Miraculous treatments, miraculous turnarounds and improvements, miracle drugs, miracle cures: the language of miracles pervades modern medicine, ironically at a time when our knowledge of the science underlying biological and pathological causation has never been greater and continues to increase each year. One perhaps could understand the appeal of assuming supernatural intervention in the past (the prescientific medical past or, more accurately, the pre-effective intervention past) when patients made an unexpected recovery. Think of the soldiers in the Civil War who somehow managed to survive heavily contaminated, unsterile traumatic field amputations or gunshot wounds fouled with dirt and animal feces.[62] How was it even possible that such grievously injured patients could survive such conditions? But some—indeed, a surprisingly large number—did. Was it due to miracles? Today, of course, we have created treatments and diagnostic tools that would be unimaginable even 75 years ago, none of which may lay claim to the form of godly intervention that people label as miracles. But patients and their families continue to express hope and pray for such amazing phenomena and attribute divine intercession when such unexpected and rare events do occur.[63] Of course, what people hope for and call miracles in medicine bears a very close relationship to the issue of statistics and rare events that I introduced in Chapter 4.

Whether "miracle talk" is being employed to indicate supernatural causative intervention or its more cynical employment as a public relations gimmick to imply that some institutions can do the unexpected and the exceptionally rare, it is commonly observed. We very casually and loosely use the language of miracles to describe almost any unexpected event as in, "it would be a miracle if such and such happened." Unfortunately, this debases the true spiritual, supernatural meaning of miracles and transmutes the usage to imply simply the extraordinary rather than true divine intervention in the affairs of people. The Children's Miracle Network (a national fundraising organization for pediatric hospitals in the United States) proclaims that "the moment a child arrives at their Children's Miracle Network Hospital, a miracle is in the making." The healthcare system in the United States and its representatives eagerly embrace this marketing approach, loudly trumpeting the latest research results as yet another miracle cure or the arrival of one more miraculous breakthroughs. Popular entertainment media, both on television and in the movies, capitalize on the drama associated with bringing people back from the brink of death, at the same time getting viewers on the edge of their seats ("will she make it?") and transmitting a totally false and overly optimistic expectation about the outcomes of interventions like cardiopulmonary resuscitation.

Other media, such as newspapers and now the Internet, also contribute to the misinformation and hype of miraculous medicine. Telling the stories of people with severe brain damage who hover at the edge between brain dead and almost brain dead, the television doctor and medical reporter Sanjay Gupta spends a great deal of time concentrating on miraculous cases or those that are extraordinarily uncommon. He blurs the distinction between the two, leading to a grave mistake of inference. Should we spend time waiting for an extraordinarily rare event or "miracle" to occur and thus continue to treat all of those patients who truly never will recover in order to discover the occasional one who will? In some ways, this is analogous to the legal precept that states that it is better that the guilty should go free than one innocent man go to jail. Recall the concept of "number needed to treat" (NNTT) I introduced in Chapter 4. This refers to the approximate number of patients who meet the clinical criteria for a given interventions (say, atorvastatin therapy for hyperlipidemia) who need to be treated to prevent (or cause) some clinically relevant (and significant) outcome. With a relatively benign intervention that may also be inexpensive and with few important side effects affecting small numbers of people, it is reasonable to accept a large NNTT to benefit the few. But we must re-evaluate the wisdom of this approach when the intervention is not benign, is very costly, and the hoped-for outcome is extremely rare. This seems extraordinarily cruel to me. First, an illustrative case:

At the age of 14 years, Bobby was a devoted fan of off-road biking. For his 13th birthday, his parents presented him with the brand new dirt bike that he had been lusting after for quite some time. He immediately put it to use, speeding off with his like-minded friends who lived near his home in a rural part of the state. They often could be seen frequenting an abandoned construction site about a mile from his house that was festooned with small hills and the sorts of obstacles in the paths that delighted them all by challenging their skills at maneuvering and taking their bikes on high jumps and in-air twists. Of course his parents insisted that he wear a helmet during his adventures, but sometimes he took it off as he felt that it obstructed the peripheral vision necessary to complete the most complicated tricks. One day—when he wasn't wearing the helmet—he miscalculated a move and crashed head first into a large boulder by the side of the path. He immediately lost consciousness. His friends noted a whitish, jelly-like material amidst the large amount of blood matting his hair and oozing out of his nose and left ear. Two of his buddies immediately called for help on their cell phones and within 10 minutes the local EMS arrived. They noted that one of his pupils was fixed and dilated, the other was sluggishly reactive to light and that he was unconscious with labored breathing. They stabilized his neck in a brace, strapped him to a board and placed an endotracheal tube in the field and loosely bandaged his head wounds. They also started a large bore intravenous line and started IV fluids. He was rushed to the local hospital Emergency Department where a stat CT scan showed a massive intracranial injury. Brain tissue (the whitish substance noted by Bobby's friends) was also seen to be extruding from the main injury site. Over the succeeding four months he underwent numerous neurosurgical procedures to attempt to manage his devastating wound. Eventually, his condition stabilized. He never regained consciousness and required a mechanical ventilator to breathe for him. He received a tracheostomy for long-term management of his airway, and a gastrostomy tube for nutritional support. Multiple neurologists were consulted and all concurred that his chance of meaningful recovery, such as regaining even minimal interactive consciousness, was remote or nonexistent. However, he did not meet the clinical criteria of the complete absence of all brain function required for a declaration of brain death. Nevertheless, throughout his hospital course he remained a full-code, meaning that cardiopulmonary resuscitation and other advanced life support measures would be provided should his condition worsen. This was done at the insistence of his parents. They were both very religious and declared that the miracle they were praying for (his full recovery) was imminent, so long as the medical and nursing staff would continue to provide everything needed to keep Bobby alive. They eventually took him home with a portable, tabletop ventilator. His mother quit her job to care for him. Over the next few years he would be admitted to the hospital 4–5 times per year for pneumonias and other infections and complications associated with people in permanent vegetative states. Most of these hospitalizations required at least some time in the ICU. Each time, Bobby's code status was addressed anew and each time his parents insisted that he must be kept alive as their hope for a miracle remained undimmed. After living in this state for 4 years, Bobby contracted influenza A during one winter and his respiratory function worsened. He continued to be a "full code" as his mother insisted as she prayed for a miraculous cure. He then suffered a cardiac arrest while in the ICU, had full CPR performed for 45 minutes without effect, and died.

There are many questions raised by this unfortunate case. One of the most salient for my purposes is whether his parents' continual insistence that he receive complete resuscitation *no matter what* as they confidently prayed for divine intervention to restore him to his pre-accident state of health would be justified under even the most liberal and generous public health care system? The fact that it is so currently in the United States is an all-too-common event for complicated reasons.[64] From a system perspective, we must ask whether the demand made by Bobby's parents was illegitimate (as I define it).

There may be other demands or requests made of doctors (or the healthcare system) that may be considered and then judged to be illegitimate in addition to those desires to wait for a miracle.[65] These could include demands for surgeries that are outlandish (perhaps for amputation of a perfectly good and functional limb), antibacterial antibiotics for a viral infection, or continued life support for patients declared dead by neurological criteria ("brain death") and the like. Even when they are made with religious rationale, we mostly feel justified (although perhaps uncomfortable at times) to refuse them, declaring them to be irrational (i.e., crazy), to have no basis in scientific fact (antibiotics for a cold), or to be against the accepted societal consensus on what physical states qualify as being dead. Irrespective of the object of the demand and whether it expresses a desire, a hope, or some combination, the situations in which these most frequently occur are heartrending for all concerned.[66]

Miracles can be viewed as unexpected and rare beneficial events that occur to help specific individuals or groups and are most frequently causatively attributed to a supernatural being (a god, for example). Unexpected bad things may also be similarly attributed but are not labeled as miracles unless they happen to the enemy and thus save the day for the group who prayed for deliverance, a typically salient story in many religious texts. The point is that we don't pray for bad things to happen to ourselves or loved ones, even if their occurrence could plausibly be labeled by other believers with a different point of view as "miraculous." It is common that miracles are believed to happen after prayers asking for help. Not surprisingly, the overwhelming majority of prayers for intercession are not successful (if they were, then these events would not be so rare and unexpected). Robert Larmer's definition is fairly comprehensive: "a miracle must not only be a physical event which would never have occurred except through the action of a transcendent rational agent, but also an event that clearly has religious significance and is of such an extraordinary nature it is either directly perceived as a miracle or immediately inferred as such."[67]

It is important to point out that miracles defined in this way are recognized only *after they have occurred* or *post hoc* and not beforehand; the expectation that one might occur is probabilistic, and even the most faithful may have hope that one *might* take place, but one cannot reasonably have the expectation that it *will* take place. Critically, the subjective part of miraculous events is the wonder they inspire; if they were quotidian happenings, they wouldn't spawn wonder, only a yawn. Indeed, the word "miracle" is derived from the Latin *miraculum,* meaning "an object of wonder."[68] So for even the most pious, a miraculous interference leading to a good outcome for a patient is an exceptionally rare and unpredictable event: it is likely as rare (if not more so) as the low probability of a spontaneous recovery against the informed predictions of experienced physicians. This therefore begs the question of how long it is reasonable to continue a (medical) intervention that is not working solely to allow the time needed for God to intervene.

Numerous dilemmas arise from these situations. Patients (or usually their families) commonly request or demand starting or continuing advanced life support interventions while they pray for and await a miraculous "cure." If these interventions could plausibly be said to be nonbeneficial (or futile), is this a legitimate request (meaning, one that deserves to be respected)? Should we obey the dictates of religion in the domain of medicine? R. F. Holland expressed his skepticism this way:

> The significance of some coincidences as opposed to others arises from their relation to human needs and hopes and fears, their effects for good or ill upon our lives. So we speak of our luck (fortune, fate, etc.). And the kind of thing that, outside religion, we call luck is in religious parlance the grace of God or a miracle of God. But while the reference here is the same, the meaning is different. . . . Whereas what happens by a stroke of luck is something in regard to which one just seizes one's opportunity or feels glad about or feels relieved about, something for which one may thank one's lucky stars. To say that one thanks one's lucky stars is simply to express one's relief or to emphasize the intensity of the relief: if it signifies anything more than this it signifies a superstition. . . . But although a coincidence can be taken religiously as a sign and called a miracle and made the subject of a vow, it cannot without confusion be taken as a sign of divine interference with the natural order.[69]

Rare and unexpected events happen all the time, albeit not very frequently, and because of their rarity, they are unanticipated in the sense that we would be surprised if they occurred (but not because they can't take place, simply because of their unusually low frequency). They key is the causal attribution. As pointed out by Richard and Enid Peschel, what they call "scientific miracles" are those uncommon events that must occur at some point in time.[70] That is the nature of probability. It is also predicated upon naturalistic explanations or causes for all phenomena in the world, no matter how little we may understand them (at present). Those people of a religious frame of mind who believe in supernatural causation and most importantly in a supernatural entity that causes things to happen, especially those events that seem counter to what we understand the laws of nature to be, accept a different kind of miracle than simply (and only) the rare and unexpected. Not to be trite or disrespect-ful, but this kind of miracle is akin to a bolt of lightning from the heavens (perhaps literally) that changes things, almost always for the better.[71] Not surprisingly, per-haps, the ability to attribute divine intervention as the cause of an unusual event has changed over the years as natural explanations have expanded their scope, range, and domain(s). Nevertheless, medicine can't cure everyone and cannot forestall death indefinitely, so there may still be room for the hopeful against the odds to pray for a miracle. Furthermore, as discussed in Chapter 4, complex biological systems (like people) are inherently unpredictable and thus our prognostic abilities are inescap-ably uncertain, probabilistic, and tentative. They can be expressed with more or less confidence, but never with absolute conviction (if one wishes to be honest). So even our most self-assured predictions of what will happen are sometimes wrong, even if most of time they are correct.

The practice of medicine (generically speaking) can be said to be composed of an often uneasy blend of the scientific and the humanistic, the objective and the subjec-tive. As such, there occasionally can be a tension between the goals, aims, and reach of medicine and those values that people hold to be important, especially in matters con-cerning the domain of faith. Demands to continue treatment or to continue to provide interventions that are not working as defined by scientific medicine but may be by the needs of the faithful (say, by simply preserving bare life) are excellent illustrations of perhaps incommensurable objectives, aspirations, hopes, and fears. I am unsure of how to resolve this clash of cultures in a manner that respects the values of each. Rather than offering some sort of facile explanation or even making the attempt to do so, I would pose the following questions to initiate a conversation: How does (can) medicine accommodate requests/demands for "waiting for a miraculous curative event" with its increasingly scientific basis? Medicine—indeed, life itself—is inher-ently probabilistic and uncertain about what might come to be. Rare things happen rarely; that is why they are rare—even unexpected perhaps—but rare nonetheless.[72]

Which are more common: miracles or rare and unexpected improvements in a patient's condition? In Jacalyn Duffin's review of miracles from the Vatican Secret Archives, she was able to interrogate records of more than 600 "documented" mira-cles from the files of individuals canonized by the Catholic Church between 1600 and 2000. In her words, "the saints whose dossiers I have examined were born from 1220 to 1922, while the miracles ascribed to them were worked from an undated medi-eval past through 1617, when dating began, to 1995."[73] While it might be a difficult task (perhaps impossible) to reliably quantify the number of people who lived (and died) during this time period and who would have been both believers and poten-tially recipients of miracles, it is still not unreasonable to assume that these events are extraordinarily uncommon. Even accounting for those occurrences that were not brought to the attention of the authorities and which could have potentially qualified as (subjectively) miraculous, the vast majority of people neither witness nor experi-ence a miracle. However, natural and no less astonishing, spontaneous remissions of human cancer and other diseases do occur, and this occurrence is likely many orders of magnitude higher that the reported rate of miracles.[74]

In many ways, miracles and medical anecdotes are similar. They both represent rare and exceptional events that impress themselves on our minds in significant ways. They nourish confirmation bias (we highlight occurrences that conform to and confirm our already held beliefs) and the "availability heuristic" of Kahneman and Tversky due to their salience.[75] They can exert unusually powerful effects on decision-making and on our views of how the world may work and especially the causation of perceptible events. Indeed, physicians often take pride in and may be awestruck by those rare cases in which they were "wrong" in their predictions and then use them to "learn" for the future whenever they might encounter a case that they classify—erroneously or not—as similar.[76] Of course, this could be an issue of a simple attribution error (in addition to the ones noted earlier) as well as the earnest motivation that almost all doctors have to want to help people in a way that they think truly matters: leading to a remission, a cure, or some condition that could count as being "better."

David Hume eloquently stated his case against the existence of miracles (and presumably also an argument against being bound by the claims and resulting demands of believers):

> A miracle is a violation of the laws of nature; and as a firm and unalterable experience has established these laws, the proof against a miracle, from the very nature of the fact, is as entire as any argument from experience can possibly be imagined. Why is it more than probable, that all men must die; that lead cannot, of itself, remain suspended in the air; that fire consumes wood, and is extinguished by water; unless it be, that these events are found agreeable to the laws of nature, and there is required a violation of these laws, or in other words, a miracle to prevent them? Nothing is esteemed a miracle, if it ever happen in the common course of nature. It is no miracle that a man, seemingly in good health, should die on a sudden; because such a kind of death, though more unusual than any other, has yet been frequently observed to happen. But it is a miracle, that a dead man should come to life; because that has never been observed, in any age or country. There must, therefore, be a uniform experience against every miraculous event, otherwise the event would not merit that appellation. And as a uniform experience amounts to a proof, there is here a direct and full *proof*, from the nature of the fact, against the existence of any miracle; nor can such a proof be destroyed, or the miracle rendered credible, but by an opposite proof, which is superior.[77]

What makes Hume's definition so remarkable is that it was written in the latter half of the 18th century, when the understanding of what caused what in the natural world was considerably less than it is today (and will undoubtedly be so again 200 years hence). Importantly, as naturalistic causal knowledge due to scientific discovery has expanded over the years, what was previously believed to be "miraculous" and unquestionably due to the hand of God, has fallen under the more mundane (but no less amazing) exegesis of natural phenomena. Recall the Reverend William Paley's argument for the existence of God (the watch must have a watchmaker) that has been used repeatedly to oppose the evidence of natural biological evolution.[78] Indeed, as the scope of scientific naturalistic explanation has advanced over the centuries, the realm over which theistical explanation reigns has correspondingly shrunk.

While William Osler cast no aspersions on the subject of faith, crediting it for profound power over the psyche of his patients and readily accepting its intersession in curing many people of what were often called "functional" disorders (or psycho-somatic maladies), he had little patience with those who sought to use faith to heal "true" disease.[79] Indeed, he regarded those who would exploit the weaknesses and desperation of the ill as quacks and worse. At the same time, he also appreciated the faith that many people held in their physicians as one that could be used respectfully and to his advantage in a search for a cure or palliation.[80]

Do "miracles" occur? Being a materialistic naturalist, I think not, but there is no question that rare events occur rarely (that is why they are rare), and they are not always amenable to simple or facile explanation (recall the story of Steven J. Gould's analysis of his chances of surviving his mesothelioma that I related in Chapter 4). Indeed, sometimes we may simply have to say, "we don't know" when queried by patients about what will happen to them. As unsatisfactory and hesitant as that might be, it does not mean that we *can't* know, just that we don't know with the available facts and knowledge of the way the world works that we possess at the current time. Of course, for those people disposed in the right way, it would be routine to resort to a miraculous explanation for a rare event, especially if it was what one was hoping and indeed praying for. The practical question is whether a publicly funded health-care system should recognize (and hence pay for) waiting for miracles, which by their "nature" can be quite unpredictable, to occur. I would think not.

Nevertheless, there are many people who do believe in miracles (in the United States, in fact, most do). This represents a fundamental difference in how one views the world and assigns causal power and how events come about. At its root, it constitutes an ontological conviction about the universe.[81] These differences have been going on for a long time, and they can have fundamental significance when they are brought to bear as constituents of arguments for starting or continuing certain medical interventions because of the role they may play in the hope for a miracle (the real kind, not simply a beneficial, fortuitous event). Most people also believe that miracles can be accomplished or be conducted via the specific activities or actions of physicians.[82] Indeed, many physicians also are believers in divine intervention into worldly affairs.[83] How should we cope with people who request or demand that we suspend our medical, scientific judgment about what might happen to them or their relatives while they pray and wait for a miraculous curative event to occur? How do we accommodate the not unreasonable and understandable patient and family desire for miraculous supernatural intervention when natural intervention appears to be unsuccessful? No one prays for miraculous cures for ear infections or appendicitis or even diabetes any more. It is not a surprise that people hope for a miracle when the doctor says she cannot fix something serious and life-threatening or make it go away. Are requests/demands to continue natural interventions indefinitely while waiting for an (affirmative) answer for supernatural intervention legitimate?

Even so, in a comprehensive questionnaire survey of the general public as well as emergency department and trauma professionals, L. M. Jacobs and colleagues found that 61% of the public "believe that a person in a persistent vegetative state could be saved by a miracle. Similarly, more of the public (57.4%) than the professionals (19.5%) believe that divine intervention from God could save a person even when the physicians have determined that treatment is futile."[84] Thus, both a large percentage of patients and their doctors subscribe to supernatural interventionist causal beliefs in extreme situations. Since this was a survey asking questions about hypothetical situations, one might expect that, in the desperate actual moment, perhaps even greater numbers of people would reach out for the hope born by a belief in miracles (although the professionals might be less susceptible to "heat of the moment" thinking because they presumably have experience in these matters).

It is not for me to quarrel or debate the nature of miracles or, for that matter, even what believers might think qualifies as such. For my purposes, it is irrelevant whether miraculous, divine interventions actually do occur, whether they are "real" events in the world. For me, it suffices that many people—including physicians and nurses—think they are. The question then becomes whether the desire or even the "deep hope" (as William Stempsey might call it) for a miracle is sufficiently important to garner the sort of respect by the health system that results in agreement for the process.[85] Are these rare events so uncommon that we cannot afford (literally) to respect them when standard hope (based on clinical information, prognostic indicators, doctors' best estimations, etc.) is exhausted? Or should they be lumped in with other requests or demands that seem unreasonable (under the circumstances and all other things being equal)?

It is certainly plausible that these sorts of demands represent a clash between opposing cultures, representing the scientific, naturalistic world of evidence-based medicine on the one hand and the supernaturalistic world of religion on the other. Of course, there are many other dimensions of culture, and the increasing diversity and ascendance of "minority" ethnic populations can add additional layers of complexity to what might be perceived as a miracle and its context.[86] Even though most doctors in the United States are people of faith, they routinely demonstrate the power of naturalism by employing the dominance of scientific medicine over the body. At the same time, they also surrender to their lack of knowledge when the current state of scientific medicine fails. That does not mean that they submit to supernatural forces; they simply concede their intermediate lack of knowledge about the world. Interestingly, religiosity in patients and families may be associated with increased demands and utilization of intensive care at the end of life,[87] but addressing the religious and/or spiritual needs of patients and their families during this time may also lead to the opposite effect: a turn to hospice and the seeming acceptance of death.[88]

Rhonda Cooper and her colleagues at Johns Hopkins suggest dealing with patients and families who express hope for a miraculous improvement in a terrible medical situation by actively engaging them in conversation using their "AMEN" protocol ("affirm, meet, educate, no matter what") as a way to bridge the gap between hoping and reality, the present and the future.[89] While both interesting and a valuable guide to engender trust and maintain the possibility for beneficial interaction, it does nothing to address the issue of how to cope with those individuals who continue to calmly demand that the patient be kept alive regardless of the prognosis, not to mention the expense and continuation of possible suffering (and, of course, the moral distress of the staff). As an alternative, Allan Brett and Paul Jersild note that the large majority of these demands come from families professing a Christian faith, and they propose employing rational theological argument to suggest alternate (and presumably widely accepted) interpretations of scripture and belief to buttress the physicians' reasoning to permit terminal patients to die without excessive prolongation of biological life.[90]

I think it is reasonable to state that "the physician does not owe the patient a miracle."[91] However, the doctor does owe patients and families compassion, understanding, and concern. Despite the extreme commercialization and commodification of American healthcare, patients and their families are not customers of the sort that buy shoes, cars, or any other commodity (nor should they be).[92] Notwithstanding the penchant of healthcare administrators in the United States to translate the practices of the marketplace and marketing to clinics and inpatient units, patients should not be able to get what they want no matter what;[93] getting what they need—financial and other conditions permitting—is a different matter. By the same token, physicians (and other healthcare providers) should not have unfettered power to accede or refuse what patients think they need without any controls or review.

Demands to continue or to initiate medical interventions with the underlying rationale being that it is vital to do so to protect the interests of the patient and/or her family while they pray for divine intercession in the form of a miraculous improvement or cure are not required to be heeded if (and only if) there is good medical, scientific reasons to believe they would be ineffective or only marginally beneficial. Interventions that can only prolong dying and suffering arguably contravene the physician's duty to help her patients, whatever their stage in life and whatever their condition might be. Maintaining intensive care life support or administering one more round of chemotherapy to the terminally ill solely to give time for divine intervention seems cruel. Of course, one should refuse to do so in a manner that attempts to maintain maximal respect for the grief, despair, and underlying beliefs that are frequently intermixed in these complex situations and that serve as motivating factors for such requests. A sympathetic and compassionate approach that utilizes resources that may not normally be components of a doctor's armamentarium (such as pastoral care experts) should be employed whenever possible. One should never dismiss a patient's or family's heartfelt beliefs (and the associated demands) as ridiculous simply because they do not conform to those held by the physician. But, as Stempsey eloquently states, "Physicians have no epistemological grounds for declaring any cure miraculous. Miracles are theological (or philosophical) entities, and not medical entities. All physicians can do is to determine whether a cure is scientifically inexplicable according to the current epistomological standards of medical science. As these standards change, what is currently unexplainable may become explainable. Unexpected observations can also force us to realize that our current explanations and laws of nature are in fact unsatisfactory."[94] To this I would add parenthetically that history has clearly shown that what were formerly believed to be miracles succumbed to the regularities of worldly materialistic explanation as we learned more how the world works. As the scope and depth of scientific, naturalistic understanding expands in medicine, this will not eliminate uncertainty or the unknown. It will, however, narrow the dominion of the natural world that people claim for miraculous happenings.

Nevertheless, we must also ask whether such demands are illegitimate on their face, not so much because of their basis in religion and supernatural causation, but due to the likelihood that they take place in situations in which it would be extraordinarily uncommon for a patient to get better. This thus takes place in that realm of futile or marginally beneficial care that I earlier marked out as one that could be considered off-limits in a rationing system. Notwithstanding this view, there may be reason to consider demands based on a religious faith to be qualitatively different from similar requests derived from other beliefs that may also not be falsifiable (such as not patently disprovable delusions or even hallucinations). We could perhaps appeal to the novel argument employed by Julian Savulescu and Steve Clarke in which they hold that a publicly funded system of healthcare must balance the rightful claims of "atheists, agnostics, and advocates of faiths that do not accept miracle claims" and those of people of faith who do have such beliefs, both of which contribute by way of paying taxes to the support of the healthcare system. They suggest that to always accede to the demands of the latter results in a form of discrimination they call "miracalism." On the other hand, they wish to give at least some respectful deference to the faithful by outlining criteria in which it might be reasonable to continue interventions to await a miracle: "the expenditure of additional resources might be justified in cases where it can be shown that particular believers have a faith-based theological justification for the belief that miracles are at least somewhat likely and have a coherent justification for the claim that keeping a person alive on life support is a way to increase the likelihood of a miracle occurring. It can also be justified, in cases where a *prima facie* case can be made for the rational plausibility of the claim, that there is evidence that a particular miracle has a not insignificant chance of occurring on the basis of a rationally based case for the occurrence of past miracles."[95]

The curious aspect of the argument about miracles is that the desire—perhaps even need—for them appears to be undiminished among the faithful over the centuries, yet the ability of modern, technological, and scientific medicine to effect cures and restore health (or at least maintain it) has never been more powerful; hence, the physical domain in which miracles would perforce be necessary to work should have been expected to shrink. But this is not so. While fewer and fewer patients succumb to their illnesses in advanced industrialized countries when perhaps 50 or 100 years ago they would have died quickly—think of common bacterial infections, trauma, diabetes, and even some cancers and heart disease—the earnest longing for a miracle has not waned. Indeed, in a somewhat counterintuitive manner, many of those of faith are more fervent than ever because of a misplaced belief that the "miracles" of medicine can surely lead to a miracle from heaven. But no matter what the public relations (and, sadly, physicians themselves all too frequently) say in their ads, the amazing products of research and science are exactly that and not miracles: they harness natural laws to produce outcomes that are readily verifiable (and commonly reproducible).

Steven J. Gould famously proposed that medicine and science represented "non-overlapping magisteria."[96] He was referring to what he believed to be their mutually exclusive domains of authority (presumably at least partially epistemic in nature, although that could be disputed). His argument has hardly been universally accepted,[97] but, for my purposes, it is useful to think of it as a premise for beginning a discussion of the authoritative jurisdiction over decision-making in medicine. In other words, can pronouncements of a distinctly theological nature that underlie demands for continuing treatments that medical science would pronounce as futile or without benefit (such as "waiting for a miracle") override what many would think would (or should) be the exclusive domain of physicians?

A needs-based system (see Chapter 4) that must draw limits somewhere should necessarily rule on what sorts of interventions or care constitute wants without associated needs. Demanding continued critical care for a terminally ill patient in the face of a unified prognosis (i.e., minimal to no disagreement among the clinically relevant physicians and nurses) and in which there is little or no reason to believe that the prognosis is tainted by morally unjustifiable bias is undoubtedly one of those instances. Claiming that continuation of ICU care is needed to allow time for a divine intervention to occur is irrelevant to the medical consideration that this sort of treatment is not beneficial. That does not mean that the healthcare team should disregard the sincerely held religious beliefs of family members and their despair and grief. As suggested earlier, spiritual counseling of the appropriate kind may indeed be very helpful, including the possibility of a peaceful, nonantagonistic resolution of the problem.[98] The fact that the demand is made in the language of religion is irrelevant to the substance of the demand (not to the emotions and social situation), which should be evaluated on its (medical and secular) face.

Could making such demands off-limits be a concern for considerations of distributive justice within a publicly funded, universal healthcare system? Of course. But I would suggest that permitting ongoing futile or nonbeneficial care—in other words, funding wants as well as needs—would lead to an inability to control costs due to the fact that fairness would dictate that clinically similar or analogous claims also be looked on favorably. A wealthy country like the United States can (and perhaps should) afford to be very generous in a national healthcare system, if for no other reasons than political and social expediency.[99] But there must be some limits (cutoffs) imposed somewhere, and I think one can argue on economic, clinical, and ethical grounds that restricting access to those interventions with a reasonable likelihood of making people better and/or relieving suffering (which may be the same thing) is both sensible and fair. Furthermore, by permitting a co-existing private market for ancillary healthcare, people would certainly be free to personally fund indefinite stays in the ICU in the same way that individuals decide that wearing eyeglasses is so cumbersome that they shell out thousands of their own dollars for corrective eye surgery. Ultimately, hope in the setting of desperation and despair and the longing for a miracle cannot be separated from the confidence that a patient and/or a family has in a physician to be the conduit for that miracle. It seems as if patients must trust that their doctor can perform the miracle they so earnestly desire and that they believe may (or will) be enabled or activated by God.

CONCLUSION

In this chapter, I discussed several important but often overlooked aspects to the practice of medicine in the United States that could pose problems for the implementation of a comprehensive, universal healthcare plan that imposed rational rationing of the kind I have suggested would be reasonable. Establishing reasonable cutoff points that define what would and would not be covered must be accomplished in such a manner that it can be somewhat flexible and able to accommodate some forms of extraordinary situations. However, the edges or boundaries cannot be so malleable that anyone so inclined can manipulate the system to get what he or she wants (or what his or her doctor wants to prescribe or do) by utilizing social media, the news media, and the like. While some may believe the saying that "rules are made to be broken," in this case permitting too much rule-breaking could lead to an erosion of the very meaning of having justifiable cutoffs. If there are too many exceptions or unique cases, their exceptionalism or uniqueness would gradually lose its force. It is not unreasonable to allow for special situations, but they should be rare.

Another consideration is the probability that there could be a disproportionate use of the means to obtain singular care or interventions, such as therapies that would normally be disallowed, by people whose other circumstances in life already bring to themselves a greater share of wealth and prestige. It is likely that those patients who would take advantage of social media as well as the mainstream news outlets would be better educated and possessed of more financial wealth and clout than others with similar clinical conditions. This could lead to a greater percentage of special cases being resolved positively for those populations who already enjoy more advantages than others. If this were the case, it would seem to violate the basic premise of fair consideration and allocation of resources, especially those at the borderlines, which is where rationing really has force and significance.

Any systematic attempt to impose rationing, even of the kind that I have suggested could be acceptable, will require that cutoffs be imposed. If they are created by consensus in a transparent manner, with fair rules governing their creation and implementation and the stipulation that they will apply to all, the chances of people attempting to get special treatment for their singular situations will be minimized. Certainly, the often impenetrable and baffling manner in which insurers exert their power over permissible covered interventions, often justifying their decisions by appealing to "medical necessity," tends to provoke anger in those denied what they feel they need. It is to be hoped that a more open and honest approach to these contested cases could diminish the distrust many people have for the nameless, faceless bureaucracies who often are the sources of rejection. In the next chapter, I will continue to discuss the subject of various problems that could tend to damage the confidence that people have in the system I am proposing.

6

LUCK

BACKGROUND

Throughout this book, I have discussed different mechanisms to establish cutoffs to accomplish a fair healthcare rationing plan (predicated, of course, on its incorporation within a system of national, universal healthcare insurance). I have attempted to distinguish between morally and medically justifiable methods of creating boundaries between the kinds of healthcare interventions that could be reasonably provided to participants in a global insurance scheme. I have focused on diverse kinds of cutoffs that concentrate on measureable parameters about patients, diseases, and the like that could be utilized to restrict access to, or the availability of, medical therapeutic and diagnostic interventions with the goal of demonstrating that they all suffer from differing degrees of methodological and/or ethical flaws. I have argued that the most morally justifiable approach would be to examine health needs, efficacy, and applicability and utilize a group decision-making design modeled on the Rand appropriateness method (RAM) with some modifications. By emphasizing evidence-based medicine, transparency, and inclusiveness, decisions could be achieved that could be plausibly acceptable. In this way—if we also assume that the system would be generously funded so that all reasonably appropriate and effective interventions would be provided and paid for all persons eligible and covered under the program[1]—then the major reasons a patient might not receive an indicated and beneficial treatment or diagnostic test would be for causes unrelated to the actual provision of the benefit and the rules governing its allocation. In the last several chapters I have raised what I think are commonly occurring situations that could serve to undermine the ability to develop and implement acceptable cutoffs. Patient, family, and even political demands for exceptions, carve-outs, and personalized or "futile" care could easily subvert systematic approaches to ration fairly and responsibly. However, I also have argued that there may be strategies to effectively counter these possibly erosive factors. But there is one more important subject that must be examined when discussing the imposition of limits. A health insurance plan, even one with the most munificent financing, cannot repair or compensate for all of the inequities that exist in a society, especially one that already tolerates the considerable inequalities of distribution in its resources as the United States. Yet, there are potentially preventable effects of the ways in which cutoffs are crafted that could minimize unintended downstream negative ramifications.

Whichever strategy is selected, it must necessarily affect individual people, possibly in fundamentally important ways. I have previously considered the effects of generalized rationing on a general group of people whom I have labeled as "losers": those persons who are negatively affected by an otherwise fair rationing plan.[2] At the time, I concentrated on how to create the rules of fairness and equity in distributing resources and put aside a detailed discussion of the possible deleterious downstream effects on how otherwise just regulations could adversely affect whole classes of people in our socially, economically, and clinically (health-wise) heterogeneous society. It is certainly conceivable that a system crafted according to legitimate and ethically defensible procedures and otherwise ostensibly fair could have differential impacts on populations of people who, in other respects, would be treated fairly *because* of the particular procedures used to create cutoffs.

A primary legacy of the Enlightenment, without a doubt, is that all people have certain unalterable, inherent, and equal political rights by virtue of their being human (among other things). However, this cannot apply to biological equality because that would be a false assertion on its face. Not only are we each reasonably unique individuals genetically (both germline and somatically due to epigenetic modification), but we are all exposed to different environments that interact with our physiology to produce the animals we turn out to be and the changes throughout our lives than can result. We each have dispositions to be more or less healthy depending on vast numbers and kinds of influences over which we may exert only limited control. Of course, some may be more fortunate than others to be born with a genetic or real silver spoon whose wealth may serve to temper (or even alter) the otherwise dismal fate set out in one's genes. This is not to say that our biology absolutely determines our lot in life, but it certainly can have a significant influence. Not surprisingly, the environment to which one is exposed contains features that are more or less immune to human alteration (consider rural or mountainous terrain) but which could be generally lumped together as a category of physical properties that can contribute to one's health in both positive and negative ways. Moreover, there are much more human-derived features of one's environment—family, psychology, social networks, education, nutrition, and the like—that may also have profound effects on individual and collective health.

It is an unfortunate truism that bad luck in life and illness is not evenly distributed throughout society, even in wealthy nations such as the United States. There are people from all backgrounds who lose the "natural lottery" due to congenital disorders, both acquired and genetic in origin, and hence start their journeys through life with the cards stacked against them. Many of these conditions tend to segregate within genetically ethnic communities (such as sickle cell disease, cystic fibrosis, and Tay-Sachs). But as devastating as these illnesses are for both those who are affected and their families, they are just an epidemiological drop in the bucket compared to the societal burden imposed by those diseases and predispositions to diseases that are due to (or complicated by) what has been termed the "social determinants" of disease. Poverty and its attendant poor housing, polluted environments with consequent multiple and sustained toxic exposures, substance abuse, crime, and the myriad other pre- and postnatal influences all combine to lead to poor health outcomes and decreases in overall well-being that compare so badly to those of the better off members of the same society.

While we cannot guarantee health or medical outcomes or even absolute fairness, we can, by the methods and rules of healthcare resource distribution we craft, potentially minimize the chances that people could suffer from unwarranted, unjustifiable, and avoidable consequences because of their circumstances in life or at least reduce the opportunities for individuals to overtly or covertly subvert the intent of the rules and thereby produce or exacerbate disparities. Therefore, we must now turn to a consideration of how these various approaches to resource allocation and allocation could impinge on different segments of society who already have distinguishing features that might predispose them to be adversely affected by these policy changes. I will concentrate on two such populations, the disabled and the poor—although it is worthwhile noting that these two not infrequently co-localize in the same people: disabled people are more likely to be less well-off than others. I will first present some background material using the overt rationing system for solid organs in which some people with organ failure are much more likely to receive a transplant than others solely because of their situation in life. Hence, the ostensibly (and arguably reasonably) fair rules are crafted in such a manner that some patients, irrespective of their medical *needs*, will never be considered for a transplant.

MISFORTUNE AND ORGAN TRANSPLANTATION

One of the best examples of tacit (and inadvertent or unintentional) discrimination in a rationing system is the allocation and prioritization that has existed for first liver, and then lung, transplantation in the United States. While few—if any—transplant physicians would acknowledge outright racial animus and prejudice, there is little doubt that fewer African-American patients with lung or liver failure historically received transplants than similarly clinically situated white patients.[3] This was primarily due to the manner in which patients not only were considered eligible for transplant, but the way in which they moved up the priority list in their geographic region and institution. It was felt to be the job of transplant doctors to advocate for their own patients and their "cause." Not surprisingly, some physicians were better advocates than others, and they were also more effective for some patients than others. It turned out that some kinds of patients and their stories were more evocative of their doctors' championing their case than others. And, not infrequently, this kind of endorsement turned on clinically insignificant characteristics of patients, such as the color of their skin. Thus, empowering doctors with the discretion to personally recommend some patients rather than others for a scarce resource led to disparities in patient candidacy for this life-saving intervention.[4] However, a simple solution was at hand that seemed to save physicians from their hidden biases. First, the liver transplant system introduced the MELD score (Model for End-Stage Liver Disease, to be followed by its pediatric correlate, the PELD score) and then, more recently, the LAS (Lung Allocation Score). Both methods replaced the former practice of using "clinical judgment" to determine who should be first in line for an organ with a simple numerical score based on quantitative laboratory values that reflected the severity of illness. Most, but by no means all, disparities of race disappeared.[5] Nevertheless, recipients of organs still reflected a skewed group with disproportionate representation of patients who were, on average, wealthier, whiter, and more urban than existed in the population with liver or lung failure.

The organ allocation and transplant systems implicitly discriminates against the least advantaged in society because socioeconomic factors are considered when evaluating the suitability of a candidate for transplantation. It is certainly not unreasonable that conditions that could sensibly be thought to have an impact on patient outcomes (and hence the survivability of the graft and, except for the case of kidneys when there is the alternative of dialysis, the patient). Indeed, there is significant evidence that a variety of what might be termed "nonmedical" (i.e., not strictly biological) characteristics about patients and their lives can both positively and negatively influence the results of transplantation.[6] And it should not be surprising that people who live complicated and perhaps messy lives may have more challenges meeting the striking demands of being a transplant recipient. Patients who have disordered families with less-than-reliable social connections, people who have marginal or no health insurance, the unemployed or underemployed, patients with underlying psychological or pre-existing psychiatric problems: all of these can lead to a negative assessment for becoming a candidate for a scarce organ that could go to someone else equally as sick but who has excellent social structural support, deep pockets, and no history of mental disorders. Both kinds of patient could potentially medically benefit from this life-saving therapy, but it would seem to represent poor stewardship of a publicly held and administered asset to award it to someone who might not be able to take care of it as well as someone else. What this means is that an individual must have sufficient resources, both financial and psychosocial, to offer the best chances for the transplant be successful. Therefore, if a patient has inadequate funds to pay for a radiological or diagnostic laboratory study (for example) or must interrupt her supply of anti-rejection medication, or has deficient housing, or an unreliable form of transportation to get to her doctor's appointments, that patient's entry onto the organ waitlist could be adversely affected. Indeed, in real life, this would almost certainly exclude patients in this situation from even being seriously considered for an organ. Of course, this means that people who are less advantaged in life will have a much lower chance of obtaining an organ. A concrete example might help to illustrate this problem.

The lung transplant program at the institution where I work requires that organ recipients live within 30 miles of the hospital for up to 1 year postoperatively. There are good and justifiable reasons for this requirement because there are many potential complications that can arise after transplant, and there are numerous outpatient visits and rehabilitation schedules that are necessary to ensure the best survivability of the organ and hence the patient. Transplant programs are regularly graded by the United Network for Organ Sharing (UNOS) and the Organ Transplant Procurement Network (OPTN), nationally accredited and federally funded regulatory organizations, on a number of metrics, including the 1- and 5-year survival of the grafts. Maximizing the chances of graft longevity entails patient participation in a rigorous program of adherence to a strict regimen of numerous, extremely expensive medications (frequently many more than the couple of immunosuppressive drugs used to prevent graft rejection, with the cumulative cost often running to many thousands of dollars per month, only a portion of which may be covered by insurance), pulmonary physical rehabilitation, and the like. Second, potential recipients must also have a full-time caregiver to assist them with the myriad associated conditions and obstacles faced by a patient who has undergone such major surgery and postoperative course. They will frequently need aid with "activities of daily living" (including physical help getting to and from to the bathroom, with meal preparation, and medication procurement and administration, and to move to the car to drive to doctors' and other medical appointments). Moreover, the vital importance of social support during what can frequently be a long, arduous, and unpredictable journey cannot be overstated. The practical effect of these common-sense and necessary requirements is that people who live farther away and cannot afford to move closer, or who have spouses or partners who work and must continue working, or who have any other impediments to meticulous adherence to a such a detailed and demanding program are locked out of access to lung transplantation. And one should not think that other kinds of organ transplants are any less burdensome; they may differ in the amount and duration of pre- and postoperative care regimens, but not necessarily the kind. It should therefore be obvious that qualifying for an organ transplant requires considerably more than simply having bad lungs or a failing liver. One must not only be sick, but must also have the financial and social wherewithal to participate. This is an example of how a rationing system—albeit one that is fair once one gains access—can adversely affect those who already are disadvantaged in life.

It might therefore be reasonable to conclude that the economic barriers might disappear if a generously funded, nationalized health insurance plan were in place. Unfortunately, the data would suggest that this is only partially true, as revealed by the results of transplantation under the auspices of the End-Stage Renal Disease (ESRD) program. Almost all the costs associated with kidney transplantation and its aftermath for up to 3 years post-transplant are covered under the Medicare benefit provided by this program.[7] Even so, the percentage of (poor) African Americans transplanted using the public, shared pool of cadaveric donors is disproportionately low compared to their fractional representation in the population of patients with ESRD.[8]

If we accept it as a given that the current state of the art of solid organ transplantation must place these sorts of requirements on potential recipients, what could be done to level the playing field and not make the socioeconomic profile of transplanted patients so heavily favor those individuals who are already better off? Short of a wholesale reordering of both the social and natural lotteries in American (or any other) society, it is difficult to imagine what could compensate for ingrained disparities, assuming that we accept inequities in economic welfare. Of course, heavier and more comprehensive expenditures on social welfare programs that have been shown to be both efficient and effective could potentially help. For example, improving overall early childhood and other education would presumably contribute to an improvement in overall population health because there is a direct correlation between educational attainment and health.[9] Increasing the amount of social welfare funds devoted to smoking cessation, obesity prevention, and alcohol abuse treatment could decrease the numbers of people with chronic obstructive pulmonary disease (COPD), diabetic nephropathy, and cirrhosis, all of which are leading causes of organ failures for which transplantation can be curative. Similarly, diminishing the ranks of the un- and underemployed could also possibly relieve some of the socioeconomic anxiety attributable to this form of chronic stress.

In the absence of these large-scale, broad, population-based interventions, could the transplant community itself take any measures to mitigate the effects of social inequities? Of course, the answer is "yes," but to do so would likely result in sacrifices in the efficacy of transplantation as a therapy. Modern immunosuppressive medications are extraordinarily successful in preventing graft rejection, but only if patients take them regularly as prescribed. Similarly, minimizing the dangers of developing opportunistic infections requires patients to assiduously adhere to regimens of risk avoidance and abatement (such as not living in homes that are in poor repair, contaminated by mold, etc.). It would be problematic to continue maintaining the posture that (cadaveric) organs comprise a shared public resource and the transplant community rightfully serves as responsible stewards of their use. It would be difficult to justify, much less maintain, support in the system if significant reductions in organ and recipient longevity were a direct result of enhancing equity in distribution. As I have previously noted, the solid organ transplant system is remarkable in that sizeable numbers of wait-listed patients die without receiving organs, yet complaints about the fairness of the system are vanishingly small.[10] Furthermore, organ donation in this country is voluntary, and the belief that the allocation of organs was somehow unfair or was biased in favor of people judged "less worthy" could jeopardize the ultimate source material that permits the program to operate. In the final analysis, I doubt if significant alterations to the current flawed, but reasonably fair, system could be accomplished without causing an even worse situation. This conclusion speaks to the challenge of attempting to mitigate the consequences of larger societal problems when they affect isolated—and relatively small—systems. One cannot repair the long-standing predicament of multigenerational poverty (for example) by altering the allocation of transplant organs. That is not to say that small corrections to systems cannot ease some of the consequences of national injustice and personal bias, such as illustrated by the implementation of the MELD and LAS methods discussed earlier. But the challenges are much greater than those amenable to mitigation with limited fixes.

SOCIAL DETERMINANTS OF DISEASE

The bulk of the global burden of disease and the major causes of health inequities, which are found in all countries, arise from the conditions in which people are born, grow, live, work, and age. These conditions are referred to as social determinants of health, a term used as shorthand to encompass the social, economic, political, cultural, and environmental determinants of health. The most important determinants are those that produce stratification within a society—structural determinants—such as the distribution of income, discrimination (for example, on the basis of gender, class, ethnicity, disability, or sexual orientation), and political and governance structures that reinforce rather than reduce inequalities in economic power. These structural mechanisms that affect the social positions of individuals constitute the root cause of inequities in health. The discrepancies attributable to these mechanisms shape individual health status and outcomes through their impact on intermediary determinants such as living conditions, psychosocial circumstances, behavioural and/or biological factors, and the health system itself. The rationale for action on social determinants of health rests on three broad themes. First, it is a moral imperative to reduce health inequities. Second, it is essential to improve health and well-being, promote development, and reach health targets in general. Third, it is necessary to act on a range of societal priorities—beyond health itself—that rely on better health equity.[11]

With these stirring words and call to action, the World Health Organization (WHO) renewed its endorsement of both the primary causes of most health inequities and the means by which they could be reduced throughout the globe in a follow-up to its 2008 report "Closing the Gap in a Generation."[12] The consensus of the WHO was that the majority of the differences in the health status of people living in wealthy/developed and poor/underdeveloped nations was attributable to differences in social conditions that both predisposed them to preventable illnesses and premature death but that were also amenable to structural and political means to relieve these burdens. Furthermore, they noted that there continued to be analogous disparities in health in rich industrialized countries, especially those that are hallmarked by significant populations of impoverished and poorly educated individuals with a relatively weak social safety net (such as the United States). It was certainly implied, if not stated outright, that these states were also responsible for permitting these disparities to continue (perhaps more so because of their ability to address them save for a failure of political, and conceivably moral, will). How much of the burden of disease is attributable to avoidable social conditions (broadly construed) may be debatable. Also controversial is the degree to which governments should be held accountable and responsible (if at all) for addressing those social and physical conditions that are causally related to poor health outcomes.[13] But there is little doubt that environmental pollution, poor education, lack of women's rights, poverty, and other circumstances that could be altered clearly play a role in how well and how long people live.

Misfortune in the social domains of life frequently has spillover negative effects on health. Whether these difficulties are in large part attributable to social conditions that could be changed either by individuals themselves or by government is a separate question. Nevertheless, there is little doubt that comprehensive health insurance available to all, such as I envision, could relieve at least some significant economic burdens and financial stress on struggling families and individuals. Indeed, there is recent evidence to support this contention from an analysis of populations who obtained health insurance coverage via the Affordable Care Act (ACA).[14] However, this has limited ability and reach to solve or mitigate other challenges in the lives of many people. The burden of untreated or preventable illness could be decreased by readily accessible, in-depth, and affordable healthcare (assuming that it is utilized), but it can do little by itself to address the structural and ingrained problems that beset most societies, but especially those with such a skewed distribution of wealth as the United States. Short of tying universal healthcare insurance to other programs designed to tackle such factors that contribute to health disparities as established and seemingly intractable as poverty, poor education, substandard housing, pockets of environmental pollution concentrated in certain geographic areas, long-term unemployment, the lack of easily available contraception, and the like, a public healthcare plan would be mostly reactive. Even a plan that stresses primary and preventive care would have mostly superficial effects on many of those elements that play instrumental roles in what diseases people are susceptible to, what conditions they develop, and even how they respond to treatment once initiated. To be sure, not having to worry about how much a medicine costs or whether a visit to the doctor would mean less food on the table could provide enormous relief, but it would not address many of the fundamental root causes underlying the sources of illness.

Even if the method of determining cutoffs is fair and the application is equitable, just, and generous (as I have argued), people occupying the lowest socioeconomic tiers of society, those living in remote and rural areas, Native Americans living on reservations, and the like, may be given short shrift. Focusing on efficacy and appropriateness is workable, practicable, and defensible but could potentially exacerbate (or certainly not alleviate) pre-existing health disparities. A clinical example will serve to illustrate this problem. Let us assume that comprehensive, universal, and generous health insurance has been implemented in the United States (of the sort I propose). There are minimal, progressively scaled co-pays for doctor visits and all interventions and medications, and there is no annual deductible. Almost everything that is clinically appropriate and effective for a condition is covered.

Ms. Smith is a 50-year-old married woman who lives in an upper middle class suburb of a major urban area. She discovers a lump in her right breast on a Monday morning and immediately makes an appointment to see her primary care doctor, who promptly schedules her for a mammogram, which is performed within 48 hours. She is easily able to take time off from her work and has existing childcare for her teenage son and daughter. She has her own car and is accompanied to her appointments by her husband (who is also able to stay home from his job). The mammogram shows a suspicious, calcified mass. An ultrasound-guided biopsy is scheduled for the next day, and, by the next week, she receives the news that she has breast cancer. A complete evaluation demonstrates that it is in an early stage and her chances for recovery with breast-conserving surgery, chemotherapy, and radiation are excellent. There is no family history of breast cancer.

Ms. Jones is a 50-year-old single mother living with her two teenage children and her daughter's infant son in a mobile home trailer park. She has two jobs: one at a fast-food restaurant and the other as a part-time helper for a disabled older man. There is only one car for the family, a 15-year-old sedan with 175,000 miles on the odometer and bald tires. She discovers a lump in her right breast on a Monday morning before she leaves for her first job at the restaurant. She is so busy and tired, she forgets about it for 6 months when she notes pain and redness in the same area. This times she calls her doctor who, immediately makes an appointment to see her that same day, but she finds that she can't get any time off from work for at least three weeks, and her doctor's office does not have evening or weekend hours. By the time she is able to get in, have a biopsy (it also shows breast cancer like Ms. Smith), and have a work-up, her disease is far advanced and has metastasized to her lymph nodes and bones. She has few therapeutic options available and will most likely die of her disease. There is no family history of breast cancer.

In these cases, both Ms. Smith and Ms. Jones developed breast cancer without obvious predisposing causes (such as a strong genetic susceptibility). But one woman should have an excellent outcome and the other likely will die of her disease relatively quickly for potentially preventable reasons. The barriers to early diagnosis and the prompt initiation of effective treatment for Ms. Jones are social: she is poor, has jobs that do not offer generous (or any) leave for medical reasons, and has substantial social obligations that cannot be addressed by hiring others to fulfill her responsibilities. Even her housing arrangements may predispose her to develop complications from her therapies if she has inadequate heating (or air conditioning in a hot summer), deficient ventilation, erratic water and sanitation, and unreliable transportation. Furthermore, if she lives in a rural area, she may have to drive long distances simply to get to the sorts of specialists needed to treat her disease (even if it was diagnosed early on when it was more amenable to successful treatment). Thus, a healthcare system that provides everything that one should need (see Chapter 3) at virtually no cost to the patient (at the point of care) will be of little benefit to a woman such as Ms. Jones whose structural and personal obstacles to taking advantage of such opportunities remain. Indeed, even in Great Britain, which has had long-standing national health insurance and a widespread network of point-of-entry accessible primary care, there have been challenges to erasing inequities in clinical outcomes due to psychosocial and economic factors beyond the control of the healthcare system.[15] It is difficult to imagine how a cutoff strategy such as I have proposed could have an appreciable impact *by itself* on the myriad societal effects on illness and the response of patients to the provision of preventative interventions. However, there is little doubt that the current system of a mostly commercialized, distorted marketplace with poorly placed regulations to rein in its most egregious excesses exacerbates existing inequities rather than moderating them.

I have concentrated my argument on cutoffs as they could apply to specific interventions. In this sense this is necessarily a focus on treatment or after-the-fact interventions. However, cutoffs would also have a bearing on such obviously beneficial and efficient activities as preventive and primary care. In all cases decisions would need to made about what (and even who) should and should not be included in a comprehensive benefits package. But, taken as a whole, a healthcare system that fails to take into account the facts about people's lives that can contribute to such gross disparities in outcome as illustrated by the cases of Ms. Smith and Ms. Jones is only taking half-hearted measures in its purported concern for the health of a population. The healthcare system in the United States as it exists has for years been faulted for emphasizing treatment rather than prevention of illness. And while the latter can (and does) include such well-known targets as universal childhood vaccinations and good and early dental care, we should not fail to recognize the more global—perhaps mundane—contributors to poor health as represented by the preceding cases and made clear in the WHO documents. How we judge eligibility for benefits, and particularly whether and how we hold people responsible or culpable for their health conditions, can have a major impact on the manner in which cutoffs are applied.

The assessment of fault or desert is common when we appraise whether an individual merits our concern and even more so if we also have to decide whether they should receive resources to which we might be required to contribute a portion. If they are believed to have brought calamity on themselves by their own imprudent choices—irrespective if this is actually true or not—we tend to have less empathy when they suffer the consequences. Many people can take a superior view and condemn such choices as a product of moral will or a personal failing, in which they abandon the sufferer to whatever fate his actions brought about. But should this sentiment affect access to healthcare services? Or is bad (or good) luck more a matter of happenstance and not completely attributable to the supposedly free choices that one makes?

LUCK

Luck comes in all forms; good luck, bad luck, hard times, good times. No matter what its appearance or course, it is often charged to some kind of accident or unexpected, perhaps unpredicted but hoped for (in the case of a good outcome) result. No one wants or looks for misfortune. When the cards get dealt, we wish for a royal flush not a "WHIP" (worst hand in poker).[16] Frequently, it seems to be almost a fluke, a matter of chance. But many people also attribute their good luck and fortune to their own personal hard work, dedication, perseverance, perspicacity, native intelligence (and the wherewithal to use it well), wisdom, and more. Those of a more religious inclination may also favor a heavenly explanation, perhaps associating their favorable lot to virtuous living according to divine law and ritual. But some believe that their prosperity is not really due to luck, but instead is earned, and hence the fruits of their labors are deserved. Conversely, these same people might also assign responsibility to the same personal qualities (and flaws) for how the lives of those less blessed with such natural and acquired endowments turned out. If good futures belong to those who merit them, then so should the bad for those who don't, or so some may believe. But how responsible are we as individuals for the events that happen to us throughout our lives that contribute to our well-being? Is the wealthy CEO, so often touted as a paragon of capitalistic success, totally accountable for all of the complex series of circumstances that culminated in her rise to the top (as is so frequently heralded to be the case, especially by their fellow captains of industry)? And is this personal power over one's fate similar for the impoverished, mentally ill man who is addicted to alcohol, which has led to chronic unemployment, cirrhosis, and now liver failure?

So far, I have discussed how social and other features of people's lives (such as environmental factors like avoidable pollution that can be deliberately or selectively concentrated in some geographic locations rather than others) can lead to preventable negative effects on health and how the mechanisms of healthcare resource distribution (cutoffs and their rules of application) can produce unintended harms. I have also suggested that a system of comprehensive, generous, and universal healthcare insurance benefits could serve to mitigate (or at least not exacerbate) some—if not many—existing health inequities. I have viewed these facets of peoples' lives as external to themselves; events and conditions over which they may have little to no control and that they are often powerless to alter. This is especially true for the genuinely downtrodden and disadvantaged, such as children born into dire poverty or women living in cultures with a long and ingrained history of gender subjugation and prejudice. Now I wish to briefly contrast other sorts of what we might call "accidents of circumstance," such as being born with a gene that predisposes one to develop a certain terrible disease—like an abnormal BRCA1 gene and ovarian and breast cancer or a mutated huntingtin gene and Huntington's chorea/disease—and those misfortunes that could arguably be thought to be attributable in whole or part to our own actions. In the latter case, one might think of the person with cirrhosis of the liver due to his chronic abuse of alcohol. Ronald Dworkin memorably referred to these two by no means easily distinguishable and dichotomous states of affairs as *brute* and *option luck*:

> I ... distinguish ... between two kinds of luck. Option luck is a matter of how deliberate and calculated gambles turn out—whether someone gains or loses through accepting an isolated risk he or she should have anticipated and might have declined. Brute luck is a matter of how risks fall out that are not in that sense deliberate gambles. If I buy a stock on the exchange that rises, then my option luck is good. If I am hit by a falling meteorite whose course could not have been predicted, then my bad luck is brute (even though I could have moved just before it struck if I had any reason to know where it would strike). Obviously the difference between these two forms of luck can be represented as a matter of degree, and we may be uncertain how to describe a particular piece of bad luck. If someone develops cancer in the course of a normal life, and there is no particular decision to which we can point as a gamble risking the disease, then we will say that he has suffered brute bad luck. But if he smoked cigarettes heavily then we may prefer to say that he took an unsuccessful gamble.[17]

Essentially, this dyadic view somewhat simplistically divides the world of human activity into two seemingly mutually exclusive camps: there are those events that result from one's natural endowments (or lack of them), such as some biological factors like innate cognitive abilities, height, good looks, perhaps physical strength. Then there is the luck that one generates for oneself by virtue of the choices one makes and the preferences one espouses. Of course, this unvarnished dualistic view is nonsensical as a description of real life. For cognitive ability to be properly and fully manifest requires good nutrition, education, social adaptation, and nurturing (at a minimum); for people to look their best and grow to the full height that their genes permit also demands decent food, vitamins, exercise, and more. Likewise, it would be absurd to believe that most alcoholics start drinking to excess as a conscious choice, fully informed of the risks to their current and future lives and health. Similarly, the 14-year-old boy who becomes addicted to nicotine via cigarette smoking doubtless does not consider the risks of getting lung cancer or COPD when he's 60; moreover, the motivation to change his behavior may be externally minimized by advertising, his social milieu, and more. Thus, pure brute luck and pure option luck as explanations for what happens in people's lives is a fantasy, a philosopher's armchair argument. Teasing out sole responsibility for a person's condition in life is no easier (or plausible) than deciding the nature versus nurture problem solely in favor of one over the other. Nevertheless, many people take this view at least partially seriously (some even more so) and hold that individuals should be held accountable for both the positive and negative results of "option luck." Moreover, this belief also informs their opinions on policy options—such as for healthcare.

A major question for a healthcare program of comprehensive insurance coverage is not simply deciding what interventions and treatments should be covered (and to what extent) but what conditions merit the protection and security of such coverage. In particular, should illnesses that could plausibly be said to be caused by behaviors or lifestyles that are under the willful control of the individual be eligible for insured diagnostic and therapeutic care? Is this a reasonable consideration to determine cutoffs? If it is, what could be the downstream effects of employing it in this manner? I have argued that the most fair and reasonable method to create cutoff points should be based on clinical need, clinical efficacy, and appropriateness. For example, we now have a number of new, albeit very expensive, pharmacologic options for curing most forms of hepatitis C.[18] They thus meet both the criteria I put forth: they are both very effective and appropriate. Furthermore, people with this chronic viral infection are at increased risk of death from liver failure, so they could reasonably be said to have a valid need for treatment (as I have characterized clinical need in Chapter 3). However, a significant percentage of hepatitis C infections are acquired via contaminated needles used by intravenous substance abusers. Should these patients be eligible for this extremely potent (and costly) treatment (hypothetically) paid for by a public health insurance program and for a disease they (arguably) brought on themselves?

Out of Dworkin's initial proposal evolved the concept of what has been termed "luck egalitarianism."[19] There are a number of different versions that vary in some details, so I am highlighting the main points of convergence. In this account, in general, it is believed that people who are moral agents and who live under conditions in which they are free to exercise choices in their lives in a relatively unfettered manner are responsible for the states of affairs that result from those choices. They are responsible for what happens to both themselves and others. According to this view I, *by right*, earn more as a university professor and physician than the person who cleans my office every morning, because I chose to go to college and then medical and graduate school, and she decided to drop out of high school and could only get her cleaning job. On the egalitarian part of this approach, because the inequality in income and welfare between the two of us was due to option luck or to choices under our control, it is just. If, on the other hand, she took this job because of a congenital intellectual disability (or some other feature about herself that she had no power to alter), then one could plausibly maintain that the inequality was due to brute luck, unjust, and therefore may be (or should be) amenable to redress. How far the state should go toward minimizing inequalities of the latter sort is debatable. Many luck egalitarians, committed to some version of equality, would also support the view that fair or unfair inequalities should only be judged after some minimum, but adequate, level of subsistence funding for food, housing, clothing, education, and (yes) healthcare were provided. Even the most strident of luck egalitarians would probably grant this.[20] Indeed, people whose misery can be reasonably attributed to their poor, ill-advised—possibly even stupid—choices should be saved (by others presumably more fortunate) from the worst effects of the results of their decisions (but not all of them). For the same reasons that we do not permit people who are destitute and cannot afford to pay the fees to die of their acute illnesses, injuries, and so on in the emergency rooms around the country, we should acknowledge and grant the psychological frailties to which we are all susceptible.

But if we accept that we do have some amount of self-control, should personal health choices, such as self-destructive (or harming) behaviors like smoking, drinking, substance abuse, and obesity be considered during the distribution of healthcare costs? How responsible (or blamed) should people be held for the consequences? Is having heart disease or lung cancer a suitable and sufficient enough "punishment" for having smoked cigarettes? Or must it also include bearing the full financial costs? Is it fair for others in society (presumably the nonsmokers) to shoulder the huge dollar burden caused by these option luck diseases? While our first intuitive impulse might be to hold accountable those people who engage in behaviors that are well-established to have deleterious effects on individual health, such as cigarette smoking and various kinds of substance abuse (alcohol being the most common), careful reflection might lead us to a somewhat different conclusion for several reasons. First, who among us is not "guilty" of some habit that is not good for us, whether it is over-indulgence in fatty (and delicious) foods or not getting enough sleep, that we should leap to condemn others for their weaknesses? Second, while it is true that some habits may be more harmful than others, we all are susceptible to their attractions (at least initially), and it might be both more beneficial and forgiving to offer help rather than censure, generosity rather than parsimony. Moreover, as a society, we permit commercial enterprises to make the things that may not be good for us as appealing as possible; even such products as cigarettes frequently draw people in by the sometimes not-so-subtle allure of danger and even sexiness. For many people, this advertising can be extraordinarily seductive and irresistible, so it would be difficult to hold people completely responsible if the ads we allow (even encourage) are successful in their goals. So it is by no means clear that people who fall prey to the wiles of social pressure and other communal external influences can be held completely responsible when they respond in the manner intended by those who are purveying these (harmful) wares.[21] At the same time, it may be reasonable to consider what might be activities that are much more plausibly construed as completely voluntary, such as many sports endeavors that can involve significant risk. Should society pay for the injuries of daredevil skiers or mountain climbers or racecar drivers? While I suppose that some may construe the "need for speed" experienced by many of these people as an addiction akin to compulsive gambling or even the highs sought by drug addicts, there appears to be a difference in degree, if not kind.[22] In addition, as I pointed out earlier, it is interesting to note that, currently, it is common for commercial insurance policies (and Medicare) to pay for treatment for adverse side effects or complications arising from uncovered services (such as elective cosmetic surgery). Therefore, in some sense, we may be expressing an amount of greater forgiveness and magnanimity than is sometimes publicly declaimed.

Finally, there are strategies to better apportion the costs of caring for the deadly side effects of dangerous habits and activities: targeted taxes. Increasing the price at the point of purchase by a combination of production and end-user taxes has certainly been demonstrated to decrease consumption.[23] If the money raised was also specifically earmarked or dedicated by law for use in supporting the healthcare of those people afflicted with disease (or injuries) related to the use of the product or engagement in the activity, it could go a long way toward offsetting the burdens on the rest of society and diminish the power of the (option) luck egalitarian argument.[24]

Richard Arneson, a proponent of a perhaps more charitable (and forgiving) version of luck egalitarianism points to what he calls the "control principle" as a feature of personal responsibility that may be used to judge what are and are not just deserts.[25] As with others who have examined what it means to have a free choice, he seems to view situations in which there are possibilities for reasonably autonomous action on the part of an individual (in which the path taken is one that is decided on, an alternate that was not a Hobson's choice) as those in which his principle would hold. In other words, one could have chosen otherwise—one could decide not to start cigarette smoking, one could have decided not to eat excessively and hence develop obesity-related diabetes, etc.—when presented with the various options. Of course, this view assumes that such choices are made free of the strong psychological and biological influences that either overtly or covertly to move us toward one option versus another. As the volumes of formerly secret tobacco company documents have demonstrated when revealed during the Tobacco Master Settlement case, manipulation of both kinds of desires and wants by manufacturers of various products can obscure the meaning of freely made choices.[26]

Holding people responsible for activities or behaviors that are reasonably believed to be causal contributors to bad health when they are complications of the social determinants of health would seem to induce a facet of double jeopardy. In some ways, this would be ignoring the brute luck argument and blaming people for their health misfortune as well as for the unfortunate circumstances that predisposed them to become sick in the first place. Rationing by creating cutoffs for service denial on the basis of "self-induced" illness would be morally unconscionable as a failure to offer comfort and help to the suffering when it is in our power to do so (to do otherwise would simply be mean-spirited) and would compound the already impoverished welfare of this population of people. Moreover, our ability to draw causal connections for certain lifestyles and the fate of an individual patient—for example, "obesity absolutely caused her heart attack"—is highly questionable and thus open to criticism as a criterion to assign responsibility with consequences of such a serious nature.[27] Finally, it is necessary to clarify that I am not implying that people do not make choices, both good and bad, in their lives. But it would be a gross misunderstanding of both my position and the reality that I believe it reflects to misconstrue my argument as one that supports a hardline sort of determinism in human behavior. We are not completely controlled by our genes, our environment, and social situation nor, as some might hold, by some external supernatural forces over which we have no control. Life is considerably more complicated than that. How our preferences come about and how they are expressed (and which ones are expressed) is both complex, open to considerable debate, and the subject of significant (and current and historical) scientific (and philosophical) investigation. Let it simply be said that the causes that contribute to what we decide to do and how and when we decide to do it are unsettled. And since our knowledge is in such an unresolved state, it seems most reasonable to be cautious.

One additional point deserves mention. Broadly assigning blame or responsibility entails judging people for the willfulness of their actions. We do this readily (albeit imperfectly) in the criminal justice system, and it is this imperfection that can be instructive. As can be easily observed from the arbitrary and seemingly capricious application of death penalty sentences (and completed executions) in the United States, meaningless superficial characteristics such as skin color and other features of "brute luck," such as lack of education and intellectual disability, are too often employed to hold some people more accountable for their actions than others.[28] Furthermore, we have a historically nasty habit of assigning stereotypical negative behaviors to racial and ethnic groups that are disfavored, such as African Americans, Latinos, and others.[29] Both social successes and failures are attributed to a confusing amalgam of ingrained and willful talents, propensities, and actions.[30]

There is also a lamentable streak of oft-expressed contempt for those less fortunate by those who enjoy more of the advantages that society has to offer. While this is not frequently voiced for those suffering from diseases or injury, it is not uncommonly observed for the poor. How else to explain the onerous obstacles that the unemployed, underemployed, and other impoverished individuals are made to overcome to simply claim some form of state-supplied welfare benefits (contributed by their fellow citizens)? How else to explain the resistance to expand Medicaid to all those people at the margins between the really poor and those eligible for subsidized health insurance through the Affordable Care Act? These expressions of scorn in many ways are pure luck egalitarianism at its most extreme.[31]

What I am suggesting is that we should place the emphasis on helping people make better choices (for their health) but not punish them for their failings if preventative measures are not completely successful. Unless we make tobacco products illegal, we should not refuse to treat or punish people by not paying for treatment of their tobacco-related illnesses such as lung cancer, COPD, emphysema, and the like. Similarly, we should put great efforts into education about the dangers of certain kinds of foods and poor diets, as well as expending funds to support physical education programs, especially for populations at great risk for obesity. But we should not totally blame and shame people for being fat along with the conditions that commonly accompany obesity; it is bad enough that these individuals suffer from shortness of breath, a decreased lifespan, diabetes, and many other ills without having to be subjected to the indignity of being pilloried for their assumed poor self-control and self-destructive choices. It also bears noting that there are wealthy smokers, alcoholics, and obese people as well as poor ones.[32] One of the consequences of a too literal interpretation of luck egalitarianism when combined with social stereotypes based on morally irrelevant characteristics (especially those that are immutable) would be to surrender to impulses to define people not as individuals but as members of a group. In this artless manner, a former smoker who mustered the fortitude (and "luck") to successfully quit but who had the misfortune to develop lung cancer many years later would be lumped in with those who continued their habit and suffered similar consequences. Attempting to distinguish degrees of "guilt" in cases such as this, and thus degrees of responsibility for the illnesses (and their costs) that result, would seem to be both a fruitless task and one rife with moral uncertainty. It would be better to be magnanimous and charitable.

Finally, I wish to bring up the situations of those who may epitomize examples of "brute (almost always bad) luck": the congenitally disabled or those whose disability (one or more) is acquired by injury or as a sequela to an illness, either past or ongoing. In the United States, discriminatory practices affecting the physically and/or cognitively disabled in accommodations, hiring and employment, and healthcare administration (among others) are prohibited by law due to the American with Disabilities Act of 1990.[33] Even so, there can be significant discretion left up to physicians and other healthcare providers, as well as systemic regulations that could be interpreted with sufficient leeway, to adversely affect those with otherwise qualifying disabilities. In this way, cutoffs by themselves or the manner in which they are applied could lead to avoidable negative outcomes for at least some people who would otherwise not be injured in this manner. The effect would then be to not only discriminate but to amplify the physical and emotional ramifications of the original disability. An example might help illustrate this concern.

Trisomy 18 is a devastating congenital disorder in which babies are born with three copies of the 18th chromosome rather than the normal two.[34] These patients can be full-term or born prematurely and have numerous characteristic skeletal and other abnormalities, including significant congenital heart disease that may be life-threatening unless surgically corrected. A hallmark of this condition is that all patients have considerable, frequently profound, intellectual deficits and, if they live, will require life-long custodial care. Many pediatricians have long considered this disorder to be "fatal," even when interventions that could prolong or even preserve life were available. It is fair to say that it was believed that these children would lead lives that were so limited that to therapeutically intervene would be clinically contra-indicated.[35] Indeed, there are some surgeons (for example) who have refused to oper-ate on these babies because of their beliefs about the futility of doing so. Therefore, most of these babies have died soon after birth while receiving only palliative care. However, the views on this condition (and another severe congenital chromosomal abnormality, Trisomy 13) are evolving, and some parents are beginning to insist upon all treatment that could save the patient's live. This altered outlook has resulted in small numbers of these patients living into their teens and even early 20s, albeit with profound disabilities and often requiring intensive and repeated medical and surgi-cal procedures.[36] While these patients may have severe cognitive deficiencies, they are still conscious and capable of experiencing suffering and, some would suggest, pleasure. While there is little doubt that some of the anatomic malformations with which these children are afflicted can be ameliorated by corrective (occasionally pal-liative) surgery, thus enabling them to even leave the hospital and go home with their families, there are significant costs, not the least of which are financial.[37] Would the minority of parents of these children who wish to have them treated and their lives saved have the "right" to insist that this be done in a public, universal healthcare sys-tem in which cutoffs (and hence payment) would be based on need, appropriateness, and efficacy, as I described in Chapters 3 and 4? Would such cutoffs adversely affect these patients? If they were not eligible for anything other than palliative, "comfort care" would this represent an unwarranted, unjust form of discrimination against the disabled? I raise these questions to illustrate the dilemmas provoked by these situations (and dependent to some extent on the advance of technology). Clearly, how we decide what qualifies as a valid medical need and what would be appropriate and effective interventions to cover in circumstances such as these would require careful thought and consideration. My suspicion is that the requirement to include some lay representation on the RAM-like committees charged with determining cutoffs would soften the possibly harsh evaluation and scrutiny of experts whose responsi-bility would be to consider evidence above all, and this would lead to greater toler-ance and compassion for patient and surrogate needs.

WHO DECIDES?

In a series of essays, David Mechanic has persuasively argued that the best way to ration health care resources is to leave significant discretionary decision-making allocation power to individual physicians who are of course trained in the art of interpreting the continuous presence of uncertainty and clinical nuance in patient care and thereby know best what is most appropriate for each patient.[38] There is little question that one's physician, with whom one has developed a close relationship, is best situated to negotiate what may be a reasonable range of options for diagnosis and therapy. However, unfettered power to order whatever tests she likes in situations hallmarked not only with uncertainty but also with a large asymmetry of information and interpretive acumen bestows on doctors the potential to be enticed by a wide variety of other allegiances that, although subtle or even unconscious, are nonetheless powerful. These include financial attractions, such as those that are widespread and pervasive in fee for service reimbursement systems, but also those like alliances with pharmaceutical and medical device manufacturers, bonuses, pay-for-performance, and other salary-at-risk payment schemes. But there are also more insidious influences that can affect what a doctor does and the sorts of decisions he makes with and for his patients, such as implicit and explicit bias on the basis of ethnicity, racial characterization, gender, sexual orientation, and the like, all of which have been demonstrated to contribute to disparities in healthcare delivery and patient outcomes.[39]

Doctors are, of course, susceptible to the same biases and prejudices as everyone else, and they not infrequently consciously or unconsciously succumb to these forces in judging the appropriateness of care for an individual patient (or even a class of patients). The evolution in how doctors in the United States are employed and the kinds of practice environments in which they find themselves may contribute to some decrease in the variability of clinical care delivery and outcomes, but the verdict is still out.[40] While more consistent standards of care and a decrease in practice variation may be thought to be a good thing, it depends on which features are brought into uniformity, and this in turn may be contingent on the incentives built into the organization(s) to which physicians bear allegiance. If the emphasis for salary bonuses, rewards, and the like is misplaced, all or some patient care could suffer.

A major argument against casting physicians in the role of gatekeepers of the sort responsible for allocation of resources within a fixed budget—similar to that intended during the short-lived infatuation with full-scale HMOs in the 1990s—was the corrosive effect it had on the doctor–patient relationship by introducing a reasonably explicit conflict-of-interest into each encounter. The suspicion that one's physician had dual loyalties and that denial of a specific service may not have been done for legitimate reasons—as opposed to a potentially personally remunerative motivation on the doctor's part—introduces a particularly damaging element into the ideal, trusting connection of the clinical encounter. Of course, in the fee-for-service environment, doctors have the opposite incentive to do more rather than to do less, but people seem to be susceptible to the allure of doing something rather than nothing as indicative of more caring rather than less, even though the negative effects of inappropriate use (in both ways) may be similar. However, it is conceivable that simply altering the mechanisms and the basis by which physicians are paid—for example, switching to a salary system with bonuses paid for certain forms of good practice or health outcomes—could go a significant way toward solving this problem.[41] Nevertheless, while this approach may remove one form of self-promoting arbitrary use of medical services, not all sources of bias are minimized.

The formal, perhaps antiquated, and nostalgic view of physicians as tireless and single-minded advocates for their patients' best interests, pursued without heed to other considerations, including in the myth family or personal life, is just that: a myth. Of course, as patients, we would like our doctors to be our indefatigable champions, no matter what, and there is little question that this is a role that doctors cherish, at least in theory. But the truth is more complex, and physicians have had to heed an increasing number of masters other than the patient's interests, for many years. Whether it is an ever-growing body of governmental and regulatory body rules or the convoluted and constantly changing Gordian knot of insurance company mandates, protocols, and guidelines, doctors are bound not only by their oath to further the welfare of their patients but also to extraneous duties that restrict that unwavering advocacy.[42] Even so, doctors may so strongly feel the impulse to help their patients as they see best that they are willing to bend the rules and even mislead, misrepresent, or even outright lie to insurance companies (for example) to get approval for some procedure or test.[43] How obvious this is to patients may influence the trust they place in their physicians to give their interests primary consideration.

The practice of medicine is messy by its very nature—due to inherent uncertainty and the always-limited knowledge available to the individual clinician and to the field in general. What is absolutely correct today may be wrong tomorrow. Furthermore, people are infinitely variable in the manner in which they and their bodies react to disease and disorder in a complex and unpredictable amalgam of distinctive personality, social context, and biology. Finally, biomedical research has discovered and successfully combated many of the common causes of illness and early death (at least in the more developed world): sanitation, early childhood infections (vaccination), clean water, antibiotics, and so on. Having conquered the "easy" and cheap stuff, medical science is now tackling the scourge of chronic illness, those disorders that take their cumulative toll on the middle-aged and older, such as atherosclerosis, type 2 diabetes, and cancer. These conditions are startling in their pathobiological complexity and demand equally complex—and expensive—solutions. Uncertainty, messiness, and complexity are the wellspring of cost. Modern, technologically advanced healthcare is unavoidably pricey. The question for luck egalitarians (as it is for me in my wider consideration and scope) is what justice requires as we create a new health system and the rules governing its application and implementation. We desire a program that is fair (as I have defined it).[44] Can that mandate accommodate those foibles and faults of peoples' lives that they will fully engage in and that produce ill health? Do they have valid claims on the health system and its funds, which are derived from public taxation? Hardline luck egalitarians might say "no." Or are our sympathies, money, and resources only extended to the prudent? I would argue for generosity both in spirit and in fact, similar to the generosity I have suggested for the system as a whole in terms of finances. Not only is no man in island but few—perhaps none—are health and lifestyle "saints" either.

Nevertheless, basing a rationing cutoff system on clinical needs and evidence-based appropriateness—even one that is generous and comprehensive—will place demands on physicians to justify what they wish to do for their patients. Undoubtedly, there will be situations when the two are at odds, with the system saying "no" and the doctor (presumably with the acquiescence or knowledge of the patient) saying "yes." As I suggested in Chapter 3 and elsewhere, a necessary adjunct to such a method of allocating resources is that there be a workable, timely, and not paralyzing mechanism of appealing decisions.[45] If this mechanism were in place and was known to function reasonably well, the impetus for doctors to evade the rules (even if for the noble purpose of advancing what they believed to be their patient's interests), would be minimized, although unlikely to be eliminated. But doctors should not retain the unlimited ability to do anything that in their judgment was for the good of the patient. This has led to much abuse by both less-than-scrupulous physicians and those whose dedication was not questioned but whose abilities might be less than optimal. Similarly, as mentioned earlier, doctors are also susceptible to the same hidden and overt biases that plague the rest of society, notwithstanding their oaths to ignore the pull of these prejudices. This can lead them to exhibit behaviors in which they advocate less for some patients than for others, a position that is just as unjustifiable as its opposite. While an appeals system may not offer a complete panacea for this problem, if it were open to challenges by patients as well as doctors, appeals may provide some relief.

CONCLUSION

Some people are "luckier" than others. For some fortunate few, everything seems to go their way; others must struggle for all they get, while still others are plagued by misfortune their entire lives. Sometimes this is due to the circumstances into which they were born, such as poverty, their genetic endowment (for better or for worse), where they were born (Beverly Hills vs. South Central Los Angeles), and, to a great extent, the mood of the day with respect to public and governmental policies—local, state, and federal—on extending help to those in need. It is a dangerous myth to believe that both success and failure in life are earned solely by the individual and not contextual. The belief that one's welfare and well-being is entirely a result of the decisions that one makes and not largely due to the circumstances in which one finds oneself may be one commonly held among those who have been fortunate in life's "lottery." But such a view is also all too frequently employed to justify a stern and reproachful attitude to those less prosperous, one that seeks to hold people accountable in a retributive way for the vicissitudes that afflict their lives. Presumably, their misery is earned in much the same manner as others' happiness.

Consider Fred, a 55-year-old man who has been drinking heavily since his later teen years and has now developed ethanol-induced cirrhosis of the liver with impending hepatic failure. Should he be eligible for a liver transplant? Many, perhaps most people, who are in this situation will die from their disease both because they can't (won't) stop drinking and due to the simple fact that there is a vast undersupply of donor organs. The latter fact is persistent despite the best efforts of the transplant community to improve donor rates; there are simply more patients than there are available organs. One way to lower the mismatch would be to *ex ante* eliminate from consideration certain entire populations of people—such as, in this case, Fred—because there is little doubt that he "caused" his liver disease from his drinking. However, transplant professionals and communities surveyed in both the United States and elsewhere have not taken this step despite what it could mean to the other, nonalcoholic patients waiting for organs.[46] Rather, they have elected to permit these patients to be eligible for transplants with the stipulation that they successfully stop drinking (usually defined as verifiable sobriety for at least 6 months). Indeed, this approach results in about a quarter of all transplants being performed in now sober former alcohol abusers.[47]

Should a compassionate and generous healthcare system exact retribution for those individual failings and foibles of people that may result in deleterious effects on their health? In other words, should a healthcare system make rules that result in retributive justice or distributive justice? The former favors punishment—although many people would frame it as a matter of holding people accountable for their willful actions—while the latter focuses on what fair and reasonable allocation of resources should be, with an emphasis on what people are owed as human beings rather than what they may deserve as individuals. The former bears a closer resemblance to the criminal justice system and the latter to various forms of social welfare programs instituted in liberal democracies. And, certainly, in many of the domains of social life we do indeed hold people accountable for the results of their actions:

> Practices of holding people responsible for their choices and actions in various ways might be justified for their instrumental or their intrinsic value (or both). One holds people responsible for choices and actions by attaching positive or negative sanctions to their outcomes. . . . Responsibility practices that are well designed can induce people to alter their behavior in ways that lead to desirable consequences. The prospect of gaining such consequences can serve as instrumental justification for establishing or sustaining the practices.[48]

Arneson goes on to reasonably conclude that "We can consider tinkering with responsibility practices at the margin, but the idea that instrumental justifications for responsibility practices might fail in some wholesale way is a nonstarter," meaning that social interactions and the essence of cooperative living is, in many senses, personal (and group) accountability. But should this view, especially with its implications for what we (society) should do to people or in response to those whose actions harm themselves and others be the norm? In the case of healthcare, the harm to others may often be in terms of the financial implications of caring for (and paying for) the results of imprudent activities by others. So, is it good policy and/or just to structure the kinds and amounts of healthcare services that would be available (and to whom) according to some form of value judgments based on the degree to which individual patients (or group of patients) can be reasonably considered to be responsible for the (medical) plight in which they find themselves? Should individual worthiness or desert, based on some arbitrary calculus of personal accountability for the circumstances in which one finds oneself, be a decisive factor in determining who gets what; can it be a justifiable way of constructing cutoffs? I think not.

One might argue that holding people accountable—or "punishing" them for their ill-advised and self-detrimental health behaviors in addition to whatever suffering and torment they undergo attributable to being sick—could serve as either a deterrent or incentive to others to mend their ways and stop indulging in junk food, smoking, and drinking to excess. This is the "instrumental" value to which Arneson refers. In addition, cutting off access to a wide variety of medical interventions specific to say, people with COPD due to cigarettes or HIV due to intravenous drug use, could potentially save an enormous amount of money (especially if we also included diabetes due to obesity along with the comorbid conditions that frequently result, such as renal failure requiring dialysis). And, after all, one of the reasons for healthcare reform of any sort is financial. Aside from the practical implications of an affirmative answer to this question, how does one systematize and organizationally approach adjudicating these sorts of matters, especially in "borderline" cases? There are both good moral and practical reasons not to do it.[49]

First, the pain and anguish associated with "self-imposed" health conditions cannot be underestimated. To abandon these people entirely to their fates simply because we have judged them to be culpable for their illnesses is not only callous, but also cruel. Even if we decided that we would provide effective palliative care for symptom relief, not to offer hemodialysis to someone in renal failure due to obesity-related type 2 diabetes *when we can afford it* and give them the opportunity to live seems inhumane and certainly disavows a cardinal tenet of medicine and nursing.[50] Second, we have no good and reliable methods for judging the degree of personal responsibility individuals may have for their conditions (even if we could operationalize such hypothetical methods). Assigning exclusive "blame" for a patient's heart disease that is most likely related to his poorly controlled hypertension ignores the many other factors that can contribute to the development of this problem. These could include genetic predisposition, including epigenetic inputs,[51] psychological and environmental influences, social structure, and more. Parsing out what percentage of a disease (especially one as complex as heart failure) is due to a "failure of personal will" (or "option luck" as Dworkin would call it) is a Sisyphean task that is inherently flawed and completely vulnerable to exploitation and arbitrary administration. Finally, while it is clear that there are some individuals who eat well, refrain from excessive intake of anything, exercise regularly, and live long and healthy lives, they are relatively uncommon. Most people, especially in America, are not so abstemious.[52] We may all be guilty in one or more ways, but to hold us accountable after the fact and punish us for our sins, rather than attempting to prevent or minimize the sins beforehand seems both mean and unfair.[53]

What I am suggesting is that a fair, reasonable, and generous healthcare system employs cutoffs that hew to these standards. The ones that meet these criteria the best, in my view, are those that I argued for previously (Chapter 3) in which the primary boundaries should be defined by clinical appropriateness and efficacy. However, as the topics in this chapter make clear, numerous factors contribute to the sorts of medical conditions that people have, how severe and complex, and how well they may respond to treatment. While one's genes undoubtedly contribute some causal percentage to the origins, development, and expression of illness, except in some extreme cases (e.g., Huntington's disease, as an example of a 100% penetrant, autosomal dominant, and genetically determined disorder), virtually all other diseases (liberally defined) owe most of their causes to environmental factors and triggers. Without question, some of those extracorporeal factors are brought about by personal choices of one sort or another and with varying degrees of willful, informed purposefulness. But others—and speaking globally, perhaps for most people worldwide—result from either happenstance or chance or by accidents of social birth: the wrong parents, an ill-favored neighborhood, dysfunctional governmental institutions, and the like. Given the complex entanglement of all these elements, it would seem foolhardy to attempt to assign *sole* responsibility most of the time to one, single cause. Not that this shouldn't be attempted in some cases; it would certainly would be reasonable—if not morally necessary—to search for the root causes and those responsible for say, toxic, disease-producing industrial chemicals that pollute a poor community. However, for the vast majority, it seems churlish and overly ethically fastidious to make individuals wholly responsible for their potentially preventable illnesses, especially *after the fact*. What is much more sensible, practical, fair, and compassionate is to devote efforts to prevent the occurrence of avoidable diseases (smoking prevention, drug treatments, alcohol moderation programs, etc.) as well as treat with generosity those who only show that they are human.

7

CONCLUSIONS

In my first book, I argued that the only plausible way to restrain healthcare costs or to limit their interminable rise was to impose some form of rationing by which *ex ante* decisions were made to restrict access to some kinds of healthcare interventions.[1] I pointed out the well-understood (by some) but not particularly well-known (by many) observation that the United States already engages in a number of different systems of both explicit and implicit rationing, the most obvious and trenchant of which is on the basis of a patient's ability to pay. Rich people can have pretty much whatever they like, those who work for companies that provide excellent health insurance as a fringe benefit and who can afford the various co-pays, deductibles, and the like also do well, and everyone else must muddle through the best they can. Even Medicare has defined caps and only covers a percentage (albeit a large one) of the total costs of one's health-care. This is not to say that the wealthy and well-insured get better care; just more of it (although the converse is definitely true: poor people get worse, less of it care and do less well for a variety of reasons, including their impoverishment).

Ronald Reagan was colloquially known as the "great communicator," presumably because of his Hollywood-honed rhetorical and speaking skills. However, it should also be recalled that he was the "great rationer" as well because it was under his watch that one of the most far-reaching and effective measures to control burgeoning hospital costs was put in place. This was the system, inaugurated by Medicare in the early 1980s, of diagnosis-related groups (DRGs) that lumped patients into distinct clinical aggregates for purposes of prospective payment for their hospital stays.[2] Hospitals were instantly provided with the negative incentive to cut costs by a variety of means, one of the most notorious (and perhaps ill-conceived) of which was the initiative to discharge women who had an uncomplicated delivery relatively shortly after giving birth.[3] Other money-based implicit rationing strategies followed, ranging from combating moral hazard with co-insurance and increasing the cost-burden to the insured to structurally limiting the drugs on a pharmacy benefits manager formulary. Of course, no one calls these actions "rationing"; rather, they are known as "cost control stratagems" or "cost savings," but rationing they most certainly are. However, we also have examples of overt, explicit rationing that are accepted, even admired, for how they have been developed and implemented.

The most notable of these is that which allocates solid organs for transplantation. Even with all of its flaws—and there are many—the transplant system in the United States is devoted to fairness and managing the inevitable tension that exists between equity and efficiency, all while attempting to maintain the confidence of the public, both those who utilize the program as potential recipients and those whose organs must be donated in order for the entire apparatus to function.[4] Indeed, it is remarkable how little controversy there is about how organs are distributed; the people who one might imagine would have the most to complain about the lack of sufficient organs for all and the rules of allocation—those who fail to get transplanted and then die from organ failure—rarely do so. Even though the system can be gamed by those who are savvy (and frequently wealthy) enough to do so, there is a sincere and concerted effort on the part of the dedicated people who run the program to make it as fair and as transparent as possible. Hence, there are always reviews and tweaks being made in attempts to improve the process. I used this, and a couple of other examples, to support my argument that rationing could be accomplished in the United States if it were done fairly and equitably. But one might say that organs are a unique, life-saving, severely limited resource; how could we apply these lessons to the entire healthcare system?

In 1910, Abraham Flexner published his report, *Medical Education in the United States and Canada*. It was a combination of a factually detailed and documented muckraking exposé of the multitude of mechanisms by which people aspiring to become doctors could do so and the lack of educational consistency or quality in the degree and certificate granting programs that enabled them to attain their goals. He included a laudatory description of what he believed to be the proper way forward.[5] He upheld the curriculum and professionalism of the faculty at the relatively young Johns Hopkins University School of Medicine as the ideal for a new era of scientific medicine that demanded the "best and the brightest" in its applicants and expected them to continue their education throughout their lives.[6] By extolling the virtues epitomized by the Hopkins faculty—whose ranks included the medical luminaries William Osler, William Welch, and William Halstead—he was also heralding the advent of evidence-based medicine, both the acquisition of data and its proper use. At the same time, he was acknowledging a fact that was becoming more obvious by the day in the early part of the 20th century: there was a clear difference between the harm that poorly educated physicians and quacks could do to patients and the increasing amount of good that properly trained doctors could offer the sick and suffering. Hospitals were transformed from warehouses for the poor and destitute with nowhere else to go to places where sick people went to be healed.[7] Recognizing that the fruits of medical research were both tangible and profitable, the federal government and pharmaceutical companies, especially during and after World War II, made biomedical research a national priority and generously funded this enterprise. The 20th century truly became the era of beneficial medicine. Not only could broad public health measures like proper sanitation and adequate nutrition improve the health of a country's citizens, but healthcare, both preventative and therapeutic, could contribute to well-being, productivity, and longevity.

Not surprisingly, all of the new things that doctors could do were expensive and potentially unlimited. They also (mostly) needed to be done in specialized facilities requiring unique equipment and supportive resources. Recognizing that hospitals (and their affiliated clinics) were no longer simply custodial establishments (as well as classrooms for medical students to practice their skills before they entered private practice to care for paying patients) and were poorly distributed throughout the country, Congress enacted the Hospital Survey and Construction Act of 1946 (commonly known as Hill-Burton) that led to an explosion of hospital building.[8] Coincident with the expansion of hospitals (and hence the need for more doctors and nurses) the National Institute(s) of Health, which had its origins in 1897, also experienced massive growth, especially with the passage of the Public Health Service Act of 1944 and the beginning of large annual infusions of money into biomedical research.[9] The discoveries came rapidly, justifying the allocation of public funds. From only sulfanilamide and penicillin at the end of World War II, there was an explosion of antibiotic drug discovery and development. The polio vaccine, introduced in the 1950s, heralded a new era of immunizations against common and feared childhood diseases. "Breakthroughs" were regularly and frequently announced in the newspapers, and the public came to expect regular results. Even cancer seemed to be conquerable, as when President Nixon created the War on Cancer and Vincent DeVita and his colleagues at the National Cancer Institute announced a drug cure for advanced Hodgkin's disease, heretofore a death sentence for anyone with this diagnosis.[10]

Who should benefit from the many advances and clear-cut good that was being regularly accomplished by medical scientists? And how should it all be paid for? Unfortunately, we have still not resolved these important questions, even though we continue to pour money into developing more and more (and sometimes even better) treatments and diagnostics, all the while raising expectations of what can be done for every ill of modern day America (including creating novel "diseases" or conditions to generate new markets for health services and products).[11] Even though the method(s) for delivering healthcare in the United States lack coordination, range from nonexistent to deluxe, from utilizing the emergency room for primary care to concierge boutique doctor-at-your-beck-and-call practices, it is a fragmented patchwork that is the most expensive and least efficient among developed countries. While we may argue incessantly about how to "fix" American healthcare (although some continue to believe we have the "best in the world"),[12] most can—and do—agree that the path we seem to be following with ever-increasing expenditures for healthcare is unsustainable.

Coincident with the post-war rise of the military-industrial complex fueled by the Cold War animus between the Soviet Union and the United States, what might be called the medical-industrial complex also experienced a massive expansion, in its case nourished first by the continuing boom in the economy and employment (along with employer-financed health insurance) and later with the expansion of social welfare programs such as Medicaid and Medicare. Piggy-backed on to the ever-productive medical research establishment (both private and government-funded), more and more patients had the ability to avail themselves of more and more drugs, devices, operations, and doctors.[13] The various sectors of the industry— insurance companies, device and drug companies, medical centers, companies to help other companies (a latest example is the electronic medical record business), and the like—were all fed by an enormous (and growing) pot of money. Healthcare had become incredibly profitable for many people (including a lot of physicians). There is an enormous amount of money to be made from sick people. Modern healthcare is a huge business. But the product that is being "sold" is not like any other product on the market today. True, it is a service. True, it utilizes equipment and disposables and requires expensive personnel and a huge infrastructure and facilities. But the "product" is of such fundamental, intrinsic importance to the lives of the people who are "purchasing" it that it must be considered qualitatively different from any other service.

It is of course possible that in modern life one could possibly choose to do without modern healthcare, and there are certainly some people who make that choice. However, the vast majority of us avail ourselves of all the potential benefits that 21st-century medicine has to offer, be it over-the-counter medications and nostrums, to seeing our doctor for aches, pains, and major illnesses. We do so because of the significant positive impact healthcare can have on our lives and well-being. Healthcare makes a major contribution to our welfare and our ability to pursue our goals and aims in life. Because of that fundamental contribution to our welfare, what is bought and sold in medicine needs to be evaluated in a qualitatively different manner from other commodities in the marketplace. Buying a stent to relieve a blockage in a coronary artery to enable one to recover from angina or a heart attack and continue to live a productive life seems substantively different from the purchase of some other "thing" that one could buy. For one, although it is true that getting the stent is elective in the sense that one could conceivably do without it, in another sense it is necessary: one *needs* it in the fundamentally important way I explored in Chapter 3. Unlike a new pair of shoes or an evening out for a dinner and movie, satisfying significant healthcare needs can bestow something of primary consequence to one's life, in much the same way that clean water, decent housing, and a good education can. We have seen fit to (mostly) not commoditize the guaranteed provision of these crucial social goods (even though the private sector may be heavily involved in servicing them), and perhaps the time has come to do the same for healthcare. Admittedly, the knowledge that clean water, proper sanitation, and a good education can lead to vast improvements in both personal and population welfare was known well before medicine acquired the efficacy emblematic of the past 100 years. But there is no longer any justification for denying that healthcare is a public good, similar to clean water, that we should regulate and provide as a function of good government for the communal welfare.

The passage of the Affordable Care Act (ACA) in 2010 was a laudable, but ultimately flawed, attempt to improve the dismal lot of the almost 50 million people (when it was enacted) without health insurance in the United States. Unfortunately, due to the numerous compromises that were part of the "normal" legislative process, especially with a law that would impact an industry that occupies almost one-fifth of the entire US economy, its ability to stem the growth of healthcare-related expenditures may be limited.[14] Moreover, even if every state expanded Medicaid eligibility and all qualified people purchased (subsidized) insurance, there would still be a sizeable group who would remain uncovered. Whether it was the give-backs to the pharmaceutical industry (prohibiting Medicare from negotiating for drug prices, plugging the "donut hole" in Medicare prescription drug benefits), the greed of doctors or hospitals (all those new paying customers), or preventing the newly created Patient Centered Outcome Research Institute (PCORI) from actually being able to fund true comparative effectiveness research in which cost was considered, what was finally enacted bore little resemblance to what many had hoped would become law.[15] Tellingly, the ACA was piggybacked onto the existing system of private commercial insurance (except for Medicaid expansion, for the most part) and thus only serves to perpetuate a system with shocking inequities in which the availability of basic but comprehensive healthcare still depends on the amount of money one earns or possesses. Thus, we find that how long one can expect to live, the chances that one's baby will live past her first year or be born extremely prematurely, or even one's probability of surviving a curable cancer can depend on factors that can be traced back to one common denominator: money.[16]

As health insurance becomes more expensive—both the sort commonly provided by employers and the kind available on the open market via federal government or state exchanges (through the ACA)—it is increasingly becoming like "real insurance," analogous to the policies people purchase for their homes or cars. Policies frequently come with high deductibles and other co-insurance costs (co-pays, for example) so that they really only become useful for catastrophic illnesses comparable to the fire that burns down the house or the accident that totals the car. In the same way that people are responsible for the costs of maintaining their homes with painting, regular repairs, and upkeep or their cars through scheduled maintenance and replacing the tires, they have also become liable for increasingly large amounts of the costs associated with regular, "routine," and preventative medical care. What people really need is not insurance designed on this homeowners or automobile model, but healthcare payment support. This is not to say that people should not bear the burden of some costs. But it seems unreasonable in a wealthy country that values the lives and welfare of its populace that their ability to stay well or get well should depend on the vagaries of the insurance markets or the amount of their paycheck.

Over the past 80 years or so, we have gradually and incrementally come to believe that not everyone in this country can provide everything he or she reasonably needs to attain and maintain a semblance of a life in which an individual can pursue personal goals and take advantage of opportunities. Furthermore, for those who fail in their attempts or who are less successful, although it is far from a universal sentiment, many believe that these people should not be punished for all of their misfortune. However, we have had a fitful and ambivalent approach to establishing a social safety net for the least fortunate among us. First with Social Security (and prior to that with experiments at providing basic healthcare to migrant and rural dispossessed farmworkers in the early 1930s)[17] and then on to Medicare and Medicaid and most recently the ACA, we have gradually, and frequently reluctantly, extended both the depth and breadth of those we care about and for.[18] It has not been easy, and various vested interest groups along the way have opposed any changes to the status quo, often defined as anything that might conceivably interfere with the generation or retention of their income or profits.[19]

Because of the slow—at times halting—accumulation of programs to provide at least some benefits for the unfortunate, poor, and others, it is reasonable at this point in time to ask whether healthcare for all—not just the few or favored or rich—should be included as an essential part of the social (welfare) contract that has slowly expanded to embrace greater numbers of people. What sorts of arguments have been marshaled against doing so? It is difficult to argue persuasively against this on the basis of efficacy or economic efficiency, for example, because we know that medicine is more beneficial for more patients than ever and is very likely to continue improving in this regard. One could hold that, as a society, we can't afford to do so, but that is specious because a reasonably well-designed and efficiently run system would undoubtedly be cheaper than what we have now, and preventive medicine can provide significant cost-savings in the long run. Another argument that has been used frequently against expanding the breadth and depth of social welfare programs—and one that has great currency in the United States—has been centered on the idea of just deserts: poor people, people down on their luck, the chronically unemployed, the homeless, undocumented immigrants—in general anyone not "like us"—do not deserve to receive something for free because they haven't earned it like "we have" (I discussed this in Chapter 6). This assertion can be countered by the line of reasoning I used in the previous chapter, as well as on the moral grounds of compassion for the suffering of our fellows.[20]

It is likely a truism that policy and money are inextricably intertwined. Indeed, expressions of good will, empathy, solidarity, and community—such as those embodied by legislative resolutions that convey approval for one cause or another—are symbolically meaningful, but only that. Unless backed up by funding, they are only vacuous statements of social harmony. And it is not only the amount of money directed toward a specific purpose, but also how it is allocated and what it is expected to purchase that are vitally important details that communicate the true motivations and intentions of a legislature. Many, perhaps most, of the laws and regulations passed by Congress that have mandates for the states and private institutions to carry out have their backbone in the power of the purse. For example, many of the regulations governing how hospitals must care for patients in a fair and equitable manner not only rely on federal antidiscrimination laws (and court rulings) but also on the threat to eliminate them from access to Medicare funding, a death knell for any hospital other than totally private organizations.[21] Thus, the willingness of the Congress, assorted state legislatures, and the like to appropriate money and direct it to healthcare resources that could arguably help the right people in the right way is a constant struggle.

Nevertheless, no matter how much money is allocated for a particular purpose and with a specific goal(s), there are usually limits to what amount is determined reasonable to spend. A notable exception is the Medicare program—even the military budget is set ahead of time—in which budgets are mostly estimates before the fiscal year outlay begins; in the end, the total annual costs are set by how much is used.

There is no provision to run out of Medicare funds, say, by the 11th month of the year, or to somehow restrict what kinds of drugs or surgeries are paid for near the end of each month. Healthcare insurance companies have a similar problem, and the premiums they charge reflect their estimates of their policyholder usage as well as their administrative costs, need for profit, and the like. The point is that, depending on the policy goals that are established, as well as any economic constraints there may be on financial outlays, somewhere, somehow there must be a mechanism to say "no" and rules in place (hopefully) on the appropriate way to say it. To do otherwise would create a free-for-all in which anyone could have anything he or she wanted with no controls whatsoever on either spending or the appropriateness—clinical or social— on what was being bought for these unlimited dollars. At the very minimum, it is not unreasonable to believe that there are some things or healthcare interventions that some people somewhere might wish to purchase for themselves that are inappropriate, no matter what, even if cost was not a consideration. However, if we accept this, then we have already accepted that it is permissible to restrict access to some things because we might have good reasons to do so.

FAIR AND RATIONAL RATIONING

As I have described, the United States has numerous different, poorly coordinated rationing strategies throughout American healthcare, except that they are not called rationing and many of them are patently unfair and opaquely created and implemented. They were not created to benefit patients, but rather established in furtive ways (see DRGs) or labeled with euphemisms (co-pays) to disguise their true intent. When commercial, for-profit insurance companies raise the co-pay or deductible, they are doing so to maintain their profit margins by discouraging people from utilizing their products, not for some noble cause. I have argued that rationing done correctly, meaning fairly and generously—rationing American style, one might call it—could possibly be both acceptable and politically palatable.[22] I went to great pains to emphasize my point about generosity, both for practical reasons—it would be important to minimize the negative impact of saying "no" to some people for some things—and for the fact that we are a wealthy country and we can and should be able to afford it if we make other systemic changes. However, while I described a process of instituting fairness, I somewhat glossed over the details of how to determine where and how to make cutoffs or where to draw the line(s). That was my goal in this book. It should first be noted that my entire argument is predicated upon several assumptions. The first and most important is that any attempt to overhaul the US healthcare system and institute some form of fair and reasonable controls on costs means that there should be one system that is available to all.[23] Second, it must be a "single-payer" plan; this would be essential in order to restrain price and demand pressures that are so prevalent in a multisupplier commercial system. Furthermore, by limiting the profit-making sector of healthcare, it would be easier to curb present and future costs due to excess administrative overhead, shareholder concerns, bloated executive salaries, and the like. A piecemeal approach that preserves the current uncoordinated system would be pointless short of declaring health insurance a public good analogous to power utilities. And third, the option to purchase additional insurance, benefits, and the like should still be available to those who wish to take advantage of such an option. This would preserve a market for these kinds of products and would offer people the freedom to supplement their coverage.[24] Nevertheless, the opportunity to buy private insurance must be regulated such that its existence (and potential popularity) does not threaten the existence or viability of the public system (see references in Note 23).

A crucial component to instituting rationing is the manner in which decisions are made about what will and will not be available as part of a comprehensive benefit package that people will accept as fair and reasonable. Of course, one could simply avoid making any difficult decisions or cloak them using technical or obscurantist language, thus making it burdensome for people to argue against what they believed to be negative decisions. Neither of these is satisfactory. The first because it will do nothing to impose any sort of fiscal restraint on the untenable growth in healthcare costs and the second because it simply continues the unsatisfactory situation we currently have. So I have based my approach on three fundamental features of decision-making that I believe are required to support a sensible kind of rationing. First, the primary goal of a healthcare system should be to adequately address medical need and thereby reduce suffering. Therefore, a methodology for defining reasonable healthcare needs must be developed. Second, the methods for dealing with needs must be based on scientific evidence, to the extent this is feasible. Where rigorous evidence does not exist or is ambiguous or conflicting, these deficiencies should serve as the stimulus for scientific research to attempt to resolve this lack. This also implies that the ability of physicians to craft treatment plans that are significant departures from the evidence base and that will be supported by the healthcare system would be limited.[25] Third, defining needs and the reasonable and appropriate means for meeting them must be done by consensus of groups comprising both experts literate and knowledgeable in relevant areas as well as lay representatives of those affected by the decisions. A cardinal rule of procedural fairness is that those who make the rules must be bound by them, and I believe it is crucially important that the committee mechanism take this into account. One of the principal causes of the mistrust and antipathy that most people have for the health insurance industry is the opaque manner in which their coverage decisions are made. It would be advisable to avoid this problem. Finally, the system chosen must focus on what really matters to people about their healthcare: the reduction of pain and suffering due to illness and disability and the prevention of avoidable causes of disease; it must focus on efficacy and appropriateness and not on irrelevant characteristics such as age.

Other than the guidelines of evidence and fairness that I have described, what other criteria could serve as moral (and practical) norms to steer the appropriateness committees (and others) in designing benefits and allocation rules? In particular, are there any (or should there be any) barometers by which to gauge success, especially to standards of social and distributive justice? Of course, there are the population metrics that we currently use: percent of the population with insurance, access to care, longevity, infant mortality, wait times for certain procedures, and the burden of medical-related debt. But it also seems reasonable to hold these committees and the system they serve to a higher standard, one rooted in a common understanding of human welfare and the role healthcare in general and medicine in particular should serve in securing it, if not advancing it. As Daniels has already persuasively argued, healthcare, like other intrinsically important products of modern society such as education, clean water, good sanitation, and decent housing, plays a vital role in permitting people—to the extent feasible—to pursue their life plans and take advantage of the opportunities made available by the communities in which they live. Indeed, without some modicum of health and the further accommodations provided to maximize the skills one has (I am thinking here of the private and public adjustments, including mechanical devices, for the disabled), the other hallmarks of a modern, just, and compassionate society are diminished accordingly. As I have remarked repeatedly throughout this book, the reasons for healthcare reform of the kind I am proposing and its institution in a manner that is fair, comprehensive, and generous are at their heart, moral ones. Abiding by rules of fairness (such as enhanced accountability for reasonableness that I previously described and endorsed) should be the watchword for reform and rationing. Such should also be the guiding principles of the allocation committees.

Not everything we might want is something we plausibly need, although I imagine that there could be some amount of argument about this on an individual level. For example, I might really want a new luxury car, or a sailboat that I can use to noodle around a large lake near my home, or a weekend house in the mountains (in addition to the one I live in the rest of the time), but it would be difficult to maintain that I actually need these items in any fundamentally important way. It would be weird to believe that I would be appreciably harmed by not having these things. I may certainly be unhappy or sad, perhaps wistful, wishing that I could have them. Indeed, if I could afford them but was denied the ability to purchase them because of a public policy outlawing say, second homes, I would likely be angry. But I would not suffer harm in the same way that I would if I could not get a medicine that could cure my pneumonia (which, if untreated, would cause me to be absent from work for 2 weeks and lose my job).

What are some of the differences between the understandings of "need" expressed in these two cases? In the first, perhaps some of my wealthy friends would agree that I definitely needed the boat or vacation house assuming that they shared the same sense of "needing" I did. In the latter, I suspect most people (perhaps all rational individuals) would accept that a sick person needs the antibiotic to cure his infection in a nondiscretionary way. And that aspect of the situation that contributes to the "neediness" and the lack of discretion would be the inevitable and possibly grievous harm to his life that would result if the item that could address his need were not supplied. This does not mean that the "satisfier" (as I labeled this in Chapter 3) must have guaranteed results, only that it has a reasonable chance of producing the desired outcome. What counts as true needs and what level of needs we are/should be willing to pay for as a matter of course is a key question. But how can we determine both the reasonable needs that people have in healthcare (and presumably other domains that contribute to individual and collective welfare) and the satisfiers available to meet them?

Most of us could probably agree on many healthcare interventions that should be illegitimate or *prima facie* not allowed (not permitted in a publicly funded social insurance program, but not outlawed a priori, although there are undoubtedly some of those as well).[26] For example, it is likely that we would concur that desires for surgical interventions that were the expressed products of a mental illness (say, body dysmorphic disorder) should have no place for system funding (for example, Medicare or private insurers). Similarly, many would also agree that so-called cosmetic surgery of a type solely designed to electively enhance one's physical appearance in the absence of gross acquired or congenital deformities that clearly interfered with physical function should also not be eligible for payment from a general fund. Of course, the borders of this second example begin to get a bit blurry because it may be a subjective evaluation about what sorts of anatomic variations—visible or not, the organ(s) affected, their origins, how severe their departure from "normal" variation, etc.—would qualify. And this last example highlights the essence of the cutoff problem: how to make justifiable and justified decisions at the boundaries where ambiguity, uncertainty, and continuous distribution variables reign.

Most of the time the human conditions that interest us the most, especially in healthcare, have fuzzy borders. Both characteristics that stand as identifiers for somewhat ill-defined concepts such as IQ and well-demarcated dimensions like height are measured by tests that have numerical scores that are both quantifiable and interpersonally comparable and thus possess this problem at the arbitrarily set boundaries. At first glance, one might think that height and IQ have little in common except for the fact that they are measured on an ordinal scale. However, although few would dispute that there are people who are smarter than others and there are those who are shorter and taller with respect to each other, the problem is applying the labels "tall" and "short," "bright" and "dull" to the numbers. Where is the distinction between someone who is tall and one who is short? How do we decide? This question and how we go about answering it has fundamental significance for healthcare and in deciding what interventions should or should not be covered and, most important, how to distinguish between the two. An example will help illustrate this conundrum.

How should insurance companies determine whether to pay for recombinant human growth hormone (rHGH) supplements for children? Should it be on the basis of height at a specific age along with growth velocity and measurements of HGH in the blood after a suitable stimulation test? Not surprisingly, all of these measurements do not yield yes/no, present/absent answers but are themselves subject to blurred or fuzzy borders at the cutoff points (which are, as one might expect, also subject to negotiation and argument about where they should be placed).[27] Most of the cutoffs with which we are most familiar in our daily lives utilize discretionary (occasionally seemingly capricious) and very narrow boundary lines to demarcate what is and is not permissible for what is and is not available for distribution. For example, the retirement age or eligibility for Social Security is 65 years of age.[28] It is not 64 years and 364 days; it's 65 years. Similarly, the age of majority (assuming that one has cognitive capacity; but remember the problem with IQ measurements) is 18 years. As I introduced in Chapter 1 and discussed in greater detail in Chapter 2, the difficulty in creating cutoffs is not so much discriminating between traits or idiosyncrasies or features that lie at the very edges when compared to others with the same *kind* of feature but on the opposite end of the scale. Rather, it's when we can hardly distinguish between two people or two conditions on a continuum of fuzziness but necessarily must draw a line somewhere. The trick is how to draw it fairly and equitably so those who fall on the "wrong" side of the boundary have little reason to complain.

Unfortunately for those who would design healthcare systems that must decide what interventions to include for coverage (and what not to include), many—if not most—conditions, especially complex ones with compound etiologies, exist on a continuum of expression and pathology. While it may be relatively straightforward to characterize, identify, diagnose, and often treat the underlying cause or the overt symptoms of diseases such as many infections, it becomes a classification nightmare to decide where illness begins for many others. This ineluctable fact about human health confounds attempts to draw boundaries between being well and being sick. Furthermore, it also poses a challenge for defining what interventions may or may not be beneficial, and for whom and for how many. Even a wealthy country with a well-endowed and generous universal healthcare plan will not be willing (nor should it) to pay for anything for anyone, leaving the conundrum of what seems reasonable to provide from the continually enlarging universe of diagnostic and therapeutic interventions, all purportedly designed to make people feel—and possibly be—better. Add to this the enthusiasm we in the United States have for enlarging both our diagnostic and therapeutic armamentarium by increasing the number of physical states we call pathologic "conditions" as well as the drugs and procedures we have to treat them, often with the latter stimulating the creation of the former, and the problem is made even more difficult. [29]

Modern medicine is immensely complex, and it is likely to become even more so in the future. If we were to engage in a wholesale remake of the US healthcare system whereby we judged payment or coverage decisions (not how much, but yes/no; I will discuss the former a bit later) on need, appropriateness, and efficacy, we would necessarily have to consider these three factors for virtually everything, ranging from childhood immunizations to platelet rich plasma therapy for degenerative joint disease, from cognitive behavioral therapy to chiropractic. This would be an enormous and daunting undertaking. But a more considered reflection would reveal that the task would not be nearly as onerous as it might initially appear. For example, there are many interventions that are currently performed routinely that would require little review; vaccinations for a variety of diseases are an excellent example (although the fact that something is commonly done or even carried out under the umbrella term "standard of care" does not necessarily mean that it is correct or supported by evidence). Almost anything that has been reviewed by the Food and Drug Administration (FDA) and approved could also pass this test.[30] However, that would still leave a number of diagnostic and therapeutic interventions, including those for which there exists excellent supporting evidence, that would require vetting (but for which FDA approval has not been sought).[31] One plausible suggestion would be to accomplish this in phases, grandfathering in many of the potentially contestable interventions (except for those that are least likely to pass muster), with their eventual elimination or replacement over time. In addition to FDA approval, one could also utilize the vast (and constantly updated) database accrued by the Cochrane Collaboration, an international, non–industry-funded association of healthcare professionals that evaluates and reviews the available evidence for and against various drugs, procedures, diagnostic tests, and more and offers considered judgments about their utility and efficacy.[32]

I have also suggested that this form of consensus decision-making could be a useful guide for contestable decisions at the blurry borders of efficacy.[33] Aside from those interventions that offer no benefit, such as mechanical ventilation for a patient who is dead by neurological criteria, there will be many cases about which there could be a great deal of emotionally laden disagreement. For example, if we intellectually agree— meaning away from the bedside and the heat of immediate passions—that supporting and paying for what are often called "marginally beneficial" interventions is something we cannot afford to do and, more important, should not do because of the minimal good that is done, then we must establish the cutoff of what distinguishes "marginally beneficial" from something that is "beneficial enough." Some authors have appealed to statistics, stating that something that has less than a 1% chance of success—usually defined as restoring a patient to some kind of meaningful, conscious life—is futile and should never be offered or maintained.[34] Others have suggested that less than a 5% chance of success is a reasonable definition of marginal benefit, and offering such an intervention (and presumably paying for it) should either be negotiable or off the table.[35] Unfortunately, as I discussed in Chapter 4, the probabilistic nature of medicine makes the ability to state definitively in a specific case that there is less than a 5% (or, for that matter, a somewhat greater than 5%) chance of benefit exceedingly problematic. Because of this, borders at this end of things are blurry and hence troublesome. Nevertheless, this could actually be an empirical question that could be experimentally addressed by carefully designed and widespread surveys of the general public throughout the country to establish what should qualify as a marginal benefit.

One approach to solving this problem at the borders might be to use *fuzzy analysis*, a complex statistical and mathematical method that could potentially help, and there is certainly no reason why the expert committees could not utilize this strategy as an adjunct.[36] However, a tool as difficult for most people to understand as fuzzy analytics might prove to be too obscure to be practical, and so, once again, I appeal to discussion, argument, and consensus-building. I suspect that careful, well-meaning, and dedicated deliberation by groups of people who are both knowledgeable and committed to resolving differences and aware of the charge to be both generous but prudent with the public's money would be able to come to agreement on almost everything. However, it is likely that there will be some decisions that will err on the side of approving interventions that could arguably be said to be unreasonable, while others could kindle the opposite opinion. If there is balance, they could cancel each other out or be amenable to repeal upon review at a later date. Flexibility and generosity tempered with circumspection must be the watchwords.

Democratic deliberation is all well and good, but in a contested and fractious political environment it may prove either too cumbersome or impossible to accomplish the monumental task of classifying everything using this method. Therefore, it must be performed by "experts" in the field with some representation of affected groups. The experts must be *completely free* of conflicts of interest (unlike many of those who serve on current clinical guidelines committees) to enhance their credibility, legitimacy, and the chances that their decisions will be viewed as unbiased.[37] Lest people think that experts in the majority weights the committees too heavily in favor of doctors (for example) making all the decisions with only token representation of others, this approach should be contrasted with what currently happens: decisions made in secret by (insurance company) committees with the heavy influence (often determinative) of the affected industries and interest groups that ignore evidence in favor of their unsupported beliefs.[38]

The expected massive increase in the elderly population of the United States, almost entirely due to the entry of the baby boomers into the ranks of the over-65 set, as well as the slowing of the birthrate, means that Medicare can expect to experience an enormous expansion in the next 10–20 years.[39] Even though Medicare has been a leader in some areas of surreptitious cost-savings (the DRG program, limits on physician reimbursement, etc.), it has also yielded to political pressure (and the influence of various lobbying groups) to not engage in price controls in which it could have major market influence, such as in the cost of drugs and devices (of interest is that the Veterans Administration, despite its many flaws and deficiencies, does negotiate for drugs and hence obtains them and offers them to patients at significantly lower prices than in the private sector). Nevertheless, the slowdown in healthcare-related inflation experienced during the recent recession is unlikely to be anything other than temporary, and the percentage of the US economy devoted to healthcare will undoubtedly continue to increase unless something is done to alter its course.[40]

Another major criticism of my proposal could be that it involves a potential monumental remaking of a major sector of the American economy, and, if implemented as I suggest, could significantly downsize the commercial insurance industry and all of the ancillary businesses that service it and feed off it. This would not be a trivial event and would undoubtedly have to take place in phases to limit the possible damaging effects and disruptions, both foreseen and unintended. At the prospect of such an upheaval, many might simply scoff at the implausibility of achieving such massive alterations, especially since it would require an extensive intrusion of the federal government into the marketplace that would produce a marked diminution (although not an elimination) of a large component of the healthcare economy.

However, there is a precedent in the relatively recent past in which the United States made a major policy decision to devote unheard of amounts of tax dollars to one program that directly led to an extensive remaking of an entire—and dominant and politically powerful—competing mega-business.

The Federal-Aid Highway Act of 1956 reached Eisenhower on June 29 in Walter Reed Army Medical Center, where he was recovering from surgery for ileitis. The bill was just one of twenty-seven he signed that day. . . . Just what had the president signed? The bill authorized $25 billion for twelve years to accelerate construction of a National System of Interstate and Defense Highways; created a Highway Trust Fund supported by increasing the federal tax on gas and diesel fuel from 2 to 3 cents; increased the federal portion of construction costs for interstate highways to ninety percent; provided for advance acquisition of right-of-way; required that the interstate highways be built to the highest standards and with the capability of handling traffic projected for 1972; and pledged to complete the Interstate Highway System by 1972.... In its conception, the Federal-Aid Highway Act of 1956 represented a triumph for all.... Motorists were happy because the legislation promised to increase their mobility over safer and better roads. Truckers approved because it provided for superhighways that allowed them to carry increased weights without paying significantly higher taxes. Mayors and managers of large cities applauded the money and jobs the urban portions of the Interstate Highway System would bring to them. Highway contractors were ecstatic because the bill demanded the best and most expensive roads imaginable.... No doubt the happiest groups of all were the manufacturers of automobiles and trucks and the refiners of gasoline.[41]

But this lavish funding for the construction of interstate highways, a direct result of a policy created by the federal government and passed into law by the Congress, issued a virtual death knell for comprehensive passenger rail transportation in the United States. Admittedly, passenger rail traffic had been declining for some time, coincident with the rise of the personal automobile. But it still reigned supreme for long-distance intercity travel. The availability of safe, fast, accessible interstates, along with inexpensive gasoline, proved irresistible to middle-class America in the post-war years. At the same time, generous government subsidies began to be offered to towns and cities to create regional airports, in a similar policy shift to build up the commercial passenger aviation industry—especially after the introduction of financially viable jet-powered aircraft—thus leading to a further decline in the railroads. Thus, planned, determined government policy led to the enhancement and creation of one set of industries at the expense of another, even one as powerful as the railroads. It is conceivable that such an effort to reformulate a sector of the economy that does not serve the public good in a manner from which most can benefit (commercial health insurance) could also work. This is not to say that those who would be on the losing end would not protest, much as railroad executives did in the mid-1950s. But history suggests that it is possible.

THE ROAD FORWARD

It is by no means a surprise nor is it an understatement to note the glaring and increasing economic inequalities that are emblematic of life in the United States. The wealthy and even the simply better off can afford to purchase goods and services that not only improve the quality and even length of their lives, but also serve to perpetuate and enlarge existing inequities into the future and across generations.

While possessing large amounts of money cannot guarantee outcomes in health, it most certainly can promise access to doctors, medicines, technology, and even care in both quantity and quality that would be unimaginable for many in the lower rungs of society. There are many reasons to radically reform and transform the American healthcare system, both medical and moral. But some of the most compelling are those offered to at least partially address and mitigate some of the most dire and tragic effects of the huge disparities of wealth and what it can buy. I would not think to deny the rich the fruits of their labors (or their inheritances), but I would urge that effort be made to not make those less fortunate in life suffer avoidable health harms solely to perpetuate a misguided and deeply unfair system.

I have concentrated on an analysis of the cutoff problem and an argument of how to approach a solution to suit a comprehensive, universal healthcare plan for America. I have also given significant consideration to the potential pitfalls and problems that could beset any reform attempt of this magnitude. But I have necessarily (until now) paid relatively little attention to the morality of this effort. What is the imperative to reform healthcare in the United States? Why ration, and why do it in the way I have suggested could work? Most of the arguments that have been advanced throughout the years have relied on economic reasons to reform healthcare, and I have not shied away from using these as well. Nevertheless, the most fundamentally significant grounds are moral. The United States is the wealthiest country on the planet, but its riches are hardly distributed equally. While I have little desire to engage in a discussion of income inequality and the vast differences between the "1%" and everyone else (nor am I qualified to do so), it is important to point out that the uneven distribution of the bounty of this country does have a bearing on healthcare. There is little question that we have the financial means to provide much more than a decent minimum of healthcare to all who live here. The unresolved issue, then, is why would we or why wouldn't we create a healthcare system that could rival those of other advanced industrialized nations? The first is considerably easier to address than the latter.

As Paul Starr has trenchantly observed, most people with employer-provided healthcare insurance, along with their dependents and those who have Medicare, comprise the majority of Americans. If not totally satisfied with what they have, these lucky people are sufficiently satisfied that they are afraid of what could replace it.[42] For many people, the status quo—what they are familiar with and accustomed to—is considerably preferable to an unknown future, even if there are reasons to believe that the future could be better. Indeed, it was this very fear that was exploited by those who set out to destroy the Clinton-era healthcare reform plan with the infamous "Harry and Louise" television ads.[43] Similarly, the public campaigns against the ACA, both before and after its passage, have attempted to stoke alarm in those people who are justly afraid of the tenuous grasp they may have on a middle-class lifestyle.[44] Hence, the impetus for a radical reform of healthcare cannot come from an outpouring of the expressive will of the people. The desire and energy must come from elsewhere, as it has for every attempt to implement a comprehensive system of national health insurance over the past 100 years.[45]

Throughout this book, I have based my argument on the assumption that the need to ration healthcare in the United States is a given for economic reasons. There are also good moral reasons to do so because not everyone should be able to have whatever he or she wants whenever he or she wants it. However, they should be able to have access to and receive all the healthcare they could reasonably need. This means that some needs are more important than others, in the same way that some people in the emergency department are more acutely ill or injured than others and must be cared for sooner. Most of the time, what people want—to live longer, be free from or have their pain minimized, to maintain physical and mental function as long as possible—can be addressed by modern scientific, evidence-based medicine. Those things that people want that they could arguably do without and that are not addressed by the realistic mission and goals of healthcare (to relieve suffering) are not true needs in the sense that I mean. But sensible rationing of the sort that I think plausible and potentially feasible must have justifiable methods for deciding where the cutoff lines will be that separate covered conditions and interventions from those that are not. Few doctors (and even fewer patients) will argue about what is included. Few will also argue in a persuasive way about unfunded interventions that are way below the cutoff line either because they are futile (continued life support for brain dead patients) or frivolous in a publicly funded healthcare system (elective cosmetic surgery). The disagreements and controversy will occur at the boundaries. How to resolve those often-blurry boundaries is the challenge I have set out to answer in this book. The solution is to determine by representative consensus or negotiated settlement where to draw the line. No longer would opaque bureaucrats working for for-profit insurance companies make these decisions arbitrarily. Rather, panels of experts (without financial or other conflicts of interest) and dedicated laypersons would examine the evidence and debate the pros and cons of clinical indications or conditions and the appropriateness of various possible treatments, diagnostic tests, and the like, and reach agreement. The committees would have to be disposed and dedicated to this form of sensible discussion and method of decision-making, but the experience with Rand appropriateness method (RAM)-like committees in experimental prototypes suggests that they could be feasible and their opinions could be viewed as legitimate if they also conformed to the cardinal rules of fairness that others and I have described.[46] Rather than drawing arbitrary lines using features about people that are either irrelevant or at best poorly correlated with healthcare needs and outcomes (such as age), this approach focuses on defining healthcare needs *as such* and considering what the best and most effective ways of meeting them would be. No doubt people might argue that what I have proposed is cumbersome, inconvenient, and a mammoth undertaking. My answer to this criticism is that it may be the only strategy to accomplish the task fairly and acceptably in a large heterogeneous democracy. But, as I have also argued throughout, it only makes sense to take this approach if it is performed under the auspices of a comprehensive, universal healthcare system.

Medicine has never been better placed to positively influence the well-being of our lives, and it will only get better. That does not mean that more is better; simply that a judicious use of what we have and will develop can truly help people live their lives better and longer. But it is shameful that the power of modern healthcare is only available in this way to those who have the money to pay for it. There is no good reason that a person born into poverty in today's America must not only suffer the burdens of being poor, but must also endure the ills of delayed diagnosis, terrible primary care (or none at all), and lack of access to the best that American medicine has to offer. There is no good reason that those people who are newly insured because of the ACA must have insurance policies with enormously high annual deductibles and co-payments (even with the federal subsidies) such that they must avoid seeking care early in an illness because of the cost. There is no good reason that people who would be eligible for Medicaid under the ACA but have the misfortune to live in one of the many states that have refused to expand this program must go without healthcare and burden both local emergency departments as well as threaten their own lives. Perhaps this is a reflection of the often poorly disguised contempt for the poor for their seeming inability to alter their circumstances—to pull themselves up by their bootstraps by sheer willpower and the desire to better their lot.[47] It is no accident that most social welfare programs that exist in this country had difficult births (and some died aborning) and have constantly been under attack, frequently by those whose wealth inoculates them from the necessity of relying on public assistance.

Ultimately, the reason to create a national and universal health insurance program is a moral one. To deny our fellow Americans the benefits of good and decent healthcare is an ongoing tragedy. Most important, it is a choice that we make *not* to do so. We could, if we chose, craft a program that was both generous and far-reaching, offering to all everything they could need. Of course, to do so would require discipline coupled with other efforts to improve efficiency and control costs.

Why do we as a nation seemingly care so little, why are we apparently indifferent to the suffering of others less fortunate when we have the means to help? Think of the wasted life opportunities that fail to be realized when we let illnesses go untreated and wounds fester. The human—and not to mention, the economic—cost is staggering. Yet all of my arguments and remonstrations are ultimately meaningless unless placed within the context of overall healthcare reform. And for that to take place would require a wholesale dedication to the idea that Americans by right deserve comprehensive healthcare; not if they can individually afford it, but as a consequence of living here and the fact that, as a nation, we can afford it. We all have the capacity to suffer—and almost all of us do at some point(s) in our lives. It is that community of vulnerability that we share with one another that makes the national failure to make the moral commitment to universal healthcare so scandalous. Modern, scientific medicine has an enormously powerful ability to improve the well-being of people. To restrict its benefits to those who have the financial wherewithal to pay for it and only grudgingly supply a modified, often mediocre or second class, form to the most disadvantaged is itself an embarrassment at best and an immoral disgrace at worst. We are not a poor country. We have the good fortune to be able to make choices on what to do with our bounty. To deliberately choose not to provide decent and generous healthcare for all is unbecoming of a country that constantly boasts of its greatness.

NOTES

Prelims

1. *National Federation of Independent Business v. Sebelius,* 2012.
2. *King v. Burwell* 576 U.S. ___ (2015).
3. Disch 1996; Thomas 1995–96; Yankelovich 1995.
4. Starr 2011.
5. Altman and Shactman 2011; Starr 2011.
6. Starr 2011; Thomasson 2002. This is the most popular narrative, but a closer scrutiny of the historical records reveals antecedents for employment-related health coverage or insurance to the country's 18th-century beginnings (Scofea 1994) as well as episodes of pre-Medicare federal government-financed healthcare (Grey 1994). Also see Dobbin (1992) for a more nuanced view.
7. Starr 2011, chapters 1 and 2.
8. Bosslet et al. 2015.
9. Hamel et al. 2016.
10. Martin et al. 2014.
11. Hartman et al. 2015.
12. Rosoff, P. M. (2015); "The Affordable Care Act is another way to ration health care." The Conversation; http://theconversation.com/the-affordable-care-act-is-another-way-to-ration-health-care-35946. February 4, 2015.
13. Katz 2013.
14. Rosoff 2014.
15. Ibid.

Chapter 1

1. Ceaser 2012; Rabkin 2012.
2. Roehrig et al. 2012; Ryu et al. 2013; Keehan et al. 2015.
3. Aggarwal 2010; Brindley et al. 2011.
4. Schroeder and Frist 2013; Tilburt et al. 2013. While it is true that steps have been taken to hold doctors and the places where they practice more accountable for the quality of some of the care they provide, little attempt has been made to control the relentless pursuit of "mission creep": expanding the populations of patients whom doctors think might benefit from receiving cardiac stents, implantable defibrillators, robot-assisted surgery, extraordinarily costly last-chance cancer drugs, etc., all despite the lack of evidence for efficacy. All that is required is evidence for payment.
5. Reddy et al. 2014; Blake 2015; Cunningham 2015.
6. See Callahan 2009; K. Baicker et al. 2012; Barbash and Glied 2010; Grimes 1993; B. Leff 2008.

7. Brownlee 2008; Cunningham 2010; Spiro et al. 2012; Stabile et al. 2013.

8. See Starr (2011) for a discussion of this phenomenon, especially chapters 1 and 2.

9. One of the problems with relying on charity to provide important social goods is that it is naturally dependent on the impulses of those with the means to dispense the charity. This extends to the amount of charity and on both whom it is bestowed and the sort that is distributed. By its very nature, it is voluntary, and, although charitable organizations have few scruples about appealing to social guilt of various kinds to engender donations, it is a far cry from that to rely on the charity of others to meet needs that all share.

10. Daniels 2008, chapter 2.

11. *Estelle, et al. v. Gamble* 1976.

12. We already do this in somewhat haphazard ways, such as by limiting access to certain medicines by the ability to pay or restricting who can even see a doctor (except in emergencies) on the basis of income by not guaranteeing and mandating healthcare for all residents, for example. The common theme of restricted access in the United States is the availability of (personal) money.

13. Rosoff 2014, especially chapter 6.

14. Rosoff 2014, chapter 7, and this book, Chapter 2.

15. Rosoff 2014, especially chapter 7.

16. Katherine Baicker and Finkelstein 2011; Daniels 1991; Hadorn 1991; Kitzhaber 1993; Lindsay 2009; Oberlander et al. 2001.

17. Hadorn 1991; Oberlander et al. 2001.

18. In their analysis of how to construct a package of essential health benefits as outlined in the ACA, an Institute of Medicine expert panel concluded (among other things) that the scope of covered benefits should be determined not only by the 10 categories specific in the ACA, but also by a defined budget. This means that, depending upon the number of people covered and the cost of services and their utilization, the amount of money allocated to the program will dictate how much can be "bought" (Ulmer et al. 201, chapter 4). This approach is very similar to that taken by Oregon Health Plan, in which a budget for the Plan was passed by the legislature and how much of the list was included in each fiscal period was dependent upon the amount of money available: see Rosoff 2014, chapter 2.

19. Gonsalkorale et al. 2013; Hummert et al. 2002.

20. Nosek et al. 2007.

21. Ratcliffe 2000; Wilmot and Ratcliffe 2002; Stahl et al. 2008; Tong et al. 2010.

22. http://www.imdb.com/title/tt0063808/plotsummary?ref_=tt_ov_pl; accessed October 10, 2013.

23. It is reasonable to mention that some might hold that there might be at least one benefit to this sort of arbitrariness, assuming it can be imposed in a justifiable and acceptable way (or even by fiat, as in the movie). The major one would be the fact that if people know when they are to be cut off from access to something at some defined age, be it freedom, influenza vaccine, or intensive care, they can prepare for that eventuality with appropriate plans. Aside from the fact that people are notoriously bad at planning for the future (all one has to do is examine the dismal state of most individuals' retirement accounts), the ability to justify one point in a person's life as determinative rather than another seems almost capricious. Why 50 years old (or 30) and not 50 + 1 month, other than we like round numbers?

24. Banaji 2013, chapter 3.

25. Jonsen 1986; McKie and Richardson 2003. The Rule of Rescue describes a psychological phenomenon by which our emotional connection to a given situation (often tragic) is triggered when an identified individual is placed at risk, as opposed to a description of statistical lives. This is irrespective of whether we actually know the person who is placed in the perilous circumstances. For example, when we hear about a child who has fallen down a well and the forces are gathering to try and rescue her, our direction empathy is evoked for that specific child (the identified individual). However, when we read about the genocide in Rwanda or chemical weapons attacks in Syria in which hundreds or thousands have died, these victims are statistical in that they represent an aggregate number without a face or name, and we do not feel the same kind of emotional tug as we do for the girl in the well. This plays out in medicine all the time: we somehow know in the background that patients are denied transplants all the time (often for perfectly justifiable reasons). But when their loved ones call the TV news and their plight is featured on the evening program, all of a sudden we have a face and a person's story to go with the background statistics that occur every day without notice by the wider public. Unfortunately, that is why using the media to alert the public to these situations can be a very effective method to get what you want even if you may have been denied it fairly. For example, see http://articles.philly.com/2013-09-01/news/ 41665225_1_adult-lungs-sarah-murnaghan-janet-murnaghan; accessed October 22, 2013. I will address the Rule of Rescue and its implications for healthcare reform and rationing in greater detail in Chapter 5.
26. Kahneman 2011. However, it is worth noting that some studies have engaged participants in discussions to explore why they chose the way they did, thus activating Kahneman's "system two," and the choices have by and large remain unchanged. This may be partly due to the fact that since we make an overt commitment or decision, we are prone to continue to endorse it even when post hoc reflection raises doubts (Greene and Haidt 2002; Haidt 2001).
27. Calabresi and Bobbitt 1978.
28. I do not mean to imply that I don't support government support for medical care and pensions for the elderly; far from it. I simply intend to illustrate the fact that under conditions of apparent resource plenty, we prioritize allocations to the elderly (presumably because they vote and do so in much higher proportions than the parents of children).
29. Peiris et al. 2007.
30. Jeffery K. Taubenberger et al. 2005.
31. Johnson and Mueller 2002; J. K. Taubenberger and Morens 2006; Barry 2004; Murray et al. 2006.
32. Ma et al. 2011; Wong and Yuen 2006.
33. Markel et al. 2007; Hatchett et al. 2007.
34. This was a different kind of "swine flu" than that which appeared in the 1970s. The latter caused a panic and the hurried production of a vaccine which may have been causally related to a slightly increased risk of developing a severe complication called Guillain-Barré syndrome (Safranek et al. 1991).
35. Osterholm 2005, pp. 32–34. With the pandemic strain of H1N1 that actually occurred (not the dreaded H5N1 that was feared), it appears as if one dose of that vaccine was sufficient to confer immunity; see Neuzil (2009). But the elderly (a major and increasing percentage of the population in most developed, industrialized nations) have a significantly decreased response rate compared to younger people, and this observation may

figure into the rationale for prioritizing the young; see Goodwin et al. (2006) and the discussion in the text.

36. Of course, it was impossible to predict how effective the vaccine would actually be because the amount of protection can vary year-to-year. For example, the seasonal influenza vaccine in the North American 2014–15 season provided protection to anywhere from 23% (Flannery et al. 2015) to about 33% of those vaccinated (Skowronski et al. 2015).

37. Bernier and Marcuse 2005; Docter et al. 2011.

38. Health 2008; Leavitt 2005; Neuzil 2009; Officials 2008.

39. Emanuel and Wertheimer 2006.

40. Harris 1985.

41. Callahan 1987.

42. Fiore et al. 2008.

43. Tsuchiya 2000; Eisenberg et al. 2011; Callan et al. 2012; Skirbekk and Nortvedt 2012; Yang and Lee 2010.

44. This assumes that there has not been a relatively recent major catastrophe that affects births and deaths, which would then distort the shape of the age distribution. For example, if everyone stopped having babies for 10 years or so, the distribution of ages would be skewed to the right because there would be fewer young people replacing the old people who died. On the other hand, if there were a major epidemic with a high mortality rate that only affected those over 60, then the opposite might be observed. Indeed, the aging of many populations in the developed, wealthy industrialized world (especially Japan and Western Europe) due to a falling birthrate is having an effect somewhat similar to (but less pronounced than) the artificial situation I mentioned first. Figure 1.1 compares the age distribution in the United States population in both 1990 and 2000. If these data were not portrayed as a histogram but rather as data points on a curve, it would appear much smoother.

45. This hypothetical is based on an assumption that the vaccine would be highly effective. As indicated previously (see Note 30).

46. And perhaps not surprisingly (but unfortunately), the committee did not address the practical aspects of the decision.

47. I have discussed this subject in detail elsewhere (Rosoff 2014). as have many others.

48. See Rosoff (2014), chapter 2.

49. This kind of distribution is also colloquially known as a "bell-shaped curve," which gave its name to the controversial eponymous book by Herrnstein and Murray (1994).

50. There is nothing magical about the number 100; the various tests were designed to be scored in this manner so that this would be the mean.

51. While vitally important for benefit eligibility, the classification of someone as being intellectually disabled can also influence whether a person convicted of murder lives or dies (if he or she is convicted in a death penalty state). In 2002, the US Supreme Court ruled that individuals found to have significant cognitive deficits (i.e., an IQ of less than 70) could not be executed (*Atkins v. Virginia* 2002). In 2014, the Court also recognized the problem with cutoffs I have been describing. They invalidated the application of a Florida statute that absolutely set the IQ test bar for execution at a score of 70. The Court stated that other factors must be taken into consideration as well as the inexactitude of IQ tests and the way they are constructed and scored (*Hall v. Florida* 2014). Also see Cooke et al. (2015).

52. MELD is an acronym that stands for "model for end-stage liver disease." It is a combination of several laboratory test values (serum albumin, bilirubin, a testing of the ability to clot the blood, etc.) that replaced the much more subjective arguments that transplant doctors previously made to try and advance the priority of their patients for the few organs available. Using the MELD led to several improvements in fair allocation, including a decrease in racial and ethnic disparities as well as the associated dependence of how good a debater or how persuasive one's doctor was. See Wiesner et al. 2003; Moylan et al. 2008; Kemmer et al. 2009; Dutkowski et al. 2011.
53. Glover 1977, pp. 126–127. Daniel Callahan alludes to this problem when he discusses what he has called the "ragged edge" of medicine, the frontier of development of therapies and interventions, the seemingly limitless "boundary" of modern medicine where uncertainty of outcomes becomes overwhelming. See Callahan 1990, chapter 2.
54. Gargus et al. 2009; Keir et al. 2014. But it is by no means zero and appears to be improving; see Patel et al. (2015).
55. Horbar et al. 2012.
56. Singh et al. 2007; Mohamed et al. 2010; Stoll et al. 2010; Patel et al. 2015.
57. Beale 2012.
58. Steven and Laudan 2013
59. Berwick and Hackbarth 2012; see also Davis and Ballreich 2014.
60. Berwick and Hackbarth 2012/
61. Melichar 2009; Bach 2013; Malin et al. 2013; Loewenstein et al. 2012.
62. Rosoff 2014.
63. Ibid.
64. Williams 1997.
65. Emanuel and Wertheimer 2006.
66. http://www.weeklystandard.com/articles/about-those-death-panels_536874.html; accessed October 22, 2013; Twight 2002, chapter 8.
67. Hyde 2014, p. 1; Allen 2012; Burnyeat 1982. Also see Whitmarsh 2015, chapter 11.
68. Of course, the inherent vagueness of terms to which the sorites paradox applies, such as needs and medical necessity (see Chapter 3) has drawn its own detractors who view this as a problem without acceptable solutions and hence are drawn toward more quantitative, tractable, and manipulable characteristics such as age: see Schultheiss (2002).
69. Callahan 2009.

Chapter 2

1. I am by no means alone in holding this view. See Cassell 1982, 1999; Lubell and Everett 1938; Pellegrino and Thomasma 1981.
2. Others recognize this problem, but I do not think pay sufficient attention to it (for example, see Fleck 2009, 2010). Interestingly, one of the main criticisms of so-called "bedside rationing" in which physicians are empowered (or empower themselves) to make resource allocation decisions for individual patients in the absence of an overarching health system allocation scheme is the inherent arbitrariness as well as the lack of any kind of guarantee that the "saved" resources would be put to "better" use elsewhere (Hurst et al. 2006; Strech et al. 2008; P. A. Ubel and Goold 1997; P. A. Ubel and Arnold 1995).
3. Norman Daniels 2008; N. Daniels and Sabin 2008.

4. For example, see Aki Tsuchiya 1999; A. Tsuchiya et al. 2005; Wailoo and Anand 2005; Sen 2002.
5. See Rawls 1999, especially chapter 2.
6. Sen 2005, 2009; Nussbaum 2000; Rawls 1999, chapter 2.
7. I need to qualify this statement by restricting the analysis to goods of vital importance to virtually all rational people. Thus, goods that would satisfy mere preferences, as opposed to the kinds of needs I discussed in Chapter 2, would not count. Therefore, it seems perfectly acceptable to give priority to people who queue up for concert tickets earlier than those who come later. While fans of a band may argue to the contrary, it is difficult to imagine that failing to purchase tickets to a specific concert will result in significant harm, as opposed to simple disappointment. However, if we allocated healthcare interventions this way, those who came later, especially because of access issues out of their control (poverty and poor information availability readily come to mind), this would not seem to be very fair.
8. For example, see Davis et al. 2014.
9. Rosoff 2014.
10. Glassman et al. 1997; Hadorn 1991; Kitzhaber 1993.
11. Morris et al. 2013; Craig 2012; Machida et al. 2013; Charlifue et al. 2011.
12. Rothwell et al. 1997.
13. Colver et al. 2012; Quale and Schanke 2010; Catalano et al. 2011.
14. Nakagawa and Obana 2014.
15. Acharya et al. 2003; Eddy 1992a, 1992b, 1992c; Gray et al. 2011; Levin and McEwan 2001; Robinson 1993.
16. M. C. Weinstein and Stason 1977, p. 717.
17. Torrance 1987, p. 594.
18. Eddy 1992b, 1992c; Fox and Leichter 1991; Glassman et al. 1997; Hadorn 1991; Kitzhaber 1993; Klevit et al. 1991; Oberlander 2007; Rosoff 2014, chapter 2.
19. P. J. S. Neumann et al. 2005.
20. Kantarjian et al. 2013; Fojo et al. 2014; Kocher and Roberts 2014.
21. This was elegantly pointed out by Harris (1987). Of course, Harris's arguments must be viewed from the perspective of his living in England with the National Health Service (NHS), thus his references to the just distribution of national resources within the context of the state's concern for individual lives and welfare (see also Soares 2012) in this regard in his discussion of the UK's NICE). In a country like the United States, without a system analogous to the NHS, it is unclear that the state's concern for individual well-being can be translated into equal distribution of resources, especially those in the healthcare domain that are heavily commoditized.
22. Nord 2005; Nord and Johansen 2014; Irving et al. 2013; Ladin and Hanto 2011; Stahl et al. 2008; Tong et al. 2010.
23. Peter A. Ubel et al. 2000.
24. Loomes and McKenzie 1989; Carr-Hill 1989.
25. Carr-Hill 1989; Sassi 2006.
26. Whitehead and Ali 2010; Drummond et al. 2009; Ollendorf, 2013 #8440; Brazier et al. 2007.
27. Turpcu et al. 2012.
28. P. J. Neumann and Greenberg 2009; Starr 2011.
29. Daniel A. Ollendorf and Pearson 2013; Rawlins and Culyer 2004.
30. Rawlins and Culyer 2004; Shah et al. 2013.
31. Shah et al. 2013. NICE has also noted the specific challenges associated with cases that evoke the so-called "rule of rescue" (Hadorn 1991; Jonsen 1986; Rosoff 2014, chapters 2

and 3). Shah et al. write "NICE SVJ guidance explicitly addresses the issue known in the literature as the 'rule of rescue' or the 'identifiable victim effect'. The second edition of the Social Value Judgements [*sic*]: Principles for the development of NICE guidance document states: 'There is a powerful human impulse, known as the 'rule of rescue', to attempt to help an identifiable person whose life is in danger, no matter how much it costs . . . NICE recognises that when it is making its decisions it should consider the needs of present and future patients of the NHS who are anonymous and who do not necessarily have people to argue their case on their behalf. NICE considers that the principles provided in this document are appropriate to resolve the tension between the needs of an individual patient and the needs of present and future users of the NHS. The Institute has not therefore adopted an additional 'rule of rescue'. . . . NICE sees these as separate issues and does not seek to favour identifiable patients who need an intervention being appraised by NICE over anonymous patients who need other forms of care" (pp. 152–153). One of the unique social justice problems presented by the "rule of rescue" is that almost everyone has someone else who can argue for them (or they can do so themselves) to evoke empathy in others. But very few of these cases become known to strangers outside of the small circle of persons who are intimately involved in the circumstances due to established relationships with the index individual. Publicity of the situation—either by accident or by design (the latter much more frequent and easier in the era of social media)—can arbitrarily elevate the importance of the case over that of the much larger number of the still anonymous similar cases. The former evokes the rule of rescue and frequently leads to the provision of resources (be they the devotion of huge amounts of attention, money, and personnel to saving a child who has fallen down a well, to the reallocation of an organ for transplant that was originally denied) that were otherwise unavailable or refused—fairly or not—to the unidentified majority. How successful NICE has been in resisting the powerful forces unleashed by publicity is unclear (e.g., see http://www.mirror.co.uk/news/uk-news/cancer-patient-denied-life-giving-drugs-3928687; accessed December 17, 2014).

32. Daniel A. Ollendorf et al. 2013; Daniel A. Ollendorf and Pearson 2010; Daniel A. Ollendorf and Pearson 2013. Also see P. J. Neumann and Greenberg 2009.

33. Beveridge 2000.

34. E. J. Emanuel 2014; Callahan 1987, 1990, 1998, 2012. Of course, neither Emanuel nor Callahan were suggesting that 75-year-old men and women be euthanized simply because they had reached that age. The simply suggested that extraordinary, heroic, and expensive efforts to keep them alive should be restricted, especially under conditions of resource scarcity or limitations.

35. Not surprisingly, he also reports the well-known fact that approximately 25% of Medicare dollars are spent in the last year of life (Halpern and Pastores 2010; Hu et al. 2012; Kelley et al. 2011; Riley and Lubitz 2010; Morden et al. 2012; Marik 2014; De Nardi et al. 2015).

36. E. Emanuel, J. 1999; E. Emanuel 2012.

37. Rosoff 2014, chapter 7.

38. Duffy et al. 2010; Schoening et al. 2013.

39. Shakespeare has his character Jacques describe this process as transgressing seven distinct periods (*As You Like It*, Act II, Scene 7):

> All the world's a stage,
> And all the men and women merely players:
> They have their exits and their entrances;
> And one man in his time plays many parts,

His Acts being seven ages. At first the Infant,
Mewling and puking in the nurse's arms.
Then the whining School-boy, with his satchel
And shining morning face, creeping like snail
Unwillingly to school. And then the Lover,
Sighing like furnace, with a woful ballad
Made to his mistress' eyebrow. Then a Soldier,
Full of strange oaths, and bearded like the pard;
Jealous in honor, sudden and quick in quarrel,
Seeking the bubble reputation
Even in the cannon's mouth. And then the Justice,
In fair round belly with good capon lined,
With eyes severe, and beard of formal cut,
Full of wise saws and modern instances,—
And so he plays his part. The sixth age shifts
Into the lean and slippered Pantaloon,
With spectacles on nose, and pouch on side;
His youthful hose, well saved, a world too wide
For his shrunk shank; and his big manly voice,
Turning again toward childish treble, pipes
And whistles in his sound. Last scene of all,
That ends this strange eventful history,
Is second childishness, and mere oblivion,—
Sans teeth, sans eyes, sans taste, sans everything.

40. He makes the point that this might differ among societies. It is also conceivable that societies that more value the aged might consider reversing this allocation scheme except for the fact that expenditures on prenatal care, childhood vaccinations, and the like have a major positive effect on longevity for more people. Thus, although spending enormous sums on the very old to keep them alive a bit longer may exhibit some sort of veneration for the elderly, it would be more prudent to enable a greater proportion of the population to reach a ripe old age by prioritizing healthcare for younger people. See Norman Daniels 1983, chapters 4–5.
41. Norman Daniels 1983, p. 92.
42. http://www.fda.gov/TobaccoProducts/ProtectingKidsfromTobacco/RegsRestricting Sale/ucm205021.htm, accessed October 28, 2014.
43. Ambrose 1989, pp. 264–266, 370.
44. Karlan 2002; Risinger 2003.
45. A typical argument utilized in this discourse is the example of spending enormous sums of money to save the life of a young child versus spending similar amounts to save the life of an elderly patient. For instance, is it reasonable to spend $100,000 to give a 15-year-old a 20% chance of cure for a metastatic rhabdomyosarcoma or the same $100,000 to save the life of a 75-year-old with colon cancer? Assume that the former patient could live to age 75 (ignore the fact that treatment for this cancer is not "free" and there can be significant late toxicities, including second malignancies caused by the therapy) and the latter patient could live to say, 82. One might view this as a bargain to treat the child and expensive per year of life gained for the senior (assuming one thought that QALYs were the most significant feature). But in a wealthy country like the United States that would not wish to make such a choice, this comparison would not

arise. What would come up is whether it would be reasonable to pay for interventions for either the child or the older person that had less than a 5% chance of success or were both palliative (i.e., noncurative) *and* expensive.

46. For interesting analyses and discussions of various aspects of age preferences or weighting, see Cruz-Oliver et al. 2010; Reese et al. 2010; Aki Tsuchiya 1999, 2000; Aki Tsuchiya et al. 2003.

47. Calabresi and Bobbitt 1978.

48. This is not to say that such tradeoffs are irrelevant to the healthcare rationing debate, only that they are of less importance in a society that would demand generosity (both politically and socially) and can afford to be generous (enough). However, in less affluent societies, where these sorts of choices would be perforce necessary because they cannot afford to treat reasonable needs of everyone, this sort of analysis is essential. For example, in many European countries, it is relatively less common to offer dialysis to elderly patients (say, over the age of 75) with new end-stage renal failure, while this is uncommon in the United States (http://www.usrds.org/adr.aspx, accessed November 26, 2014). There are a numbers of reasons why this therapy is offered liberally in the United States, including the fact that Medicare pays for most of the costs via the End-Stage Renal Disease Program, and dialysis and ancillary services can provide a substantial portion of income for nephrologists (Wish et al. 2014; http://www.nephrologynews.com/articles/109383-changes-in-practice-size-revenue-sources-mark-rpa-benchmarking-survey, accessed November 26, 2014).

49. Saving lives per se, without due consideration for the kind of life being saved, would seem not only shortsighted, but foolish: saving the life of an 80-year-old man with progressive, severe dementia means that one has saved the life of someone whose life span is not only quite limited but also may be unappreciated. Similarly, saving the life of a profoundly intellectually disabled 25-year-old (say, with a mental age of less than 6 months) or in a permanent vegetative state would be to restore someone to the minimal existence she had previously. Minimizing pain—even in those whose ability to experience pain may be minimal itself—would seem to be a priority in these kinds of cases, irrespective of age. Of course, if we were forced to choose between saving the life of a vigorous elder or an otherwise normal child, then it would seem reasonable to emphasize fair innings and others sorts of equalizing arguments.

50. I will discuss this and other forms of uncertainty in greater depth in Chapter 4.

51. Hacker 2010, tables 1 and 2.

52. Eichler et al. 2004; M. Weinstein, C. 2008; P. J. Neumann et al. 2014. Also see Sendi and Al 2003.

53. Rosoff 2014, chapter 6.

54. Braithwaite et al. 2008.

55. Peter A. Ubel and Loewenstein 1996; Peter A. Ubel et al. 2000; Stolk et al. 2002; Stolk et al. 2005.

56. Larson 2013.

57. C. J. L. Murray and Lopez 2013, p. 449.

58. (Vos et al. 2015)

59. Struijk et al. 2013.

60. C. J. Murray et al. 2013.

61. For example, see Oostvogels et al. 2015.

62. Despite numerous and repeated studies demonstrating how poorly the United States compares to other wealthy industrialized nations on standard arbiters of

population health, mere embarrassment has not seemed to provide sufficient motivation to Congress and others to make any substantive moves to address these problems (Davis and Ballreich 2014; Davis et al. 2014).

63. Marrow and Joseph 2015.
64. Rosoff 2014, chapter 6.
65. Reimers 1998; Schrag 2010.
66. Lee et al. 2001; Ziv and Lo 1995.
67. Indeed, the Affordable Care Act expressly forbids government healthcare funding for undocumented people. See Patient Protection and Affordable Care Act of 2010, §1312f.
68. For example, see the website of the Federation for American Immigration Reform (FAIR): http://www.fairus.org/issue/illegal-immigration-is-a-crime or that of the Citizens for Immigration Law Enforcement (CICE): http://www.citizensforlaws.org/index.php?option=com_content&view=article&id=76&Itemid=101, both accessed December 19, 2014.
69. *Estelle et al. v. Gamble* 1976.
70. McKneally and Sade 2003; Meyers 2002; Santiago-Delpin 2003; Schneiderman and Jecker 1996. Also see http://auburnpub.com/news/local/inmate-gets-organ-transplant-evaluation/article_be90ddbc-6d58-11e0-b7cb-001cc4c03286.html, accessed December 19, 2014.
71. Afendulis et al. 2011; Finkelstein and McKnight 2008; J. McWilliams et al. 2003; J. M. McWilliams et al. 2007.
72. Alexander 2010; Stevenson 2014.
73. Griffin and Prieto 2008.
74. Rosoff 2014.

Chapter 3

1. In this chapter, I am going to intermingle and at times conflate the terms "healthcare" and "medicine." This is more out of convention than to convey any kind of deeper meaning. When I speak of the goals of medicine, I am referring more specifically to the kinds of intervention that doctors (and to a certain extent nurses) perform and control. This does not mean that I wish to diminish what have been called the social determinants of disease or human welfare as they contribute to human suffering. When I speak of healthcare, I am more often reflecting on a system or structure.
2. I do not count the Affordable Care Act as comprehensive healthcare reform for several reasons: it is unlikely to result in significant savings or decreases in escalating healthcare costs, it leaves intact the hybrid public–private healthcare delivery structure in which the fee-for-service model will continue to dominate, and it still leaves indefensible numbers of people uninsured. While it is a major improvement, it will do little to solve either the fiscal or moral defects in American healthcare.
3. Davis et al. 2014; Davis and Ballreich 2014.
4. Philip M. Rosoff 2014, especially chapters 1 and 7.
5. Wennberg 2002; Anthony et al. 2009; Song et al. 2010; Brownlee 2008; Berwick and Hackbarth 2012; Welch 2011; Cassel Ck 2012; Hoffman and Pearson 2009; Tilburt and Cassel 2013; Brody 2012. Also see Callahan 2009.
6. However, it is also valuable to bear in mind that the numbers of people who adhere to the most strict, conservative libertarian convictions are relatively few. Many who loudly profess their allegiance to small and limited government are also the first to defend

their "right" to have tax breaks that affect them or their livelihoods (such as the home mortgage interest deduction or the tax-free health insurance premiums paid by businesses for their employees) or their entitlements such as Social Security or Medicare (i.e., "keep your goddamn hands off my Medicare!"; see http://www.huffingtonpost.com/bob-cesca/get-your-goddamn-governme_b_252326.html).

7. Atkinson et al. 2014

8. Kahn et al. 2014

9. Best and Scott 1923; Simoni et al. 2002.

10. Banting et al. 1922.

11. Dart et al. 2014; Zoungas et al. 2014.

12. Saran et al. 2015.

13. Tenner 1996, especially chapter 3.

14. B. W. Ward and Schiller 2013; Schneider et al. 2009.

15. Vogeli et al. 2007.

16. Leff 2008; Dixon-Woods et al. 2011.

17. While some types of cancer can be cured (especially in children), many types can be turned into chronic conditions, similar to HIV, with newer kinds of drugs. For example, chronic myelogenous leukemia, formerly a uniformly fatal disease that could only be treated by sibling tissue-matched bone marrow transplantation, can now be successfully controlled with imatinib (or one of its newer "relatives"). See Mathisen et al. 2014

18. Hanson 1999, p. 144.

19. Tappero and Tauxe 2011.

20. Hanson and Callahan 1999; Special Supplement: The Goals of Medicine: Setting New Priorities 1996; Cassell 1982; Nordenfelt 2001.

21. See the McMath and Munoz cases for the absurdity of these situations (Gostin 2014).

22. In their seminal paper on medical futility, Schneiderman, Jecker, and Jonsen argued that one criterion for continuing to provide intensive care—and hence meeting a need for it—would be that there was some realistic probability that the patient would be able to be maintained outside of an ICU setting, as well as not being permanently unconscious (Lawrence J. Schneiderman et al. 1990). This does not mean that advances in supportive care technology have not enabled some people to live productive lives outside of the ICU. For example, when they published their paper 25 years ago, portable, tabletop ventilators did not yet exist and the ability to administer medications at home via permanently implanted intravenous catheters had yet to be developed to the level of sophistication we see today. Concomitant with these technical advances has been the wholesale growth of a homecare industry that can help care for the medical and equipment needs of these patients. Thus, many people who would previously have been confined to permanent residency in an ICU due to the lack of capabilities to deliver their supportive care requirements outside of such a setting can now be supported. This also means that the patients remaining in the ICU with incurable—and usually multiorgan—dysfunction are sicker than ever and cannot be transitioned to the sort of outpatient care that is currently available. Will further advances in supportive care enable even more patients to make this transition? Perhaps that does not challenge the validity of their assertion.

23. As Pellegrino writes in his essay on the ends of medicine, "it means that proposed public policies regarding medicine must ultimately return to the ends of medicine. Societal policy must not frustrate the ends of medicine—healing, helping, curing, caring and cultivating health—but rather enhance those ends. If these distinctions are kept clear, a

valid relationship can be established between the ends of medicine essentially defined [meaning, inwardly or internal to itself as a profession and human activity], and the purposes and goals that society may wish to attain through medicine." (Pellegrino 1999 p. 65)

24. Frankfurt gives a very nice explanation of this form of urgency (he calls it necessity) and "precedence"; see Frankfurt 1984.

25. Smith (1994) on necessities versus luxuries book, 5, chapter 2, part 2, pp. 938–939.

26. Nevitt 1977, p. 115.

27. For example, see Brock 1998.

28. "We can never survey our own sentiments and motives, we can never form any judgment concerning them; unless we remove ourselves, as it were, from our own natural station, and endeavour [sic] to view them as at a certain distance from us. But we can do this in no other way than by endeavouring to view them with the eyes of other people, or as other people are likely to view them. Whatever judgment we can form concerning them, accordingly, must always bear some secret reference, either to what are, or to what, upon a certain condition, would be, or to what, we imagine, ought to be the judgment of others. We endeavour to examine our own conduct as we imagine any other fair and impartial spectator would examine it. If, upon placing ourselves in his situation, we thoroughly enter into all the passions and motives which influenced it, we approve of it, by sympathy with the approbation of this supposed equitable judge." (Smith 1969/1759 pp. 162–163.

29. Cohen 1996, p. 269.

30. Frankfurt gives the example of someone with a life-threatening disease who can have his life prolonged by surgery but decides to use his time and resources to go on a cruise he has always wanted to take; see Frankfurt 1984, p. 1. Arguably, many would not make this choice, seeing the "need" for surgery to be much more significant than the "desire" for the cruise, but it is his to make. However, as a practical matter, it is not uncommon for others (especially family members and health care providers) to question the wisdom of such choices, even to the point of suggesting that the person may be cognitively disabled and therefore should undergo testing to see if he is "competent." This is especially true when patients refuse the advice of their doctors. Indeed, it is an old truism that patient capacity to make healthcare decisions is rarely questioned when the patient agrees with the doctor (even if it's a possibly demented person simply nodding her head in acceptance and smiling somewhat vacantly), but when the doctor's recommendation is refused, then the patient "must" be incompetent.

31. Throughout this book, I will often refer to elective cosmetic surgery (itself a statement about the "neediness" of it) as an example more of a want or desire rather than a healthcare need of the sort that can exert a claim power on a nationalized health system to be met. But there are many other examples to which we could turn as well, including things like tattoo removal, recombinant human growth hormone treatment for constitutionally "short" children, and testosterone supplementation for older men. All raise similar questions about necessity as well the challenges of cutoff decisions.

32. See Philip M. Rosoff 2014, chapter 6.

33. Daniels 2008.

34. Thomson 2005.

35. Wiggins and Dermen 1987.

36. Daniels 1983, pp. 70–71.

37. Thomson 2005, p. 177.

38. Doyal and Gough 1991, chapter 4.
39. Daniels 2008, chapter 2.
40. Nussbaum 2000, chapter 1; and Sen 2005; Nussbaum and Sen 1993. Of course, what satisfiers are required to meet basic health needs and what exactly those needs may be remains to be described; the blanks must be filled in. McGregor et al. attempt to global-ize Doyal and Gough's theory of needs and try to use local quality-of-life assessments to distinguish between needs (and their satisfiers) and wants; they succeed somewhat, but I am not sure how this helps us here (McGregor et al. 2009). Of course, they utilize the main definition of needs in which the absence of satisfaction leads to grave harm.
41. Rivers 2008.
42. Frankfurt 1984; Braybrooke 1987; Wiggins 1998; Wiggins and Dermen 1987.
43. Cassell 1982, 1983, 1991, 1999a, 1999b.
44. Cassell 1999b, p. 106. I make this statement only in reference to healthcare for humans because this is what this book is about. This does not mean in any way that sentient, nonhuman animals cannot suffer and therefore do not deserve our moral empathy and compassion (and, to the extent that it is feasible, the relief or avoidance of inten-tional imposition of suffering). As Bentham so notably wrote: "The French have already discovered that the blackness of the skin is no reason why a human being should be abandoned without redress to the caprice of a tormentor. It may come one day to be rec-ognized, that the number of the legs, the villosity of the skin, or the termination of the *os sacrum*, are reasons equally insufficient for abandoning a sensitive being to the same fate? What else is it that should trace the insuperable line? Is it the faculty of reason, or, perhaps, the faculty of discourse? But a full-grown horse or dog, is beyond comparison a more rational, as well as a more conversible animal, than an infant of a day, or a week, or even a month, old. But suppose the case were otherwise, what would it avail? the question is not, Can they *reason*? nor, Can they *talk*? but, Can they *suffer*?" (Bentham 1970, p. 283b, emphasis in the original). This statement underscores the relevant and significant point that what is required to suffer is consciousness of a sort that can have the experience of suffering. Verbal ability and advanced, developed cognition are not necessary. Thus, earthworms, which are assuredly conscious in some sort of minimal-ist neurological sense, do not suffer in the way that concerns us (although I imagine it may concern some, but their numbers must be very few indeed). But normal babies, the intellectually disabled either congenitally (e.g., Down syndrome) or acquired (e.g., Alzheimer's disease) *can* suffer and deserve (*need*) to have their suffering relieved.
45. This statement also entails that nonhuman animals (or at least vertebrate animals) that are sentient can also suffer. That they may do so in a manner that may be different or alien to we humans does not matter to the fact of the existence of their suffering and the duty we have to neither cause unnecessary suffering and to relieve it if feasible. This brings to mind Jeremy Bentham's the famous statement about extending the umbrella of moral concern to animals by virtue of their capacity to suffer: "the question is not, Can they reason? nor, Can they talk? but, Can they suffer?" (Bentham 1970, p. 311). This does not mean that conscious animals should be afforded equivalent respect, rights, and privileges as humans. Rather, it strongly argues that the suffering of animals in this class should be taken sufficiently seriously to acknowledge and merit our compassion and hence intervention.
46. Importantly, this does not include persons who are temporarily unconscious, such as those receiving general anesthesia or patients for whom there is reason to believe their unconscious state may be transient (either in its duration or depth).

47. The case of Sunny von Bulow is illustrative. Ms. von Bulow's family could pay for her to be kept alive for decades at Columbia-Presbyterian Medical Center, but the public financing would not. Ms. von Bulow was maintained in a coma (permanent vegetative state) for many years after she suffered an event after an overdose of insulin. Depending on which story one wishes to believe, it was either an accident or an attempted murder at the hands of her husband, Claus. He was tried in a sensational case (sensational enough to be made into a TV movie, the *sine qua non* for these sorts of events) but was acquitted with the assistance of his attorney, Alan Dershowitz. See Dershowitz 2013 and http://www.nytimes.com/2008/12/07/nyregion/07vonbulow.html?pagewanted=all.

48. This is an important point and essential to my argument. Many people are under the mistaken impression that modern medicine possesses the capability of curing many more diseases or conditions that it actually does. Many people believe that many more therapeutic interventions are considerably more effective than they actually are, perhaps from their depiction in popular culture or perhaps simply from the expressed hope that they are (Diem et al. 1996; Lapostolle et al. 2013). Nevertheless, while it may certainly be understandable that patients with diabetes *want* a cure for their illness, they do not *need* one since that currently does not exist. What they can definitely need is treatment for the suffering (both experienced and potential) attendant to diabetes. The potential suffering is what could occur if the disease is not well managed (i.e., blindness, peripheral neuropathy, heart disease, kidney failure, etc.). Therefore, one should not equate the relief of suffering with cure, although occasionally the two are approached by identical means.

49. Liss also points out the fundamental importance of framing healthcare needs within an overall theory of the goals of healthcare (Liss 2003).

50. Sheaff 2002.

51. For example, see A. Buchanan 2008; Allen Buchanan et al. 2000.

52. Sheaff 2002, pp. 9809.

53. Ozar 1983.

54. Of interest is the fact that he does not cite Maslow, who can be reasonably be said to be the originator of the idea of a "hierarchy of needs." See Abraham H. Maslow 1948.

55. Daniels 2008, especially chapter 2.

56. Hasman et al. 2006; Hope et al. 2010. Niklas Juth wrote an interesting paper in 2013 in which he mostly endorsed the "prioritarianism" views of healthcare needs proposed by Hope et al. (see above) as well as Crisp, but with certain caveats and cautions (Juth 2013; Hope et al. 2010; Crisp, 2002 (In this paper Crisp revisits the standard three forms or theories of accounts of well-being: hedonism, desire satisfaction, and objective list explanations as ways of stating what worthy objectives for need satisfaction are thought to be (he ends of by trying the mash the three together in a somewhat messy way for healthcare-related needs). Interestingly, he does not mention relief or avoidance of suffering or harm as an end for need satisfaction (unlike many others: see earlier discussion). In this way, he takes a more positive view: well-being as something to be maintained or improved as opposed to a state in which it is to be restored (or maintained):

> I have suggested that the characteristic feature of principles of needs is that they are sufficientarian, saying that we have a right to a minimally acceptable or good life or health, but nothing more (or at least much weaker claims beyond that level). Accordingly, principles of needs must answer two distributive questions: (1) when do we have sufficient, that is, when do further claims to health care lack normative

force (or cease to be legitimate)? And (2) how should we prioritise [sic] among those who do not yet have sufficient? I also argued that Crisp's version, which combines sufficientarianism with prioritarianism below the threshold of need, is the version best equipped to answer these questions as well as meeting the challenges formulated by Hope, Østerdal and Hasman. . . . A principle of need must be complemented either with a theory on the human good or a theory about the proper goals of health care, or so I have argued. Second, it has to say something about where the threshold should be set, that is, what is minimally good. . . . I think therefore that prioritarianism in principle allows us to adopt plausible principles of need in practice, principles that then can be adjusted to changes in situations: in a very affluent society (or world) public health care can spend more resources on problems that are, relatively speaking, trivial. However, then we have left sufficientarianism behind and we have to formulate principles of need outside a sufficientarian framework. (p. 13)

There are some problems with his approach, as with many others who try to measure health gains by improvement in some metric. But if an important component in well-being is feeling well, then there must be room for putting palliative and end-of-life care in a central place for healthcare benefits. Interestingly, he mentions Crisp's threshold issue and seems to refer to it as a boundary or cut-off problem (as it undoubtedly is): "The plausibility of any principle of need seems conditional on where more precisely the threshold lies. However, any attempt to make the threshold more precise seems to run into problems. This becomes especially apparent when considering those close to the threshold" (p. 12). I don't think one needs some sort of comprehensive theory of the good or the good life to come up with a plausible concept of healthcare needs. One can (simply) frame it within an understanding (be it common or philosophical) of what the goals of medicine are (or should be). It is not unreasonable to propose the following:

- To prevent, relieve, or reduce suffering.
- To restore and/or preserve (to the extent reasonable or feasible and/or desired by the patient) function (whatever that may be; this could also possibly include the restoration and/or preservation of biological life, with or without the caveat that it should be a life capable of being experienced, i.e., one with some reasonable level of consciousness that some reasonable number of people would endorse as acceptable to themselves if they were in that position).

This should enable one to determine needs based on the degree to which a person is suffering and/or has diminished function that medicine is capable to addressing or satisfying. Furthermore, it permits one to fill in the needs function formula: A needs X to satisfy Y, where Y should fall under the umbrella of (I) and (ii) above. It should be noted that both (i) and (ii) refer to conditions to which all (rational) humans are liable to experience and wish to avoid. Furthermore, (ii) refers to a condition that all (rational) humans wish to pursue or obtain. This confers the normative force on those kinds of needs that can be met by healthcare and thus exerts a claim on all of us to help each other to the extent that we can (e.g., by paying taxes to support a healthcare system and voting to have universal, single payer healthcare). See Gustavsson (2013) for an interesting take on this. Her proposal formulates healthcare needs as a special version of the instrumental needs formula: "X has a *health care need* for y in order to z: y *can benefit* x in order to z." Unfortunately, he leaves open what he means by benefit that is a glaring deficiency in his theory.

57. Hadorn 1991.
58. Boorse 1977.
59. That being said, there are likely some people—undoubtedly rare—who are naturally resistant to this bacterium and do not (or cannot) be infected with it. A good example of this situation are those rare individuals who naturally carry a variant of the cell surface protein that is vital for attachment and internalization of the human immuno-deficiency virus (HIV). These people are thus innately immune to HIV (Liu et al. 1996). The important point is that biology and pathobiology are complex, and they may not be absolutes that can categorically distinguish between disease and health.
60. Boorse 1977, p. 555.
61. Kingma 2007; Krag 2013.
62. Krag 2013, p. 8.
63. The story of the evolution of the views by the American psychiatric community of whether homosexuality is a "mental illness" or not is instructive in this matter (De Block and Adriaens 2013; Greco 2015; Cooper 2006).
64. Sandel 2012; Satz 2010.
65. "What constitutes suffering or wretchedness or harm is an essentially contestable matter, and it is to some extent relative to a culture, even to some extent relative to people's [sic] conceptions of suffering wretchedness and harm" (Wiggins 1998, p. 11).
66. Braybrooke 1987, chapter 2, § 2.
67. See Magi and Allander (1981) for a nice discussion of the differences between one's perceived need(s) and those perceived by others about someone else. Also see Jeffers et al. 1971. The denomination of "patient-centered care" (Barry and Edgman-Levitan 2012) has led some to suggest that needs should primarily be defined by patients themselves, rather than by some other arbitrary power (Starfield 2009).
68. The exact circumstances of her original medical condition have not been revealed in the public press, so we do not know why it was felt that she needed this surgery. Photographs of her before the events that followed surgery show a smiling young teenager who was overweight. Hence, it seems reasonable to believe that perhaps the operation was indicated for sleep apnea, a common condition in the obese. For a detailed chronology, see http://en.wikipedia.org/wiki/Jahi_McMath_case, accessed June 13, 2014. For commentary see Magnus et al. 2014; Gostin 2014. Both these articles also refer to the Munoz case in Texas in which a pregnant young woman who suffered anoxic brain damage and met neurologic criteria for death was maintained on "life" support despite the wishes of her husband and family (and her physicians). The decision to remove her from mechanical ventilation was finally ordered by a court.
69. All the cases I discuss in this book use pseudonyms unless the case is publicly known (such as that of Jahi McMath or Helga Wanglie). I have also changed some of the details to preserve anonymity.
70. In a "pulseless electrical activity" condition, there is discernable electrical activity in the heart as determined by an ECG, but there is no pulse (so the heart is not pumping effectively for circulation). Not infrequently, PEA arrests have a nonshockable rhythm, meaning that defibrillation (the paddles one sees applied to the chest with almost 100% positive effect on TV shows) would be ineffective; similarly, the implantable defibrillator would probably not fire. These events have a poor prognosis (Mehta and Brady 2012).
71. I will discuss miracles and other requests for interventions based on similar phenomena in chapter 5.

72. This case has remarkable similarities to the famous Helga Wanglie case from Minnesota, except that, in this case, the courts were not involved. See Angell 1991; Golenski and Nelson 1992; Miles 1991.
73. L. J. Schneiderman and Jecker 2011.
74. Botter et al. 2014.
75. Luetke et al. 2014.
76. P. D. Jacobson and Parmet 2007, p. 205.
77. *Abigail Alliance for Better Access v. Von Eschenbach* 2007.
78. Pittler et al. 2011.
79. Campbell et al. 2013; Menchik and Jin 2014
80. Manning et al. 1987.
81. van Dijk et al. 2013.
82. The way I use "necessity here" and throughout the remainder of this chapter and the book is different from the manner in which the term was employed by Frankfurt (1984).
83. See https://www.nextgen.com/SEO/RCM.aspx?cm_mmc_o=7BBTkwCjCq24CjCPyBz pCjC4BEftkY&gclid=CPT3r9eZuL4CFUMF7AodtUAAzQ, for example; accessed May 19, 2014).
84. Taitsman 2011.
85. This story also illustrates the trap that exists when prescribing what is good for others without necessarily taking into consideration whether you would view the situation differently if you were the recipient of the prescription (or proscription). In other words, any attempt to implement universal rules must employ a Kantian "universalizability" directive or imperative. Indeed, it may be useful to have those empowered with the initial decisions on coverage to place themselves in a theoretical Rawlsian "initial position" with a "veil of ignorance" so that they don't know what their own medical condition is or will be. It is interesting that it is often stated that one of the unique things about healthcare is that we are all susceptible or vulnerable to getting sick (and almost all of us will be at some time or another), and hence it evokes a special sense of harmony among us. That should also be true for the "need" for clean air and water and a decent climate, but we have loads of people who think we should compromise on water, air, and climate change for short-term economic gratification. This shortsightedness will undoubtedly plague any attempt to come up with a "one-size-fits-all" definition for need or necessity.
86. See Philip M. Rosoff 2014, especially chapter 7. The importance of the lack of any negative impact on the average recipient of commercial insurance in the United States cannot be overestimated, as Starr (2011) has emphasized.
87. (Kirch et al. 2012)
88. Gaskin et al. 2014.
89. Chahine et al. 2011; Dwyer-Lindgren et al. 2014; Cerdá et al. 2010; Lee et al. 2014; Levine 2011.
90. Philip M. Rosoff 2014. Although, it should be pointed out that the less-well-funded NHS came out quite well in the most recent Commonwealth Fund report on the state of health and healthcare outcomes in the major industrialized countries (Davis and Ballreich 2014). Also see Chapter 6 in this volume.
91. Crisp 2002.
92. For example, see Bergthold 1995; Hall 2003; A. Ward 2007; A. Ward and Johnson 2013; Singer and Bergthold 2001. Morreim (2001) speaks about the "futility of medical necessity" and refers to its history as emerging coincident with health insurance itself

in the 1940s and 1950s. She calls it too vague and variable to have much utility, as well as being clinically "artificial," unreliable, and restrictive. She suggests that "[health-care insurance] plans should jettison the notion of medical necessity and the vague promises of providing 'all the care you need.' Instead, plans should turn to guidelines-based contracting: they should lay open to consumers the clinical guidelines by which they make benefit determinations, explain the procedures by which the guidelines will change over time, describe the procedures they use to adjudicate disputes and resolve ambiguous cases, and then make those guidelines and procedures the explicit basis on which they contract with enrollees. Put simply, plans should say to consumers, 'If you buy this plan, here is what you will receive'" (p. 25). Of course, this proposal has the limitation of guidelines themselves. Of course, this proposal suffers from the intrinsic limitations of clinical guidelines themselves – not only the many conditions or clinical situations for which guidelines do not exist or where the evidence base is minimal (so-called Class C or Class D evidence) – but the fact that they are or can be heavily influenced by conflicts of interest amongst the guideline writers, thus skewing their recommendations.

As described by Bergthold (somewhat previewing the later paper by Morreim), the history of the term "medical necessity" as operationalized by insurers changed over time as cost pressures increased (Bergthold 1995). Initially, it was a term of art to describe in general terms what should be covered in a standard insurance contract, leaving to physicians to fill in the blanks of what was medically indicated. As medical or healthcare costs started to skyrocket, and especially with the introduction of Medicare and Medicaid in the 1960s and 1970s, it became increasingly used to limit what would be covered by narrowing the definition of what was "necessary." She cites *Doe v. Bolton* as the Supreme Court case that established the precedent that physicians have the legal mandate to determine what is necessary for their patients. Notwithstanding this case, doctors' recommendations are not absolute and have frequently been successfully contested. Courts have also been sympathetic to patients claiming that their pleas of medical necessity for a treatment were unfairly denied, even if there existed little evidence for efficacy at the time (*Doe v. Bolton* 1973).

93. https://www.healthcare.gov/glossary/medically-necessary/, accessed April 10, 2014). This is also the definition used by Medicare for payment.
94. Card et al. 2004; Duggan et al. 2014; Baiker et al. 2012.
95. P. Shekelle 2004, p. 228.
96. Abbott and Stevens 2014. Also see P. Shekelle 2004; Park et al. 1986.
97. D. M. Eddy 1997.
98. Hadorn 1991; Oberlander et al. 2001.
99. But perhaps worthwhile? In a sense, this approach is also somewhat similar to clinical guidelines prepared by specialty societies (for example).
100. Lawson et al. 2012.
101. Brouwers et al. 1997; Higgins and Green 2009.
102. There is an uneasy but time-honored usage of anecdotes or personal "clinical experience" in medical decision-making; see Aronson 2003; Aronson and Hauben 2006; Butterworth 2009; Kosko et al. 2006; Nunn 2011; Phillips 2009; Stuebe 2011. However, as Tvesrky and Kahneman's work demonstrates, anecdotes may operate via the "availability heuristic" in which notable events can be recalled easily and quickly and hence overly influence decision-making (Tversky and Kahneman 1973, 1974; Kahneman 2011). Anecdotes gain their authority by having an impact on the participant(s) who

remember the special or unique aspects of the situation and its context. When confronted with a similar (or similar enough) set of circumstances, the clinician immediately recalls the prior event (but now it is an anecdote) and attempts to match it with the current situation. Unfortunately, the anecdote may represent a "one-off" condition and hence may exert undue influence. Almost any physician or nurse can remember patients and events that made a huge impression upon them and are easy to recall many years later. Introspective or reflective clinicians will admit how these experiences influence how they approach similar cases. Undoubtedly, anecdotes also employ the "risk as feelings" effect for negative-outcome experiences (Hemmerich et al. 2012; Goldstone et al. 2004; also see Woolf 2012).

103. Andrew Hutchings and Raine 2006; Carpenter et al. 2007; Taffé et al. 2004. To quote from the literature review and analysis of Hutchings and Raine: "We found that practitioners who perform a procedure tended to emphasise [sic] the appropriateness of the procedure compared with non-performing practitioners, and that individuals from groups that were subject to performance criteria are more critical of those criteria than individuals from other groups. These findings may be secondary to practitioners having greater knowledge in their own field, or because they only see a subset of patients with a given condition whom the referring physicians deem are appropriate for the clinical intervention offered by that practitioner. Finally, the research evidence that participants have knowledge of may be based on selected patients rather than all those with the relevant condition. We also found evidence that participating in a mixed rather than single-specialty group, even without face- to-face contact, has a moderating effect on these differences. This suggests that participants learn from colleagues in other specialties during the consensus process. Multi-specialty groups are therefore preferable to single-specialty groups" (pp. 178–179).

104. Sanmartin et al. 2008.

105. Krahn and Naglie 2008; David M. Eddy et al. 2011; Owens 2011; Qaseem et al. 2012.

106. Perhaps one of the biggest real-life practical challenges would be the firestorm of political opposition for both ideological and self-interest reasons. For example, see the stories about the Agency for Healthcare Research and Quality (AHRQ; neé, the Agency for Health Care Policy and Research [AHCPR]) in Gray et al. 2003; Sorenson et al. 2014.

107. P. Shekelle 2004.

108. Bogdan-Lovis et al. 2012; Sinclair et al. 2013; Qaseem et al. 2012; *Clinical Practice Guidelines We Can Trust* 2011.

109. Fitch et al. 2001, pp. 2–3; Brook et al. 1986.

110. Kahan et al. 1994, p. 359 (emphasis in the original).

111. Cupler et al. 2012; Kishnani et al. 2006.

112. Moraes Vinícius et al. 2014.

113. Undoubtedly, there will be strong advocates for these treatments or interventions, both professional (some orthopedic surgeons, for example) and from the lay public (such as patients who will swear that they were helped by the intervention). Indubitably, they will serve as formidable opponents to either restrictive regulation or worse, elimination from payment by a nationalized health scheme. However, the burden should be on them to present evidence supporting their claims to the RAM panels (or some other analogous mechanism that is adopted) to argue their case. One of the major challenges will be to minimize the corrosive effects of politics in judging the veracity of benefit

claims; hence, the panels will have to be immunized—to the extent possible—from undue influence from these groups.

Interestingly, the IOM reports on essential health benefits does a great deal to define a process for the Secretary of Health and Human Services to make a list (it should be similar to the average list of covered benefits of a typical small employer plan), how it should be open to revision, appeals, etc., but it doesn't actually try to define what is meant by "essential" (Ulmer et al. 2012*a*, 2012*b*). By approaching it this way, they are basically begging the question by saying that essential benefits are those that are already deemed essential. No new ground is being broken. On the other hand, the AHA itself, by mandating the 10 major categories of EHB does state the major categories (without filling in the details).

They also stated that they "did not recommend specific service expansions beyond the 10 categories required by the ACA because these, together with the requirement for the scope of services of typical employers, were seen as sufficiently broad and adding categories beyond these, although not precluded, might prove difficult under the committee process that requires consideration of the overall cost of the package" (Ulmer et al. 2012*b*, p. 81).

That being said, the report does make a very nice presentation on the importance of community engagement as a method for public notification and review with (hopefully) endorsement and buy-in (Ulmer et al. 2012*b*, chapter 6). Of note is a policy statement from the American Academy of Pediatrics (AAP) about the potential impact of possible changes in the functional definition of "medical necessity" during the implementation of the ACA (from the reading of the statement and the lack of referencing, they apparently did not read the IOM reports). They are concerned (as I imagine other specialty society are as well) about the effect of this on their practices and, one would hope, children. They make the following statement: "If patient-centered or scientific evidence for children is insufficient, then professional standards of care for children must be considered. The AAP, other pediatric medical specialty societies, and consensus expert pediatric opinion could serve as references for defining essential pediatric care in the context of medically necessary services. Hence, the pediatric definition of medical necessity should be as follows: health care interventions that are evidence based, evidence informed, or based on consensus advisory opinion and that are recommended by recognized health care professionals, such as the AAP, to promote optimal growth and development in a child and to prevent, detect, diagnose, treat, ameliorate, or palliate the effects of physical, genetic, congenital, developmental, behavioral, or mental conditions, injuries, or disabilities." (Financing 2013, p. 400)

114. I will discuss the problem of doctors acceding to demands or wishes of their patients to meet what could be viewed as inappropriate treatment (and not infrequently having it paid for by insurance companies or Medicare) later in this chapter as well as in Chapter 5. Suffice it to say that procedures would have to be developed to discourage doctors from prescribing inappropriate treatment (i.e., for which there exists little supporting evidence) but, at the same time, taking care not to insert an inadvertent wedge between doctor and patient that could erode trust and the essence of the physician–patient relationship. Part of the solution could be to remove any financial incentives that physicians have to prescribe more drugs (for example), as in the case of oncologists who have significant portions of their incomes tied to prescribing expensive chemotherapy (Philip M. Rosoff 2014, chapter 7; Bach 2013; M. Jacobson et al. 2006.

115. Aronson 2003; Aronson and Hauben 2006; Butterworth 2009; Nunn 2011; Phillips 2009.
116. Tversky and Kahneman 1973, 1974.
117. Leveque 2008; Bazzano et al. 2009; Chen et al. 2009; P. M. Rosoff and Coleman 2011.
118. Bloche 2011, 2012; Callahan 2009.
119. Zuckerman et al. 2011; Basu and Hassenplug 2012; Sorenson and Drummond 2014; Resnic and Normand 2012.
120. Schleifer and Rothman 2012; Carman et al. 2010; Gerber et al. 2010a, 2010b; Emanuel and Fuchs 2008.
121. Bleustein et al. 2014; Zgierska et al. 2014. However, not all agree; see Tsai et al. 2015.
122. Kravitz et al. 2005; Macfarlane et al. 1997.
123. Fenton et al. 2012; also see Sirovich et al. 2008. In a study with a Veterans Administration population it was found that patient satisfaction was very high, even in those patients who came to the doctor's visit with preconceived expectations or desires for something, except for those who wanted certain medications and were denied them (Peck et al. 2004).
124. The Belmont Commission, formed in response to public revelations of the sordid Tuskegee syphilis study, was charged with developing definitions and guidelines for the conduct of clinical research in humans. Their 1978 report and its accompanying essays exploring what kinds of enterprises should be regulated was notable for their definition of research as activities in which the goal is the pursuit of "generalizable knowledge." They distinguished between clinical care utilizing "innovative" methods—essentially something that could be considered to be a one-time event in an individual patient and deemed by the practicing physician to be for the sole benefit of that patient—and research that was appraised as a more broad-based enterprise. They admitted that there could be overlap between the two, but they emphasized the distinction between them based on their goals: either the benefit accruing to one person versus society as a whole. However, in practice, physicians use fairly loose criteria to try something new for their patients and frequently rely on both their clinical judgment and their experience with the same therapy in similar past patients and apply their prior observations (i.e., data). It can be argued that this may qualify in some respects as research. See Biomedical and Behavioral Research 1978; P. M. Rosoff and Coleman 2011.
125. S. D. Ellis et al. 2012 Kircher et al. 2011.
126. D. M. Eddy 1996.
127. D. M. Eddy 1996 p. 653.
128. Ritsinger et al. 2014; Nathan et al. 2005.
129. L. M. Ellis et al. 2014.
130. D. M. Eddy 1997.
131. (Eddy 1997)
132. Guyatt et al. 2010; Jones et al. 2012; Kung et al. 2012; Mendelson et al. 2011; J. Neuman 2011; Norris et al. 2011; Steinbrook and Lo 2012.
133. M. D. Neuman et al. 2014; P. G. Shekelle 2014.
134. Pronovost 2013.
135. Graham et al. 2011. For a different point of view see Jones et al. 2012.
136. (Eddy 1997)
137. Sirovich et al. 2008.
138. Callahan 1991, p. 30.
139. Tomlinson and Brody 1990.

140. Blackhall et al. 1999; Brandon et al. 2005; Fairrow et al. 2004; Barnato et al. 2009; Hanchate et al. 2009.
141. see Sharpe 1997 for an early perspective on this tension.
142. Klein 1994, 1995.
143. Simoens et al. 2013; Rombach et al. 2012.
144. Screening for Breast Cancer: US Preventive Services Task Force Recommendation Statement 2009; Hendrick and Helvie 2011; Squiers et al. 2011; Volk and Wolf 2011; Detsky 2012; Catalona et al. 2012.
145. Starr 2011, p 280.
146. Lott 1992, p. 84.
147. Paul G. Shekelle and Schriger 1996; A. Hutchings et al. 2005. Nevertheless, some pessimism (or realism) is warranted, as pointed out more than 20 years ago by Blustein and Marmor. For many reasons, they urged caution before placing much hope in waste-cutting by making rules to control healthcare costs. One of the most significant reasons was the professional "duty" they found in physicians' devotion to what they believed to be their patients' welfare, irrespective of cost (or, for that matter, data). They write:

> The "professional imperative" will prevail unless powerfully constrained. While many physicians will refrain from performing procedures known to be ineffective, most will not be willing to unilaterally cut other "wasteful" activities (practices of uncertain effectiveness, activities that are ethically problematic, and therapies that are not allocationally efficient). If doctors will not say "no" to their patients, then we can expect that payers will begin to say "no" to doctors. And indeed they have begun to do so. A new coalition has promised to cut health expenditures by making rules forbidding wasteful treatment. But it is doubtful that "cutting waste" is as straight forward or as painless as the most voluble members of the coalition have suggested. And it is certain that cutting waste by making rules will mean different things to different people. (Blustein and Marmor 1992, p. 1569)

> I suspect that physicians may be somewhat less resistant to this form of rule-making if for no other reason than the creeping incrementalism of "third-party" control over reimbursement for medical services that has produced the result that many doctors have become inured to what might have been previously viewed as loss of professional independence. Whether it is clinical guidelines, prior authorization by insurers, limitations on prescribing by pharmacy benefits managers and formulary inclusion/exclusion, etc., time and irresistible change may have taken its toll and prepared the ground for easier implementation and acceptance of more intrusive rule-making of this sort.

148. Frankfurt 2015.
149. Rawls 1999, pp. 18–19, 42–45.

Chapter 4

1. These and other clinical cases described in the text have been altered to the extent that any identifying features of the patients or families have been removed, but the essential facts and features of the stories have been maintained. When public cases are described or cited, I have retained the identifiers. I would like to thank Dr. Hope Uronis of the Gastrointestinal Malignancy group of the Duke Cancer Institute for her advice on the second case.

2. Aronson 2003; Butterworth 2009; Kosko et al. 2006; Nunn 2011; Phillips 2009. However, it is worth noting that so-called "n-of-1" clinical "trials" may have great utility in optimizing treatment for individual patients when there is real uncertainty about the efficacy, safety, or value of a particular intervention. Admittedly, to truly learn something worthwhile about a specific intervention in a specific patient requires a formalism—not to mention the expertise, interest, and time—that few physicians possess, but it can be tremendously helpful in some clinical situations. See Hankey 2007; Wolfe et al. 2001; Nikles et al. 2005.

3. A. B. Hill 1952; Rothwell 2007.

4. This has been a recurring issue ever since the dawn of statistics in medicine. While the official stance of modern organized medical science embraces the singular and pre-eminent (and correct) role played by statistics, and it is rare indeed that a doctor would claim not to wholeheartedly endorse the basis and practice of evidence-based medicine, reconciling dogma with its real-world application is on shakier ground. Indeed, an anonymous mid-20th-century author writing in the *British Medical Journal*'s collective summary of the previous 50 years' accomplishments of British medicine somewhat acerbically commented (with respect to the general view of the practitioner of the use and significance of medical statistics) that "The mathematical methods develop there in by Pearson and applied by him to biology were undoubtedly slow in influencing scientific thought in general and slower still in entering the medical field. . . . These applications were mainly limited to, however, to the problems of public health and social medicine—the analysis, for instance, of infant mortality in relation to environmental conditions, the study of the epidemic curve, and so on. Clinical medicine was but little influenced, and the method of choice was still too often based upon a handful of uncontrolled cases and 'my personal experience.' To some extent, too, there was antagonism. The medical man charged with the responsibility for the patient was contemptuous of the statistician's fundamental approach through the group; and the statistician took a jaundiced view of the conclusions light-heartedly [*sic*] drawn by the practitioner from a handful of cases without allowance for the play of chance" (Statistics in Medicine 1950, p. 68).

5. Seely 2013.

6. R. C. Fox 1957.

7. Davis 1960. This is an interesting longitudinal study of children with paralytic polio (and their families) from their initial diagnosis through their rehabilitation. During this period, prognosis transitions from being uncertain to quite certain, and the understanding of certainty changed for the families. Initially, they were as knowledgeable about the unknown future outcome as the physicians. However, several months later, the doctors knew what the future would hold as far as disability, but they did not share this with the families. In his interviews with the medical team, Davis believed that uncertainty was maintained to avoid emotionally laden and time-consuming discussions with the families when the prognosis was grim. While it is true that this took place in the heyday of physician paternalism, something similar still exists today when (for example) doctors frequently hold out hope for a brighter future than they "know" is true for the patient's actual prognosis. For example, see Apatira et al. 2008; Baergen 2006; J. Lantos 2006; Mack et al. 2007; Nurgat et al. 2005; Widera et al. 2011.

8. Montgomery 2006.

9. A. B. S. Hill 1984. Quotation in Horton 2000, p. 3152.

10. Donald A. Redelmeier and Tversky 1990.

11. However, this could take anywhere from 24–48 hours; most primary care practices nowadays utilize a so-called "rapid strep test" that detects one or more of the proteins associated

with the organism and can be performed quite quickly in the practitioner's office (Nakhoul and Hickner 2013). The sensitivity and specificity of these test kits is quite good and have mostly (although not completely) eliminated the use of throat cultures (Lean et al. 2014). However, if the history, symptoms, and physical examination are "classic," some doctors may simply make the diagnosis and forgo the test, assuming that the risk of antibiotics is very small (this may or may not be a completely reasonable assumption).

12. In common medical parlance, treating a patient without firm evidence of the cause(s) of the problem(s) is somewhat confusingly known as "empiric" therapy.

13. Ronald M. Epstein and Gramling 2013.

14. As I argued previously (Philip M. Rosoff 2014), such a healthcare system should also be predicated upon removing many of the perverse incentives that currently exist, including the fact that many nephrologists make a substantial percentage of their living based on prescribing dialysis and its associated medicines. In addition, commercial dialysis centers have been a source of substantial profits almost since the End-Stage Renal Disease Program was added to Medicare in 1972. Diminishing or deleting the profit motive for initiating and keeping people on dialysis might lead to more considered decisions about which patients can benefit most from this often difficult treatment. See Gabbay et al. 2010; Feroze et al. 2011.

15. See H. G. Welch 2011; Brownlee 2008.

16. A good example of this are the drugs used in advanced pancreatic cancer, which remains a fatal disease; see Conroy et al. 2011; Rahma et al. 2013.

17. Gould 1985.

18. One of the papers he assuredly would have seen to bolster his confidence in his statistical analysis was published by his Harvard colleagues (Antman et al. 1985). I suspect he was not bothered by the problems present in single institution studies of this type, with their inherent selection bias.

19. Djulbecovic et al. 2011.

20. Han et al. 2011.

21. Han 2013, p. 17S.

22. Error as I mean it here is an "honest" mistake due to uncertainty. The risk of errors of all causes can be vastly increased when inherent uncertainty combines with ignorance—willful or not—or negligence. I am referring to what might be called "benign" or unavoidable errors due to the sort of intrinsically probabilistic nature of medicine.

23. Kohn et al. 2000.

24. Pinsky et al. 2013; Johnson and Kline 2010; Singh et al. 2013; Lee et al. 1987; Cadieux et al. 2011. Relying on newer technology to decrease human error may not be perfect either (see Bae et al. 2012), although intensive education may help in some circumstances (see Geller et al. 2014).

25. Baiardini et al. 2009.

26. There is a large literature demonstrating that there can be little correlation between a physician's overall skill and the risk of getting sued for alleged negligence. Although there are some exceptions, in general, caring, nice doctors don't get sued, even if they may be less than competent (even dangerous). See Ho and Liu 2011; Tamblyn et al. 2007; Cydulka et al. 2011.

27. Arawi and Rosoff 2012.

28. Powers et al. 2010; Rothman et al. 2006; Galesic and Garcia-Retamero 2010; Berkman et al. 2011; Manganello and Clayman 2011; Marden et al. 2012. Even though the data

are derived from a 2003 survey and hence are more than 10 years old, there is little reason to believe that the performance of Americans has improved on the comprehensive
National Assessment of Adult Literacy. This survey found that 14% of the survey population had below basic skills, which were defined as "no more than the most *simple
and concrete* literacy skills," and an additional 29% had only basic skills ("can perform
simple and everyday literacy activities"). Source: http://nces.ed.gov/NAAL/kf_demo-
graphics.asp, accessed July 9, 2014. Nevertheless, there may be ways to avoid confusion
and increase mutual understanding of clinical probability through, for instance, using
qualitative terms rather than numbers or other adaptive approaches (R. M. Epstein
et al. 2004; Mazur and Hickam 1991).

29. Galesic and Garcia-Retamero 2010.
30. Berwick et al. 1981; Lisa M. Schwartz et al. 1997; Rao and Kanter 2010; Wegwarth et al.
    2012; Virginia A Moyer 2012.
31. Gigerenzer 2009; Wegwarth et al. 2011, 2012.
32. Daniels and Sabin 2008; P. M. Rosoff 2012, 2014, chapter 3.
33. K. Kaiser et al. 2011; Nguyen et al. 2009; D. E. Jones et al. 2012.
34. L. S. Zier et al. 2008, 2009, 2012. It is also important to note that not all responsibility
    for looking at the future through rose-tinted glasses lies with patients and their fami-
    lies. Indeed, the failure of physicians to adequately explain poor prognoses and enable
    patients to prepare for bad outcomes is well known. For a particularly evocative explo-
    ration of this problem, see the beautiful essay by Wolf and Wolf (Smith 2013; Wolf and
    Wolf 2013).
35. For example, exploiting Reyna's "fuzzy trace theory," in which the most effective way to
    get across information—especially numerically based—is to transmit the "gist" or the
    bottom line (the "bullet points" if you will). See Reyna 2008; Smith and Hillner 2010.
36. Brase 2009; Garcia-Retamero and Hoffrage 2013; Garcia-Retamero and Cokely 2013.
    Unfortunately, these approaches may do little to enable the illiterate and/or innumer-
    ate to understand medical information, especially when it is complex; see Zarcadoolas,
    2011 #8194; Aboumatar et al., 2013 #8193
37. Djulbegovic and Paul 2011.
38. P. M. Rosoff and Coleman 2011.
39. Callahan 2009.
40. McKenna et al. 2013.
41. Bernstein and Bernstein Peter 1996, p. 207. It should be noted that he was writing
    about decision-making under the uncertainty of capital markets investing, but the
    analysis is the same.
42. Goodman 1999; Kahneman 2011; Steiner 1999; Tversky and Kahneman 1981.
43. I discuss this phenomenon in detail in Chapter 5.
44. Quill 1993; Diem et al. 1996; Gupta 2009; Kruskal 1988; Manning and Schneiderman
    1996; Stempsey 2002; Larson et al. 2005; Schenker et al. 2014; Vater et al. 2014.
45. Callahan 2009.
46. The sad and somewhat sordid story over myeloablative chemotherapy with autologous
    stem cell rescue (colloquially and inaccurately labeled as "autologous bone marrow
    transplantation") for advanced breast cancer, a major *cause celebe* in the 1980s and
    early 1990s, was a blatant example; see Rettig et al. 2007.
47. H. G. Welch 2011.
48. Lisa M Schwartz et al. 1997, p. 620. P_C = the percentage experiencing a specified
    event in the control group (it could be a side effect of the medication or an event the

treatment may reduce, for example); P_T = the percentage of study subjects in the exper-imental or treated group who experienced the event. If the treatment is effective, then there should be a reduction in the number of events in the treated group (assume they are bad, and the treatment is designed to decrease them). While it is true that for many complex, multifactorial diseases—meaning illnesses that have a number of causative elements that interact in often unpredictable ways to produce signs and symptoms (a good example is coronary artery disease)—the number needed to treat is rarely close to 1, it often is so for infectious diseases. For instance, one of the triumphs of modern medicine has been the multiplicity of effective vaccines that can almost completely prevent many childhood (and now adult) infections that prior to their introduction caused millions of deaths and horrendous morbidity throughout the world. Indeed, one of these diseases—smallpox—has been eradicated due to universal vaccine. Polio may be the next to be eliminated. While not all children vaccinated with, say measles, mumps, and rubella vaccine (MMR) are immunized against these three viruses, the overwhelming majority are, thus the number needed to treat—the percentage of vac-cinated patients who become immune—is very close to 1. See Demicheli et al. 2012.

49. For the many people in the United States who are religious and who believe in super-natural causation and intervention, especially when they or a loved one are sick, and who fervently and passionately pray for a miraculous cure, explaining the disutility of praying for very rare events (such as cures for advanced metastatic cancer or terminal heart failure) may prove futile. I will discuss this more fully in Chapter 5.

50. Perneger and Agoritsas 2011.

51. Ronald M Epstein et al. 2010; Wells and Kaptchuk 2012; Clark 2009; Jha et al. 2007; Mehta et al. 2010; Mayberry 2014.

52. Politi et al. 2011. For a somewhat different outlook, see Henry 2006.

53. Cousin et al. 2013.

54. Aronson 2003; Fagerlin et al. 2005; Kosko et al. 2006; Nunn 2011. I think the problems with relying on these kinds of "data" are the inherent arbitrariness, bias, and the poor reliability of one's memory of clinical response.

55. Lillie et al. 2011.

56. Tversky and Kahneman 1973, 1974.

57. H. G. Welch 2011; Boggs 2014; Badcott 2013; Churchill and Churchill 2013; Bloss et al. 2014; Howard Brody 2007.

58. Conrad et al. 2010; Thorpe and Philyaw 2012; Brennan et al. 2010; Kenkel and Wang 2013.

59. Wiechers et al. 2013; Slashinski et al. 2012; Vidal et al. 2012.

60. Graf et al. 2013.

61. Niederdeppe et al. 2013. For a different view analyzing and extolling the benefits of such advertising, see Liu and Gupta 2011. A personal note: I had a profoundly upset-ting experience in 2012 when I was approached by an administrator of my institution who wished to discuss with me the role of clinical ethics in patient care. This was part of a larger effort on behalf of the hospital to apply for an award for excellence in administrative governance and organizational quality bestowed by an association of major businesses. However, she did not actually use the word "patient" in describing the people whose care we supervised in the clinics or the wards of the hospital. She called them "customers," which is how they were described in all of the documents submitted in support of the award application. Increasingly, patients are labeled and portrayed as buyers of healthcare goods and services (which is itself both ironic and incorrect because patients themselves rarely pay *in toto* for healthcare), and hospitals

and clinics are designed to cater to their whims (http://www.cbsnews.com/news/
michigan-hospital-goes-luxe-ceo-explains-patient-centered-approach/). When I told
this woman that I was offended by her reference to patients as customers, she had
no idea what I was talking about (I am sure this is where I was transformed from
curmudgeon to crank). I suggested that my Hippocratic devotion to people was on
the basis of my relationship to them as patients, not as customers of goods that my
institution or I had for sale. Sadly, she still did not understand and, I suspect, neither
would legions of her like-minded colleagues, a clearly expanding field as confirmed by
their professional organizations (http://www.aaham.org/ and http://www.ahcap.org/
and http://www.ache.org/) and the proliferation of master's degree programs (https://
www.cahme.org/Background.html). All websites accessed July 8, 2014.

62. Spence et al. 2005. See also R. Moynihan and Cassels 2005; Lane 2007.

63. Liu and Gupta 2011.

64. N. J. Fox and Ward 2008; Kontos and Viswanath 2011.

65. Drosten et al. 2003; Pepin 2011; de Groot et al. 2013.

66. Examples of the former include those powerful patient groups—often openly or sur-
reptitiously sponsored by drug companies who stand to profit if these conditions (and
the supposed treatments) are acknowledged as bona fide diseases—arguing for the
existence of chronic Lyme disease and chronic fatigue syndrome. The former has
failed (to date) in being recognized, whereas the latter is closer to the goal: see Feder
et al. 2007; P. M. Lantos et al. 2013; Holgate et al. 2011.

67. In this category, one usually thinks of infectious diseases, and they certainly are prototypical, but there are some illnesses that also are due to single causes, such as diabetes
(lack or insulin or insulin resistance) and chronic myelogenous leukemia (the bcr-Abl
mutant protein caused by a chromosomal translocation).

68. These problems plague the field of chronic pain management (Solanki et al. 2011;
Dworkin et al. 2012; Kerns et al. 2011).

69. Arnold and Oakley 2013; Mackey and Liang 2012; Humphreys 2009.

70. Jong et al. 2004.

71. Danika Valerie Hall et al. 2011.

72. R. Moynihan and Cassels 2005, p. 9; emphasis in the original.

73. See Bowker and Starr 1999.

74. Greene 2007, chapter 2.

75. There is an interesting history behind the genesis of this convention. It appears that
it began as a "misunderstanding of the hypothesis-testing technique of Neyman and
Pearson. The latter is a common method of making decisions when the absolute probability of an event is unknown; conditional probabilities only can be given" (Edmond
A. Murphy 1965, p. 343. Since the convention was adopted in statistics a p value of
< 0.05 (i.e., < 2 standard deviations from the mean), this was somehow bastardized
onto clinical laboratory medicine (as well as other aspects of newly measureable and
thus statistically analyzable medical data). See also Benson 1972; King 1945; Lyon
1942; McCall 1966; Edmond A. Murphy and Abbey 1967; Sunderman 1949, 1975.

76. Parry 2003.

77. Woloshin and Schwartz 2006; Hadler 2008. One of the more heart-rending examples of
the "treatment" for a benign condition that has thankfully passed out of favor was the
attraction of giving high-dose estrogen (or synthetic estrogens) in the 1950s through the
late 1980s to adolescent girls who were perceived as "tall" or were predicted to become
tall as they approached adult height. The rationale for this was that "excess" height was
deemed by some to cause great distress to young women as it somehow detracted from

their attractiveness to boys/men. Therefore, closing their epiphyses (boney growth plates) and hence halting their linear growth would prevent this distressing condition (Rayner et al. 2010). Aside from the fact that there was little to no actual evidence that such a psychological or somatic "disease" existed or that tall women were anything other than tall, this became a fairly common practice, at least among families who could afford the intervention and cared about such things. Lest one think that this obsession with adult height has been lost, we now have treatments for constitutional short stature with the advent of genetically engineered human growth hormone (huGH). Initially approved by the FDA (and reimbursed by insurance companies for laboratory-proven GH deficiency), it now finds its largest market in children who are normal but short (Sotos and Tokar 2014; Allen and Cuttler 2013). These examples suggest that much of this sort of medicalization, or using traditionally regarded medical treatment or interventions to alter a physical body state, is more in the line of fashion than disease. Some people certainly "suffer" if they cannot keep up with the latest clothes or other expressions of currency in fashionable statements (or have the "right" size or shape nose or be sufficiently tall), but that doesn't entail that they have a disease and all of the socially and economically associated accouterments.

78. It is interesting to note that Medicare will pay for diagnosis and treatment for complications arising from uncovered procedures such as cosmetic surgery, and many (most) commercial insurers follow Medicare guidelines in their own coverage policies. For example, United HealthCare (UHC) states that it will cover (pay for) services "When a member is admitted to the hospital for a non-covered service: (a) Complications of non-covered procedures develop after the member has been formally discharged from the hospital providing the non-covered service. Example: A member undergoes a non-covered cosmetic procedure and, following discharge, develops an infection at the surgical site. Services to treat the infection are covered. This includes subsequent inpatient stays or outpatient treatment ordinarily covered under the member's health plan" (UHC MA Coverage Summary: Non-Covered Services, p. 3).

79. Danika V. Hall et al. 2011.

80. Woloshin and Schwartz 2006.

81. See http://www.rls.org/. I should state clearly that I am not passing judgment on the accuracy or reality of any of these conditions or seeking to deny or denigrate the suffering experienced by people who have these symptoms or have been diagnosed. I simply wish to indicate that the recognition and naming of clusters of signs and symptoms as a bona fide illness or disease is not simple and is constantly open to scrutiny and amendment. Occasionally, new diseases are recognized that were previously unknown, most often due to novel infectious causes such as HIV, SARS, and, more recently, MERS. When an etiologic agent is discovered and known to be causative, it is rather straightforward to "invent" a disease label to accompany it. At other times, it is quite complex, if not controversial. The people who have or claim to have these symptoms clearly are distressed both mentally and physically by them, and the failure of mainstream medicine to recognize them as truly sick can be both frustrating and heartbreaking. These individuals are also prey to the hucksterism of phony practitioners who are more than willing to take advantage of their suffering to enrich themselves. The unsavory story of "chronic Lyme disease" may be an excellent example of this phenomenon (Feder et al. 2007; P. M. Lantos et al. 2013; Cameron 2010; Auwaerter et al. 2011).

82. Ball et al. 2006; K. Jones 2008; Hemminki et al. 2010; Colombo et al. 2012.

83. Larson et al. 2005; Schenker et al. 2014; Vater et al. 2014; Volpp et al. 2012.

84. Gilens 2012, especially chapter 5.
85. Naughton et al. 2009; J. W. Yackee and Yackee 2006; S. W. Yackee 2006, 2012; McKay and Yackee 2007.
86. http://www.futuremedicine.com/page/journal/pme/aims.jsp.
87. While "personalized medicine" as an area of scientific and clinical inquiry is a very sexy area of investigation, I have told my students and younger colleagues for many years that doctors are supposed to deliver personalized medicine to all of their patients and have been expected to do so for millennia. There is no question that their responses—especially those from the more jaded—indicate that I have not kept up with the times.
88. David A. Price Evans et al. 1960.
89. David A. Price Evans 1968.
90. Lunde et al. 1977.
91. Sharis et al. 1998.
92. Cruden et al. 2013.
93. Scott et al. 2013; Holmes et al. 2011.
94. Lala et al. 2013.
95. L. R. Hoffman and Ramsey 2013.
96. J. Kaiser 2012.
97. Balfour-Lynn 2014; Dickenson 2013; O'Sullivan et al. 2013.
98. Braun et al. 2010; Largent and Pearson 2012; Meekings et al. 2012.
99. The current state of such projects is exemplified by the National Cancer Institute's MATCH program (for Molecular Analysis of Therapy Choice; see Chau et al. 2016; McNeil 2015). Its goal is to perform detailed genetic, proteomic, and other profiles of tumors to match their acquired mutations with the latest drugs that are directed at those targets. The prototype is chronic myelogenous leukemia (CML) that is caused (initially) by a mutant fusion protein caused by a translocation between chromosomes 9 and 22 to create the so-called Philadelphia chromosome. The drug imatinib directly targets the abnormal enzyme created by this event and has transformed what was formerly a disease that was difficult to manage—and then only with very toxic drugs— into one that is either a chronic condition or curable. Since the introduction of the revolutionary (and extraordinarily expensive) medicine, many, many more have been introduced that target different identified mutations in cancer. Unfortunately, very few of the most common cancers have only one mutation that causes the disease like CML does (at least initially). Furthermore, the experience with CML has shown that cancer, like bacteria, can be much smarter than we are and frequently evolves resistance mutations.
100. Dickenson 2013.
101. It is worthwhile noting that the commercial genetic testing services (and others) emphasize that the value in knowing more about yourself and your risks for developing some malady is that it helps you change behaviors that could then lead to diminishing (although not eliminating) the risk. The idea thus counters pure determinism in which our fate is already written and decided. It simply attempts to control for that portion that is not flexible and hence immune to lifestyle modification (or surgery, such as prophylactic removal of the breasts for those patients who carry the mutations for BRCA 1 or 2). See Dickenson 2013, pp. 13–18.
102. Begun and Kaissi 2004.
103. Villanueva 2015; Verdin and Ott 2015.
104. Heard and Martienssen 2014.

105. Arah 2009.
106. Arah 2009, p. 238. An interesting variation on this view is provided by Mackenbach 2006.
107. Donne 2010.
108. http://www.secondgenome.com/go/microbiome-profiling/?_kk=microbiome&_
     kt=be2e198c-66df-4cdb-95ff-78d166a05385&gclid=CIeFsomT2b8CFSMV7AodKGs
     AJQ. The microbiome is the huge variety of microorganisms that inhabit our body in
     a steady-state commensal arrangement; see Blaser et al. 2013 for a review.
109. Kenkel and Wang 2013.
110. Philip M. Rosoff 2014, chapter 7.
111. Greene 2007, p. 231. See also Eddy 1984.
112. H. Brody 2005, 2007; Angell 2004; Kassirer 2005.
113. H. G. Welch 2011.
114. H. G. Welch and Black 2010; Virginia A. Moyer 2012; Esserman et al. 2013.
115. Canguilhem 1991; Szasz 1961; Illich 1976; Greene 2007; H. G. Welch 2011.
116. As mentioned elsewhere, it will be vitally important to ensure that any committees or
     groups charged with developing treatment and diagnostic guidelines and what should
     and should not be included in a comprehensive healthcare coverage plan be free from
     conflicting interests, especially financial (R. N. Moynihan et al. 2013). The history of
     clinical guideline committees has been rife with members having multiple economic
     ties to the industries directly affected by the outcome of their decisions (Mendelson
     et al. 2011; Norris et al. 2011; Lenzer 2013). It is unclear and probably unlikely that sim-
     ply open disclosure or transparency of these conflicts will be sufficient to eliminate
     their effects, much less the suspicion of inappropriate influence. While many academic
     physicians argue reasonably that all benefit from a close association between academic
     and industry due to the productive intellectual cross-fertilization of such associations,
     it remains an unsolved problem how to manage these arrangements successfully to
     minimize (or better, eradicate) improper leverage (Gallin et al. 2013; Califf et al. 2013;
     Dzau et al. 2010; Harrington and Califf 2010). Similarly, it has been argued that guide-
     line committees will be unable to find experts because so many are consultants for the
     drug and device industries. Nevertheless, any future arrangements will need to take
     the current situation into account to suitably compensate experts for these tasks and to
     maintain the beneficial aspects of industry–academia ties without the taint of corrup-
     tion that is so pervasive today. Another interesting view is presented in a short piece
     from an industry insider, touting the advantages to be had by smart marketing and
     promotion strategies and ignoring the salient fact that he is discussing selling prod-
     ucts to people who either are truly sick or who the manufacturers want to persuade are
     sick so that they will "consume" (i.e., purchase) more stuff (see Freiherr 1995).
117. Ryle 1961, p. 138, 140.
118. L. M. Schwartz et al. 2011; Berlin 2011; Berland 2011; J. R. Hoffman and Cooper 2012.
     Sometimes, an aggressive approach is recommended, although the data support-
     ing this are somewhat questionable (Pituitary Incidentaloma: An Endocrine Society
     Clinical Practice Guideline 2011).
119. Now, some might argue the third point, costs. They might say that, in many cases, it
     is actually quite cost-effective to treat an at-risk population, even if the risk of any one
     patient developing the problem treatment is designed to prevent is low. For instance,
     let us assume it costs $1 million to prophylactically treat a population with say, a
     statin drug, to prevent five heart attacks or strokes over a period of 10 years. The cost-
     effectiveness experts would want several important pieces of information: how much

on average does it cost to treat those five patients who have heart attacks or strokes (including both immediate medical costs as well as lost wages, life-long therapies now needed, etc.), how much might it cost to cope with the anticipated harms to x number of people who have adverse reactions to the statin, and how would these two compare to the $1 million we are spending on the drug? For expensive, brand-name drugs on patent, sometimes these numbers don't add up in favor of prophylaxis unless one tightens up the treatment criteria to focus on a much higher risk group.

120. H. G. Welch 2011; H. G. Welch and Black 2010.
121. D. A. Redelmeier and Shafir 1995; Donald A. Redelmeier et al. 1995.
122. P. G. Shekelle et al. 2000. How this approach might be integrated with the "fast and frugal" decision heuristics advocated as both efficient and accurate by Marewski and Gigerenzer (2012) is an interesting and unanswered question.
123. P. Shekelle et al. 2012.
124. This is a very complex issue, and to be addressed in this manner must be enveloped in a comprehensive, inclusive redesign of the healthcare system so that it does not conflict with other goals. See also Gagliardi et al. 2011; Vandvik et al. 2013.
125. H. Welch et al. 2011; Zhang et al. 2010; Brooks et al. 2013; Song et al. 2010; Franzini et al. 2010.
126. Emanuel 2002.
127. Ahmed et al. 2012, p. 1. The most effective way(s) this should be done is open to question; see Woloshin and Schwartz 2011; Garcia-Retamero and Cokely 2013; Garcia-Retamero and Galesic 2010; Garcia-Retamero and Hoffrage 2013; Politi et al. 2007.
128. Interestingly, this is similar to what currently exists when an individual's insurance plan does or does not cover something that his physician believes is clinically indicated and thus should be covered (see the discussion on insurance definitions of medical necessity in Chapter 2). Doctors constantly grouse (often with good reason) about trying to argue with insurers to provide what they believe to be a needed service and complain about the time they spend on the phone attempting to convince a nurse or a company-employed physician of the rightness of their cause (Kocher and Sahni 2011; Dyrbye et al. 2012; Bendix 2013; Morra et al. 2011; Shipman and Sinsky 2013). If the debate about what will be covered (and presumably applicable and available to all) occurs upfront at the time the decisions are being discussed, then later appeals will either be moot (or nonexistent) or must take place in some sort of formal setting established for this purpose: see Philip M. Rosoff 2014, chapter 3.
129. Philip M. Rosoff 2014, chapter 3.
130. Brill 2015; Starr 2011.
131. Gigerenzer 2002, 2009; Gigerenzer et al. 2007.

Chapter 5

1. http://www.nytimes.com/1987/10/17/us/toddler-is-rescued-after-2-1-2-days-in-a-texas-well.html.
2. http://www.nytimes.com/2010/10/13/world/americas/13chile.html.
3. Jonsen 1986.
4. Schelling 1968; Fried 1969.
5. Fried 1969. A recent edited volume discusses many of the philosophical issues with the Rule and some of its practical implications as well (I. G. Cohen et al. 2015).

6. See Kogut and Ritov (2005, 2007) for interesting psychological studies of this phenomenon that highlights the critical significance of identification with a real (even
if idealized) person who is defined by her misfortune. Also see Small and Verrochi
(2009) for another interesting take on this issue. In this regard, it was not simply an
accident that the National Kidney Foundation had a patient with kidney failure testify
before Congress while receiving dialysis to emphasize the urgency and plight of those
with this condition, all while arguing for passage of amendments to the Medicare
Reauthorization Act that would create the End-Stage Renal Disease Program in 1972
(Blagg 2007; Levinsky 1993).

7. Beach et al. 2005; Honeybul et al. 2011; Kohn et al. 2011.

8. Redelmeier and Tversky 1990; Asch and Hershey 1995; Haque and Waytz 2012; Kohn
et al. 2011. See also Dekay et al. 2000 for a different (and contrary) view.

9. Brody and Bonham 1997; Daniels and Sabin 1998; Melichar 2009; Thom and
Campbell 1997.

10. Peter A. Ubel and Arnold 1995; Largent and Pearson 2012; Hurst and Danis 2007;
Schoen et al. 2010.

11. Gerber et al. 2014; J. Cohen et al. 2009; Werner et al. 2004.

12. For example, see Blackburn and Thompson 2012; Wastfelt et al. 2006.

13. Largent and Pearson 2012; Quigley and Harris 2008. Also see McKie and
Richardson 2003.

14. Schelling touches on this in his essay; see Schelling 1968, pp. 142–144.

15. Hope 2001.

16. Soares 2012; Shah et al. 2013. See also http://www.nice.org.uk/about.

17. See Hadorn 1991 and Philip M. Rosoff 2014, chapter 2.

18. Sheehan 2007.

19. Courtney and Maxwell 2009; Neuberger 2012; Segev 2009; Tong et al. 2013; Wells 2009;
Williams et al. 2015.

20. Peter A. Ubel and Loewenstein 1996 a, b.

21. Akpinar et al. 2009.

22. Scott W Biggins 2012; S. W. Biggins et al. 2014; P. A. Ubel et al. 1993.

23. See policies of the Organ Procurement and Transplantation Network (OPTN), available at http://optn.transplant.hrsa.gov/governance/policies/, accessed March 4, 2015).

24. http://www.politico.com/story/2013/06/sarah-murnaghan-lung-transplant-donor-
92643.html.

25. http://www.cnn.com/2014/06/24/health/murnaghan-lung-transplant-policy/.

26. One of the better known exceptions was the publicity generated by breast cancer advocacy groups to generate publicity to shame insurance companies to fund so-called
"bone marrow transplants" for advanced breast cancer in the 1990s (actually, the use
of the patient's own bone marrow to replenish that destroyed by high-doses of chemotherapy designed to kill any residual breast cancer cells). Not only was this a broad-
based movement of generally better-educated women and their doctors with a massive
campaign waged in the press, but there was also a parallel effort on the legal front
with numerous lawsuits filed against insurance companies in an attempt to force them
to pay for the procedure even though there was little convincing evidence to support
its efficacy. Nevertheless, these plaintiffs formed a very compelling group, and, after
several high-profile cases were won with multi-million dollar payouts, the insurance
companies capitulated and started funding them (Rettig et al. 2007, chapters 3 and
4). Unfortunately, the clinical trials that were eventually performed showed that the

treatment was heroic, toxic, and ineffective (Rettig et al. 2007, chapters 8 and 9). This experience demonstrates that the Rule of Rescue may satisfy our empathic desire to help those who appear to be in need even if the help we have to offer is misplaced or even harmful, as it was in this very tragic case.

27. Rettig et al. 2007; and see the story of Amelia Rivera following.
28. For example, the annual telethon appeal in the United States for the Muscular Dystrophy Association.
29. Largent and Pearson 2012.
30. Andersen et al. 2014, p. 464.
31. http://www.dailymail.co.uk/news/article-2088148/Mia-Rivera-Doctors-deny-sick-toddler-kidney-transplant-mentally-disabled.html, accessed August 3, 2015.
32. I wouldn't begin to speculate on the reasons that the hospital used to deny this patient a transplant. In public statements after the hospital relented following the deluge of negative publicity that was a consequence of its somewhat tin-eared responses to the initial stories appearing in the press, the staff were at pains to declare that they do not discriminate on the basis of cognitive function when considering patients for transplant. However, they alluded to this patient's many other comorbidities as well as her need for life-long custodial care, suggesting that—as with many of these cases—the subtleties and nuances of complex patient care are lost in the sound bite mess that comes from public debate in the news media. It is also likely that the explosive growth of the Internet and its ability to publicize virtually anyone's unfiltered point of view contributed to the tenor and tone of the hullabaloo and no doubt was instrumental in convincing Children's Hospital to alter its stance.
33. Although one could make the argument that, in the Coby Howard case cited earlier (Note 19) within the confines of the inclusive Oregon Health Plan, the money saved by not doing his transplant actually could have been allocated to some other worthwhile healthcare-related endeavor (although it is unclear if that actually would have occurred). However, even in this case, there is some reason for skepticism. Since the OHP covered only poor people, a large but minority part of the entire healthcare enterprise in the state, and since the money came from general tax (and some other) revenues and was budgeted at the whim of the state legislature, it is certainly conceivable that the money saved from doing high-risk expensive interventions could have been used to fix roads or give a tax cut to wealthy people (not that the former is unimportant).
34. See, for example, the story of Coby Howard in Oregon; Hadorn 1991; Philip M. Rosoff 2014, chapter 2.
35. See Philip M. Rosoff 2014.
36. http://www.pbac.pbs.gov.au/section-f/f3-other-relevant-factors.html, accessed February 4, 2014. Also see Whitty and Littlejohns 2015
37. http://www.pbac.pbs.gov.au/section-f/f3-other-relevant-factors.html, accessed February 4, 2014.
38. Cookson et al. 2008.
39. The report can be found at https://www.nice.org.uk/get-involved/citizens-council, accessed February 4, 2015. It is dated January 2006.
40. Cookson et al. 2008, pp. 541–542.
41. The situation closest to this scenario is when Medicare chooses not to pay for a given drug or device. Of course, the Medicare rule that states that it must pay for all FDA-approved devices and drugs when used appropriately limits the ability to show this kind of discrimination. I suspect that the demand for marginally effective drugs would

dry up if the criteria for insurance payment were based on the demonstration of substantive benefit.

42. Philip M. Rosoff 2014, chapter 3.

43. This would be something like a negative Rule or perhaps a Rule of Disregard or Rule of Refusal; see P.M. Rosoff 2012; P. M. Rosoff et al. 2012; Philip M. Rosoff 2014, chapter 3.

44. Resnick 2003; Schneiderman and Jecker 1996.

45. Schöne-Seifert 2009.

46. Johansson 2005.

47. Quigley and Harris 2008.

48. Nancy Jecker (2013) argues this point very well, although not from the perspective of the effects rampant "rescues" may have on a healthcare system. See also Sheehan 2007.

49. *Estelle et al. v. Gamble* 1976.

50. http://www.cbsnews.com/news/prisoner-gets-1m-heart-transplant/, accessed March 11, 2015.

51. Resnick 2003; Wailoo et al. 2006. See also Philip M. Rosoff 2014, chapter 6.

52. http://www.oed.com/view/Entry/7367?rskey=VxPM5C&result=1#eid, accessed February 24, 2015.

53. Tversky and Kahneman 1973, 1974.

54. Fagerlin et al. 2005.

55. Bazzano et al. 2009; Donna et al. 2009; Leveque 2008.

56. P. M. Rosoff and Coleman 2011.

57. It is worth noting one of the most infamous recent examples of this and the terrible consequences that can result. I refer to the prolonged fight over autologous stem cells rescue after myeloablative chemotherapy for advanced breast cancer during the 1980s and early 1990s. The reader interested in the complete story of this fiasco should consult the excellent book by Richard Rettig and his colleagues (Rettig et al. 2007). The desperate patients and their willing enablers (their doctors, the medical centers seeking the highly profitable transplant business, and the news media looking for good stories) also made excellent use of the Rule of Rescue (as well as, on occasion, the courts) to force insurers to pay for this expensive treatment.

58. It is important to clarify this point. It should be obvious on its face (and, I suspect, in the personal experience of many readers) that patients who have either public or private insurance (or a hybrid) cannot simply get any healthcare service they want or their doctors recommend for them. Sometimes this is due to the (medical) worthiness of the test, procedure, drug, etc. Many other times it is because the test, drug, procedure, etc. is not specifically covered under the policy and will thus be denied for payment. Nevertheless, it is true that there is little control over the numbers and kinds of diagnostic tests that physicians order and insurance companies pay for if there is an "appropriate" matched indication. So, while it is technically correct to say that Americans cannot get whatever they (or their physicians) might want, it can come terribly close.

59. Fang et al. 2014.

60. For example, see Miller et al. 2014.

61. I realize that this may be controversial since the Baby K case in Virginia (Bopp and Coleson 1994; Flannery 1995), but it would be a rare physician or nurse who would imagine any reasonable goal of life support in such an infant. See also Clayton 1995.

62. Schroeder-Lein 2008.

63. My institution, like most others in the United States, is certainly not above accepting the excellent public relations that accompanies patient claims of miraculous events. See

the March 29, 2015, broadcast of the CBC television show *60 Minutes* for an example (http://www.cbsnews.com/news/polio-cancer-treatment-duke-university-60-minutes-scott-pelley/).

64. There are probably many, complex, and interacting reasons that numerous physicians and their institutions believe that they have no choice but to accede to the demands of patients and families in these situations. Fears of litigation, a perverse misunderstanding of the meaning of patient (and surrogate) autonomy, and an avoidance or abdication of professional responsibility all probably play some role.

65. It should be noted that both New York and New Jersey have amended their laws governing the declaration of death by neurological criteria to attempt to accommodate religious objections (such as those by Orthodox Judaism and some Muslims) to this category of death. The pertinent section of the New Jersey statute reads: "The death of an individual shall not be declared upon the basis of neurological criteria pursuant to sections 3 and 4 of this act when the licensed physician authorized to declare death, has reason to believe, on the basis of information in the individual's available medical records, or information provided by a member of the individual's family or any other person knowledgeable about the individual's personal religious beliefs that such a declaration would violate the personal religious beliefs of the individual. In these cases, death shall be declared, and the time of death fixed, solely upon the basis of cardio-respiratory criteria pursuant to section 2 of this act" (NJ Rev Stat § 26:6A-5; 2013). In New York, the law reads that institutions must establish "a procedure for the reasonable accommodation of the individual's religious or moral objection to the determination as expressed by the individual, or by the next of kin or other person closest to the individual" (10 N.Y.C.R.R. § 400.16, part 3).

66. For example, see Green 2015.

67. Larmer 1988, p. 12. Interestingly, he also argues that miracles do not have to contravene the laws of nature (see chapter 2 in this reference).

68. Oxford English Dictionary referenced at http://www.oed.com/view/Entry/119052?rskey=d9PvGv&result=1#eid, accessed March 31, 2015.

69. Holland 1965, p. 44. I wish to acknowledge Robert Larmer's book for making me aware of this reference (Larmer 1988).

70. Peschel and Peschel 1988. See also Shermer 2004; Charpak 2004, chapters 2 and 3.

71. Of course, scripture and historical tales are filled with accounts of the one group of godly people asking their supernatural being to smite their (presumably different-godly) enemies against overwhelming odds and attributing the unlikely success to miraculous intervention.

72. It is of interest that in the modern-day United States, we have resolved to ignore some of the demands of the faithful when the results of respecting them could lead to predictable (and avoidable) harm to the vulnerable. For example, it is common to transfuse blood products into anemic children over the protestations of their Jehovah's Witness parents, often with the power and protection of a court order. Similarly, parents professing faiths that condemn (modern) Western medicine have been successfully prosecuted for criminal negligence or manslaughter when they fail to seek medical help for their ill children who then suffer unnecessary, preventable harm (see, e.g., *State v. Neumann*, 832 N.W.2d 560, 2013 WI 58 (2013). Of course, competent adults (and, in some states, so-called "mature minors") are free to accept or refuse recommended care. The issue under consideration here is whether the tenets of religious faith can be used to demand or dictate certain types of care that are counter to medical advice: must doctors (and

their hospitals, and thus the "system") comply with such demands supported by these sorts of reasons?

73. Duffin 2007, p. 706.

74. Sarkar and Banerjee 2005; Wong et al. 2000; Vesely et al. 2011.

75. Tversky and Kahneman 1973, 1974.

76. For example, see Glod 2014.

77. Hume 1999, Section 10, page 173. Also see Mackie 1982, chapter 1. It should be noted that at least one modern theologian (and bioethicist and physician) dismisses this (and similar definitions) as overly simplistic; see Sulmasy (2007). Hume, being an empiricist, had a radically different view of what constituted "evidence" of a miracle, and unsupported faith that one had occurred was insufficient for him. He also had a healthy skepticism for the veracity of human perception and its fallibility, even though our senses are all we have to go on to substantiate our beliefs about the workings of the world.

78. Paley 2006. While there continue to be significant religious communities that take the Biblical account of human (and geologic) origins literally, major faiths, such as the Roman Catholic Church, have accepted the facts of evolution (for example) for many years.

79. Osler 1910.

80. Not everyone agreed with Osler or other scientifically minded physicians or subscribers to "medico-materialistic monism," as most politely noted by the Reverend Francis Boyd (1910).

81. Pawlikowski 2007. For a short exegesis of the orthodox Christian (Catholic) view of miracles and the "order of nature" (as opposed to what he dismissively refers to as the erroneous "laws of nature"), see Sulmasy (2007).

82. Mansfield et al. 2002. Also see the results from a Pew survey from the late 2000s:

> The Landscape Survey finds that belief in miracles and supernatural phenomena are widespread among U.S. adults. Nearly eight-in-ten adults (79%), including large majorities of most religious traditions, believe that miracles still occur today as in ancient times. More than eight-in-ten members of evangelical (88%) and historically black (88%) churches, Catholics (83%) and Mormons (96%) agree that miracles still occur today. However, relatively narrow majorities of Jews and the unaffiliated express belief in miracles, and among Jehovah's Witnesses, only about a third (30%) believe in miracles. In fact, nearly half of all Jehovah's Witnesses (48%) say that they completely disagree with the statement that miracles occur today as in ancient times. Two-thirds of U.S. adults (68%) believe that angels and demons are active in the world. Significant majorities of members of Christian traditions agree with this statement, including about nine-in-ten members of historically black and evangelical Protestant churches, Jehovah's Witnesses and Mormons. Less than half of Buddhists and Hindus, and less than a quarter of Jews, say angels and demons are active in the world. Although relatively few atheists and agnostics believe in angels and demons, nearly a third of the secular unaffiliated (29%) and more than two-thirds of the religious unaffiliated (68%) believe angels and demons are active in the world. http://www.pewforum.org/ 2008/06/01/chapter-1-religious-beliefs-and-practices/, accessed April 1, 2015.

> For an interesting discussion of what constitutes hope in healthcare and how it might be better expressed, see W. Stempsey (2015).

83. Catlin et al. 2008; Curlin et al. 2005, 2006. Although scientists are considerably less religious than doctors; see this study from the Pew Research Center on Religion and

Public Life: http://www.pewforum.org/2009/11/05/scientists-and-belief/, accessed April 1, 2015. One of the most well-known scientists who is also a believer is Francis Collins, the Director of the National Institutes of Health (as of this writing); see Collins (2006).

84. Jacobs 2008, p. 734.
85. W. Stempsey 2015.
86. Smith et al. 2009.
87. Phelps A. C. and et al. 2009.
88. Balboni et al. 2010. See also Alcorn et al. 2010. Unfortunately, the issue may be considerably more complex and less clear as shown in the work by Shinall and colleagues (Shinall Jr 2014; Shinall Jr and Guillamondegui 2015; Shinall et al. 2014). See also Johnson et al. (2005) for an interesting look at the ethnic diversity dimensions of spirituality in the very ill.
89. Cooper et al. 2014.
90. Brett and Jersild 2003. See also Widera et al. 2011.
91. Schneiderman and Jecker 2011, p. 10.
92. Bostan et al. 2007.
93. Powers et al. 2013; Hartzband and Groopman 2012; Goldstein and Bowers 2015.
94. W. E. Stempsey 2002, p. 7.
95. Julian Savulescu and Clarke 2007, p. 1262. Interestingly, part of their argument supporting giving some due weight to the hope for a miraculous cure after they admit to both being nonbelievers, presumably bolstering their bona fides as even-handed evaluators, is that they do not philosophically or even scientifically rule out the possibility, as remote as it may be, that miracles actually do, in fact, occur and exist as part of the natural world. Hence, to categorically rule against families who are praying for a miracle is a mistake. See also Brierley et al. 2013; Clarke 2012.
96. Gould 1997. For a contrasting, up-to-date view, see Biggar 2015.
97. For example, see Evans and Evans 2008; Ecklund and Park 2009.
98. See Buryska 2001; J. Savulescu 1998 for interesting analyses, as well as Bracanovic 2013; Childress 2007; Orr and Genesen 1997. Bock tries to thread a very narrow needle in trying to bridge this gap by presenting "valid" qualifications that would command that doctors respect the wishes of people grounded on religious belief. Unfortunately, except for the most idiosyncratic, outlandish, and perhaps even delusional beliefs, his formula would endorse the vast majority of such demands. See Bock 2008.
99. Philip M. Rosoff 2014, chapter 7.

Chapter 6

1. As I have stated throughout this volume and elsewhere, such a healthcare insurance plan must be both comprehensive and universal. Whether "universal" would include some populations at the margins of society for reasons of prejudicial social exclusion— such as undocumented immigrants ("illegal" aliens) and incarcerated prisoners—is more of a political question to be determined by the tolerance of the electorate and the leadership ability of their elected representatives (see Rosoff 2014, chapter 6).
2. Rosoff 2014, chapter 5.
3. Mathur et al. 2010; Harrington et al. 2014; Chidi et al. 2015.
4. See also Joshi et al. 2013; Kucirka et al. 2012.

5. Mathur et al. 2010; Kemmer et al. 2009; Moylan et al. 2008; Wiesner et al. 2003; Wille et al. 2013. There is evidence that gender disparities in access to liver transplant persist (Mathur et al. 2011).

6. Baker et al. 2009; Singh et al. 2010; Coglianese et al. 2015. For a view from a European country (Italy) that demonstrates minimal influence of psychosocial factors for transplantation outcomes see Sponga et al. (2015).

7. A. W. Williams 2015.

8. Lipworth et al. 2012; Monson et al. 2015; Vranic et al. 2014. A new allocation system for kidneys may mitigate some of this disparity. See Israni et al. 2014; W. W. Williams et al. 2015.

9. Finer and Zolna 2011; Montez et al. 2012; Olshansky et al. 2012.

10. Rosoff 2014, chapters 2, 3.

11. World Health Organization (WHO) 2011, p. 2.

12. WHO 2008.

13. Braveman et al. 2011; Daniels 2015; Preda and Voigt 2015; Sreenivasan 2015. A more libertarian view would be that it is not a legitimate role for governments to concern themselves with such things, especially for those factors that are conceivably attributable to personal attributes and/or behavior.

14. Collins et al. 2015. On the other hand, an analysis of hospital admissions and discharges after the full implementation of the Massachusetts state health insurance plan (upon which the ACA was based) demonstrated that racial and ethnic disparities, which might be thought to have been amenable to mitigation by the wide availability of insurance that would lower any perceptible barriers to access, remained mostly unchanged (McCormick et al. 2015). While one might state that these data are preliminary and applicable to only one state with a relatively small minority population, they are cause for concern and they support an argument that providing good health insurance may not be sufficient to remove all obstacles to care. More recent data from a Kaiser Family Foundation survey suggests that the issue of medical debt as a significant contributor to financial stress remains a major problem (Hamel et al. 2016).

15. Ellis et al. 2012; Scholes et al. 2012.

16. There is even a modern blues song with the lyrical lament,

> Born under a bad sign
> Been down since I began to crawl
> If it wasn't for bad luck
> You know, I wouldn't have no luck at all.

Copyright, Cotillion Music Inc., East Memphis Music Corp; written by Booker T. Jones and William Bell.

17. Dworkin 1981, p. 293.

18. Rice and Saeed 2014; Linas et al. 2015; Leidner et al. 2015.

19. Elizabeth Anderson coined the term, and it has been adopted by many others (although she is one of its leading and, in my opinion, most eloquent and articulate critics; see Anderson 1999). See also

(Albertsen 2014; Albertsen and Knight 2015; Arneson 2004; Marchman Andersen et al. 2013; Saul 2008; Segall 2007).

Interestingly, Ronald Dworkin himself has taken care to refute any claim to embrace at least some forms of at least part of this view: see Dworkin (2003).

20. Anderson suggests that Rakowski might be an exception (Anderson 1999; Rakowski 1991).
21. Brown 2013.
22. See Kelley (2005) for an interesting argument relating physician paternalism and the movement to hold patient's responsible for their health-related (causal) behavior. Feiring (2008) mounts a related argument that also endorses a moderate form of personal responsibility that is not tied to retrospective blaming (and punishment by withholding treatment, for example), but tying prospective consideration to some metrics of compliance with a program to alter the behavior that has contributed to a specified health condition.
23. Jha and Peto 2014; Chaloupka et al. 2012; Callison and Kaestner 2014.
24. This suggestion should be contrasted with how many states utilize cigarette and alcohol taxes. Frequently, the money raised is deposited in general revenue accounts and is not devoted to either tobacco addiction prevention or disease treatment (Saul 2008).

    However, the possible downside is that only those people wealthy (and perhaps foolish) enough to afford the increased costs would engage in these activities. For many harmful habits, that would be tolerable (as in tobacco addiction, for example). But for those pursuits that are already viewed as the somewhat exclusive domains of well-off, such as downhill skiing, this approach could further limit access. Whether that is good or not is arguable.
25. Arneson 2004, pp. 2–4.
26. For example, see Hilts 1996; Proctor 2011.
27. Golan 2010.
28. See Levinson et al. 2014; Steiker and Steiker 2015; Alexander 2010; Stevenson 2014.
29. Pickett et al. 2014.
30. Higham 1957.
31. Anderson 1999, p. 311. See also Eyal 2011; Katz 2013.
32. It is worth noting that this argument also applies to many other differences between people that both affect their health and could arguably be related to "choices" they make in life. For example, should people who commit crimes and are convicted of them and then sentenced to prison have access to medical care commonly denied to law-abiding citizens? By ruling in favor of this position, the US Supreme Court has also endorsed universal free healthcare for incarcerated people, an entitlement that does not exist outside of jail (*Estelle et al. v. Gamble* 1976). This is not to say that the healthcare that prisoners receive is either comprehensive or excellent (in many cases and states, the opposite is true), but, in principle, they are supposed to. This is also not to say that people commit crimes to obtain medical care. The point is that society is filled with people who have many innumerable choices throughout their lives that can affect their health in one way or another, and it would be both impracticable and inhumane to tally up a balance sheet for each and every one.
33. See http://www.ada.gov/, accessed July 15, 2015.
34. Pont et al. 2006.
35. Although this is by no means a uniform view; see Hurley et al. 2014.
36. Bruns and Campbell 2014; Janvier et al. 2012; Nelson et al. 2012.
37. Boss et al. 2013.
38. Mechanic 1992, 1995, 2004. To be fair, in the 1992 paper, Mechanic does acknowledge the fact that physician's loyalty to their patients' interests has never been total

(pp. 1729–1730). In his argument for what he calls "implicit rationing," Mechanic writes, "Thus, initially, the threshold decision of whether to provide a new entitlement is clearly an issue with political implications and consequences. However, once the entitlement is available, the most constructive way of controlling the cost of the entitlement is to constrain supply and allow expert professionals to allocate treatment. This is not to say implicit rationing does not have some serious difficulties. Allocation of services through clinical judgment of patient condition and motivation requires built-in safeguards for resolving contested cases, but as a medical care rationing approach it offers the most *realistic* model for dealing with the complexities and uncertainties of clinical situations" (p. 1737; emphasis in the original). Also see Chapter 3.

39. Mayberry 2014; Gaskin et al. 2014; Joshi et al. 2013; Sondak et al. 2012; Bustamante et al. 2012.
40. Mantel 2013.
41. Hennig-Schmidt et al. 2011; Robertson et al. 2012; Shafrin 2010. However, some data suggests that caution may be advisable; see Green (2014).
42. Matthew K. Wynia et al. 2003; Meyers et al. 2006.
43. Freeman et al. 1999; Werner et al. 2004; M. K. Wynia et al. 2000. Indeed, some have argued that it is a physician's duty to lie to an insurance company if done for the welfare of her patient; see Tavaglione and Hurst (2012).
44. Rosoff 2014.
45. Rosoff 2014, chapter 3.
46. Neuberger 2007; Ratcliffe 2000; Secunda et al. 2012; Tong et al. 2013.
47. These data vary somewhat from year to year, but this recent analysis pegs it at 27% for 2009 (Singal et al. 2013).
48. Arneson 2004, pp. 5–6.
49. See Chapter 3 and Rosoff 2014, chapter 3.
50. This is not a state of affairs in which the resources needed to help people are in finite short supply, such as kidneys or livers. I am not suggesting that we renounce careful efficiency and equity screening procedures for allocation of solid organs (for example). A smoker with bad lung disease who could potentially benefit from a lung transplant but who refuses to quit smoking should not be eligible for a transplant, but it is not unreasonable to offer her ICU care and a ventilator for a flare of her COPD when she gets pneumonia or influenza (assuming that there are good reasons to believe she could get better).
51. For example, see Murray et al. 2015; DeMarco et al. 2014.
52. While Winston Churchill is often viewed as a paragon of leadership virtues, self-abnegation was not part of his character: not only was he obese, he smoked huge cigars constantly and drank like a fish. He died at age 90.
53. It is important to note that my forgiving position does not depend on any negation or acceptance of beliefs about (moral or other) personal agency, free will, determinism, and the like. I readily admit that we are responsible in some way and to some indeterminate degree for many of our actions. But since it is virtually impossible in the healthcare sphere, except in some very isolated and perhaps unique cases, to assign complete responsibility for the cause of an illness or condition to a single individual act over which a person had complete control, it seems both extraordinarily difficult and impractical to make the attempt. The reason why I specify and restrict this view to the field of healthcare is that I well realize that we have developed sophisticated (although by no means foolproof) methods for adjudicating guilt and innocence in the

sphere of criminal law. But I would maintain that the system of juries, judges, courts, lawyers, laws, and lawbreakers bears little relationship to the world of disease, where most conditions have numerous contributing causes, only some of which may be under volitional control. This is not to say that we should ignore the contribution(s) of personal behavior to the development and exacerbation of disease. But, rather than punish people for their behavior by denying treatment, I suggest that we focus our attentions on creating conditions that are more prophylactic, preventive, and mitigating rather than retributive.

Chapter 7

1. Philip M. Rosoff 2014.
2. Geist and Hardesty 2014; Iglehart 1982.
3. Stern and Epstein 1985.
4. Philip M. Rosoff 2014, chapters 2 and 3. I discuss more of the flaws and the competing interests generating this moral and practical tension in Chapter 5 in this volume.
5. Flexner 1910.
6. Ludmerer 2015.
7. Thomson 1997.
8. A little-known clause in the law also provided for (some) desegregation of newly constructed hospitals (see Reynolds 1997). However, there was also a notorious "separate but equal" section in the act that permitted simple maintenance of the status quo in existing institutions and allowed it in new construction as well. However, this clause was found unconstitutional in 1963 in a ruling by the 4th Circuit Court of Appeals (*Simkins v. Moses H. Cone Memorial Hospital* 323 F2nd 959).
9. http://history.nih.gov/exhibits/history/index.html, accessed August 10, 2015.
10. Mukherjee 2011; DeVita et al. 1970.
11. Welch 2011; Moynihan and Cassels 2005.
12. Louis Jacobson, "John Boehner says U.S. health care system is best in world," July 5, 2012 at http://www.politifact.com/truth-o-meter/statements/2012/jul/05/john-boehner/john-boehner-says-us-health-care-system-best-world/, accessed August 10, 2015.
13. P. Starr 1982, book 2, and Paul Starr 2011.
14. Blumenthal et al. 2015.
15. Steven Brill's book, while not an academic treatise, gives an excellent day-by-day account of the ACA (Brill 2015). The "horse-trading" so patently evident in the creation of the ACA is by no means unusual in American law-making; see Redman 2001.
16. McGee et al. 2013; Niu et al. 2013; Ngo-Metzger et al. 2012; Rowley and Hogan 2012; Chan et al. 2012; Davis et al. 2014.
17. See Michael R. Grey 1989, 1994.
18. See Dobbin 1992; P. Starr 1982 2011 for excellent historical analyses.
19. See McGoldrick (1945) for a fascinating (and disturbing) view of the American Medical Association in the (unanimous) opposition to a continuation and expansion of the Emergency Maternal and Infant Care Program after World War II. Also see Best 2012; Goldsteen et al. 2001; Keller and Packel 2013; Yackee 2012.
20. Of course, some people might then counter this by stating that this is what charity is for, meaning that individuals should not be compelled to contribute to funds to provide for the welfare of others (in the form of say, taxes) but should only do so out of their own

free (charitable) will. For example, see http://www.cato.org/blog/fundamental-fallacy-redistribution, Pilon 1995.

21. One of the most effective over the past 50 years has been Title VI of the Civil Rights Act of 1964; §200d states "No person in the United States shall, on the ground of race, color, or national origin, be excluded from participation in, be denied the benefits of, or be subjected to discrimination under any program or activity receiving Federal financial assistance" (http://www.justice.gov/crt/about/cor/coord/titlevistat.php). On the other hand, the federal rule-making operation, which mandates an open comment period prior to the crafting of the final rules, can be heavily influenced by heavily financed outside actors that have a major stake in the outcome of the process; see Gilens 2012.

22. Philip M. Rosoff 2014, chapter 7.

23. What percentage of the population—if any—would be excluded from such a plan would be susceptible to the vagaries of democratic debate. I have previously suggested that de Tocqueville's "tyranny of the majority" could dictate that some socially marginalized populations could be sacrificed for political expediency. For example, unless there is some major sea change in the animus against undocumented immigrants that appears to be prevalent among many members of Congress, it is unlikely that any feasible plan would embrace all residents of the country, rather than just citizens and permanent residents. See Philip M. Rosoff 2014, chapter 6.

24. In some ways, this could be analogous to current Medicare Advantage commercial insurance plans that supplement the basic Medicare benefits. In my proposal, people who chose to buy such insurance could opt out of the main health insurance program but only if they could prove that they were replacing it with equal or better coverage. In this sense, it would be analogous to public schools: even if one chooses to send one's children to private school, one still must pay the taxes to support public education. Where it becomes complicated is when the percentage of people who opt out becomes so large that the dedication to the public system wanes. In a nationalized system, isolated pockets of affluent people who decide to opt out should not jeopardize the entire system. One could also look to the situation in Great Britain where utilization of the National Health Service (NHS) is quite high, even among the affluent, but the growth of a private—often supplemental—health insurance market has also grown. Of course, one could argue that the existence of the private market takes some financial pressure off the NHS to improve services. See Lostao et al. 2014; Hamilton et al. 2013; Brekke and Sørgard 2007.

25. We should not underestimate the resistance to this idea by organized medicine, such as the American Medical Association (AMA) and other professional societies that represent various medical specialties such as the American Society for Clinical Oncology (ASCO) and the American Heart Association (AHA). While the much vaunted lobbying power of the AMA is justifiably feared, in truth, the AMA represents fewer than 30% of practicing doctors, most of them members of the ever decreasing group of private practitioners. Nevertheless, unless care is also taken to alter the way in which doctors are paid, especially those who still derive significant (and large) amounts of their income from fee-for-service models, the obstacles could possibly be insurmountable. Physicians would have to be reassured that both their independence and their salaries would not be seriously jeopardized. The reality argues for wholesale restructuring to align incentives with policy and patient care in mind. As important will be how the message to physicians is crafted. The goal of creating cutoffs is not so much to reduce discretionary decisions by doctors (it is that, as well), but to set limits on the variability

to minimize arbitrary, unique, notional, and unsupportable (by evidence) medical decisions. Ever since Flexner, doctors' unfettered freedom to practice as they wish with their patients with minimal interference has been steadily eroded.

26. Although some "pure" libertarians might argue that there should be no restrictions on what one might wish to purchase for oneself as long as no one else was harmed by the transaction and there was a willing seller.

27. Cohen et al. 2008; David et al. 2011; Savage et al. 2010; Bidlingmaier et al. 2014.

28. This is not exactly true because some people can elect to retire later or earlier than age 65 with corresponding increases or decreases in benefits (ssa.gov/planners/retire/1943/html).

29. Lane 2007. I do not intend in any pejorative way to pick on psychiatry or psychiatrists by citing this example except for the fact that the various editions of the *Diagnostic and Statistical Manual of Mental Disorders* make such a tempting target. One could readily find other examples in more commonplace and conventional areas of medical practice, often typified by a drug whose patent is about to expire and whose manufacturer is looking for new indications that it could also patent, thus extending the life (and sales) of the drug. See Doan et al. 2011; Oprea et al. 2011; Organization 2012; Moriyama et al. 2011.

But one should not be lulled into complacency about so-called "organic" disorders because they, too, fall prey to the "inclusion creep." One has only to examine the confusion sown by the repeated expansion of what serum cholesterol, LDL, and HDL levels constitute "hypercholesterolemia" or "hyperlipidemia" and thus receive a recommendation for pharmacologic treatment (if diet and exercise are not successful) to correct the problem (Welch 2011, chapter 2).

30. I use the qualifier "almost" because the FDA has had an increasing tendency over the past 15 years or so to approve medications, especially enormously expensive anti-cancer or anti-inflammatory drugs, that either improve the clinical conditions of patients only temporarily (such as increasing median life expectancy by just a few months) or utilize biological surrogates (such as lowering or increasing the amount of a specific chemical in the blood, in which the relationship of the laboratory change to clinically significant outcomes is tenuous).

31. P. M. Rosoff and Coleman 2011.

32. http://www.cochrane.org/.

33. Leonard Fleck (2009) has also argued that democratic deliberation can be key to acceptable decision-making in the creation of limits.

34. Schneiderman et al. 1990, 1996.

35. Gilmer et al. 2005; Pearson and Bach 2010; Sabbatini et al. 2014; Tilburt and Cassel 2013; Leonard M. Fleck 2011.

36. Bellman and Zadeh 1970; Reyna 2008; Sadegh-Zadeh 2000.

37. Ransohoff et al. 2013; Vandvik et al. 2013; Shekelle 2014; Tibau et al. 2015.

38. For example, see the contentious debate over the Preventive Services Task Force reports on mammography and prostate specific antigen (PSA) testing. Not surprisingly and despite the data reviewed by reasonably unbiased experts in the field, there was an enormous and immediate outcry by groups with little evidence to support their counterclaims. Arguing in favor of early-age mammography were both radiologists (who stood to lose income if the recommendations for mammograms were changed) and breast cancer advocacy groups who appealed to emotions. In the case of the PSA kerfuffle, it was mostly urologists who were upset, perhaps seeing that they could perform

fewer prostate surgeries if the PSA guidance was observed. See Block et al. 2013; Moyer 2012a; Guallar and Laine 2014.

39. Annual Report of the Boards of Trustees of the Federal Hospital Insurance and Federal Supplementary Medical Insurance Trust Funds (2014), available at https://www.cms.gov/Research-Statistics-Data-and-Systems/Statistics-Trends-and-Reports/ReportsTrustFunds/Trustees-Reports-Items/2012-2015.html?DLPage=1&DLEntries=10&DLSort=0&DLSortDir=descending, Appendix B.

40. Dranove et al. 2014.

41. Lewis 2013, pp. 121–122.

42. Paul Starr 2011.

43. Goldsteen et al. 2001.

44. Brill 2015; Quadagno 2011; Skocpol 2010. Also see Leonard 2011; Marmor and Sullivan 2015.

45. Leonard 2011; P. Starr 1982, 2011.

46. N. Daniels 2000, 2008; P. M. Rosoff 2012; Philip M. Rosoff 2014.

47. Katz 2013.

BIBLIOGRAPHY

Abbott, R., & Stevens, C. (2014). Redefining medical necessity: A consumer-driven solution to the U.S. health care crisis. *Loyola of Los Angeles Law Review,* 943–965

Abigail Alliance for Better Access v. Von Eschenbach (2007). *F. 3d* (Vol. 495, pp. 695): Court of Appeals, Dist. of Columbia Circuit.

Aboumatar, H., Carson, K., Beach, M., Roter, D., & Cooper, L. (2013). The Impact of Health Literacy on Desire for Participation in Healthcare, Medical Visit Communication, and Patient Reported Outcomes among Patients with Hypertension. *Journal of General Internal Medicine, 28*(11), 1469–1476, doi:10.1007/s11606-013-2466-5.

Acharya, A., Adam, T., Baltussen, R., Evans, D., Hutubessy, R., Murray, C. J. L., et al. (Eds.). (2003). *Making choices in health: WHO guide to cost-effectiveness analysis.* Geneva: World Health Organization.

Afendulis, C. C., He, Y., Zaslavsky, A. M., & Chernew, M. E. (2011). The impact of Medicare Part D on hospitalization rates. *Health Services Research, 46*(4), 1022–1038. doi:10.1111/j.1475-6773.2011.01244.x

Aggarwal, S. (2010). What's fueling the biotech engine, 2009–2010. *Nature Biotechnology, 28*(11), 1165–1171. doi:10.1038/nbt1110-1165

Ahmed, H., Naik, G., Willoughby, H., & Edwards, A. (2012). Communicating risk. *BMJ, 344*(7862), 40–44.

Akpinar, E., Selvaggi, G., Levi, D., Moon, J., Nishida, S., Island, E., et al. (2009). Liver retransplantation of more than two grafts for recurrent failure. *Transplantation, 88*(7), 884–890.

Albertsen, A. (2014). Luck Egalitarianism, social determinants and Public Health initiatives. *Public Health Ethics.* 8(1), 42–49.

Albertsen, A., & Knight, C. (2015). A framework for luck egalitarianism in health and healthcare. *Journal of Medical Ethics, 41*(2), 165–169, doi:10.1136/medethics-2013-101666.

Alcorn, S. R., Balboni, M. J., Prigerson, H. G., Reynolds, A., Phelps, A. C., Wright, A. A., et al. (2010). "If God wanted me yesterday, I wouldn't be here today": Religious and spiritual themes in patients' experiences of advanced cancer. *Journal of Palliative Medicine, 13*(5), 581–588.

Alexander, M. (2010). *The new Jim Crow: Mass incarceration in the age of colorblindness.* New York/Jackson, TN: New Press/ Perseus Distribution.

Allen, D. B., & Cuttler, L. (2013). Short stature in childhood—Challenges and choices. *New England Journal of Medicine, 368*(13), 1220–1228. 10.1056/NEJMcp1213178

Allen, J. (2012). Carneades. *The Stanford encyclopedia of philosophy.* Available at http://plato.stanford.edu/archives/win2012/entries/carneades/.

Altman, S. H., & Shactman, D. (2011). *Power, politics, and universal health care : the inside story of a century-long battle.* Amherst, N.Y.: Prometheus Books.

Ambrose, S. E. (1989). *Nixon: Volume II. The triumph of a politician 1962-1972.* New York: Simon and Schuster.

Andersen, E. F., Carey, J. C., Earl, D. L., Corzo, D., Suttie, M., Hammond, P., et al. (2014). Deletions involving genes WHSC1 and LETM1 may be necessary, but are not sufficient to cause Wolf-Hirschhorn Syndrome. *European Journal of Human Genetics: EJHG*, *22*(4), 464–470. doi:10.1038/ejhg.2013.192

Anderson, E. S. (1999). What is the point of equality? *Ethics*, *109*(2), 287–337.

Angell, M. (1991). The case of Helga Wanglie. A new kind of "right to die" case. *New England Journal of Medicine*, *325*(7), 511–512. doi:10.1056/NEJM199108153250712

Angell, M. (2004). *The truth about the drug companies: How they deceive us and what to do about it*. New York: Random House.

Anthony, D. L., Herndon, M. B., Gallagher, P. M., Barnato, A. E., Bynum, J. P. W., Gottlieb, D. J., et al. (2009). How much do patients' preferences contribute to resource use? *Health Affairs*, *28*(3), 864–873. doi:10.1377/hlthaff.28.3.864

Antman, K., Klegar, K., Pomfret, E., Osteen, R., Amato, D., Larson, D., et al. (1985). Early peritoneal mesothelioma: A treatable malignancy. *The Lancet*, *326*(8462), 977–981. doi:hTtp://dx.doi.org/10.1016/S0140-6736(85)90526-4

Apatira, L., Boyd, E. A., Malvar, G., Evans, L. R., Luce, J. M., Lo, B., et al. (2008). Hope, truth, and preparing for death: Perspectives of surrogate decision makers. *Annals of Internal Medicine*, *149*(12), 861–868. doi:10.1059/0003-4819-149-12-200812160-00005

Arah, O. A. (2009). On the relationship between individual and population health. *Medicine, Health Care and Philosophy*, *12*(3), 235–244. hTtp://dx.doi.org/10.1007/s11019-008-9173-8

Arawi, T., & Rosoff, P. M. (2012). Competing duties. *Journal of Bioethical Inquiry*, *9*(2), 135–147.

Arneson, R. J. (2004). Luck egalitarianism interpreted and defended. *Philosophical Topics*, *32*(1/2), 1–20. doi:10.2307/43154426

Arnold, D. G., & Oakley, J. L. (2013). The politics and strategy of industry self-regulation: The pharmaceutical industry's principles for ethical direct-to-consumer advertising as a deceptive blocking strategy. *Journal of Health, Politics, and Policy Law*, *38*(3), 505–544. doi:10.1215/03616878-2079496

Aronson, J. K. (2003). Anecdotes as evidence. *BMJ*, *326*(7403), 1346.

Aronson, J. K., & Hauben, M. (2006). Anecdotes that provide definitive evidence. *BMJ*, *333*(7581), 1267–1269. doi:333/7581/1267 [pii]10.1136/bmj.39036.666389.94

Asch, D. A., & Hershey, J. C. (1995). Why some health policies don't make sense at the bedside. *Annals of Internal Medicine*, *122*(11), 846–850. doi:10.7326/0003-4819-122-11-199506010-00007

Association of State and Territorial Health Officials. (2008). *At risk populations and pandemic influenza: Planning guidance for state, territorial, tribal, and local health departments* (Executive summary). Arlington, VA: ASTHO.

Atkins v. Virginia (2002). *U.S.* (Vol. 536, pp. 304): U.S. Supreme Court.

Atkinson, M. A., Eisenbarth, G. S., & Michels, A. W. (2014). Type 1 diabetes. *The Lancet*, *383*(9911), 69–82. http://dx.doi.org/10.1016/S0140-6736(13)60591-7

Auwaerter, P. G., Bakken, J. S., Dattwyler, R. J., Dumler, J. S., Halperin, J. J., McSweegan, E., et al. (2011). Antiscience and ethical concerns associated with advocacy of Lyme disease. *The Lancet Infectious Diseases*, *11*(9), 713–719. http://dx.doi.org/10.1016/S1473-3099(11)70034-2

Bach, P. B. (2013). Reforming the payment system for medical oncology: Reforming the payment system for medical oncologyviewpoint. *Journal of the American Medical Association*, *310*(3), 261–262. doi:10.1001/jama.2013.8127

Badcott, D. (2013). Big Pharma: A former insider's view. *Medicine, Health Care and Philosophy, 16*(2), 249–264. doi:10.1007/s11019-012-9388-6

Bae, M. H., Lee, J. H., Yang, D. H., Park, H. S., Cho, Y., Chae, S. C., et al. (2012). Erroneous computer electrocardiogram interpretation of atrial fibrillation and its clinical consequences. *Clinical Cardiology, 35*(6), 348–353. doi:10.1002/clc.22000

Baergen, R. (2006). How hopeful is too hopeful? Responding to unreasonably optimistic parents. *Pediatric Nursing, 32*(5), 482, 485–486.

Baiardini, I., Braido, F., Bonini, M., Compalati, E., & Canonica, G. W. (2009). Why do doctors and patients not follow guidelines? *Current Opinion in Allergy and Clinical Immunology, 9*(3), 228–233. doi:210.1097/ACI.1090b1013e32832b34651

Baicker, K., Chandra, A., & Skinner, J. S. (2012). Saving money or just saving lives? improving the productivity of US health care spending. *Annual Review of Economics, 4*(4), 33. doi:10.1146/Annurev-Economics-080511-110942

Baicker, K., & Finkelstein, A. (2011). The effects of Medicaid coverage—Learning from the Oregon experiment. *New England Journal of Medicine, 365*(8), 683–685. doi: 10.1056/NEJMp1108222

Baker, K. S., Davies, S. M., Majhail, N. S., Hassebroek, A., Klein, J. P., Ballen, K. K., et al. (2009). Race and socioeconomic status influence outcomes of unrelated donor hematopoietic cell transplantation. *Biology of Blood and Marrow Transplantation, 15*(12), 1543–1554. doi:10.1016/j.bbmt.2009.07.023

Balboni, T. A., Paulk, M. E., Balboni, M. J., Phelps, A. C., Loggers, E. T., Wright, A. A., et al. (2010). Provision of spiritual care to patients with advanced cancer: Associations with medical care and quality of life near death. *Journal of Clinical Oncology, 28*(3), 445–452. doi:10.1200/jco.2009.24.8005

Balfour-Lynn, I. M. (2014). Personalised medicine in cystic fibrosis is unaffordable. *Paediatric Respiratory Reviews, 15*, Supplement 1(0), 2–5. http://dx.doi.org/10.1016/j.prrv.2014.04.003

Ball, D. E., Tisocki, K., & Herxheimer, A. (2006). Advertising and disclosure of funding on patient organisation websites: A cross-sectional survey. *BMC Public Health, 6*(1), 201.

Banaji, M. R. (2013). *Blindspot: Hidden biases of good people.* New York: Delacorte.

Banting, F. G., Best, C. H., Collip, J. B., Campbell, W. R., & Fletcher, A. A. (1922). Pancreatic extracts in the treatment of diabetes mellitus. *Canadian Medical Association Journal, 7,* 141–146.

Barbash, G. I., & Glied, S. A. (2010). New technology and health care costs—The case of robot-assisted surgery. *New England Journal of Medicine, 363*(8), 701–704, doi: 10.1056/NEJMp1006602.

Barnato, A., Anthony, D., Skinner, J., Gallagher, P., & Fisher, E. (2009). Racial and ethnic differences in preferences for end-of-life treatment. *Journal of General Internal Medicine, 24*(6), 695–701. doi:10.1007/s11606-009-0952-6

Barry, J. M. (2004). *The great influenza: The epic story of the deadliest plague in history.* New York: Viking Press.

Barry, M. J., & Edgman-Levitan, S. (2012). Shared decision making—the pinnacle of patient-centered care. *New England Journal of Medicine, 366*(9), 780–781.

Basu, S., & Hassenplug, J. C. (2012). Patient access to medical devices—A comparison of U.S. and European review processes. *New England Journal of Medicine, 367*(6), 485–488. doi:10.1056/NEJMp1204170

Bazzano, A. T., Mangione-Smith, R., Schonlau, M., Suttorp, M. J., & Brook, R. H. (2009). Off-label prescribing to children in the United States outpatient setting. *Academic Pediatrics*, 9(2), 81–88.

Beach, M. C., Meredith, L. S., Halpern, J., Wells, K. B., & Ford, D. E. (2005). Physician conceptions of responsibility to individual patients and distributive justice in health care. *Annals of Family Medicine*, 3(1), 53–59. doi:10.1370/afm.257

Beale, A. V. (2012). The evolution of college admission requirements. *Journal of College Admission*(214), 20–22.

Begun, J. W., & Kaissi, A. A. (2004). Uncertainty in health care environments: Myth or reality? *Health Care Management Review*, 29(1), 31–39.

Bellman, R. E., & Zadeh, L. A. (1970). Decision-making in a fuzzy environment. *Management Science*, 17(4), B141–B164. doi:10.2307/2629367

Bendix, J. (2013). Curing the prior authorization headache: you probably can't avoid having to get upfront approvals, but you can reduce the hassles and costs they bring. *Med Econ*, 90(19), 24.

Benson, E. S. (1972). The concept of the normal range. *Human Pathology*, 3(2), 152–155. Retrieved from http://dx.doi.org/10.1016/S0046-8177(72)80068-6

Bentham, J. (1970). *An introduction to the principles of morals and legislation*. London: Athlone Press (University of London).

Bergthold, L. A. (1995). Medical necessity: Do we need it? *Health Affairs*, 14(4), 180–190.

Berkman, N. D., Sheridan, S. L., Donahue, K. E., Halpern, D. J., & Crotty, K. (2011). Low health literacy and health outcomes: An updated systematic review. *Annals of Internal Medicine*, 155(2), 97–107. doi:10.7326/0003-4819-155-2-201107190-00005

Berland, L. L. (2011). The American College of Radiology strategy for managing incidental findings on abdominal computed tomography. *Radiologic clinics of North America*, 49(2), 237–243. Retrieved from http://dx.doi.org/10.1016/j.rcl.2010.10.003

Berlin, L. (2011). The incidentaloma: A medicolegal dilemma. *Radiologic Clinics of North America*, 49(2), 245–255.

Bernier, R. H., & Marcuse, E. K. (2005). Citizen voices on pandemic flu choices. A report of the Public Engagement Project on Pandemic Influenza. Keystone, CO: The Keystone Center.

Bernstein, P. L., & Bernstein Peter, L. (1996). *Against the gods: The remarkable story of risk*. New York: Wiley.

Berwick, D. M., Fineberg, H. V., & Weinstein, M. C. (1981). When doctors meet numbers. *American Journal of Medicine*, 71(6), 991–998.

Berwick, D. M., & Hackbarth, A. D. (2012). Eliminating waste in US health care. *Journal of the American Medical Association*, 307(14), 1513–1516. doi:10.1001/jama.2012.362

Best, C. H., & Scott, D. A. (1923). The preparation of insulin. *Journal of Biological Chemistry*, 57(3), 709–723.

Best, R. K. (2012). Disease politics and medical research funding: Three ways advocacy shapes policy. *American Sociological Review*, 77(5), 780–803. doi:10.1177/0003122412458509

Beveridge, W. (2000). Social insurance and allied services. 1942. *Bulletin of the World Health Organization*, 78(6), 847–855.

Bidlingmaier, M., Friedrich, N., Emeny, R. T., Spranger, J., Wolthers, O. D., Roswall, J., et al. (2014). Reference intervals for insulin-like growth factor-1 (igf-i) from birth to senescence: Results from a multicenter study using a new automated chemiluminescence IGF-I immunoassay conforming to recent international recommendations. *Journal of Clinical Endocrinology & Metabolism*, 99(5), 1712–1721.

Biggar, N. (2015). Why religion deserves a place in secular medicine. *Journal of Medical Ethics, 41*(3), 229–233. doi:10.1136/medethics-2013-101776

Biggins, S. W. (2012). Futility and rationing in liver retransplantation: When and how can we say no? *Journal of Hepatology, 56*(6), 1404–1411.

Biggins, S. W., Gralla, J., Dodge, J. L., Bambha, K. M., Tong, S., Barón, A. E., et al. (2014). Survival benefit of repeat liver transplantation in the United States: A serial MELD analysis by hepatitis C status and donor risk index. *American Journal of Transplantation, 14*(11), 2588–2594. doi:10.1111/ajt.12867

Biomedical, N. C. f. t. P. o. H. S. o., & Behavioral Research, B., MD. (1978). *The Belmont report: Ethical principles and guidelines for the protection of human subjects of research*: ERIC Clearinghouse.

Blackburn, M. R., & Thompson, L. F. (2012). Adenosine deaminase deficiency: Unanticipated benefits from the study of a rare immunodeficiency. *Journal of Immunology, 188*(3), 933–935. doi:10.4049/jimmunol.1103519

Blackhall, L. J., Frank, G., Murphy, S. T., Michel, V., Palmer, J. M., & Azen, S. P. (1999). Ethnicity and attitudes towards life sustaining technology. *Social Science and Medicine, 48*(12), 1779–1789.

Blagg, C. R. (2007). The early history of dialysis for chronic renal failure in the United States: A view from Seattle. *American Journal of Kidney Diseases, 49*(3), 482–496. doi:10.1053/j.ajkd.2007.01.017

Blake, V. (2015). Narrow networks, the very sick, and the patient protection and Affordable Care Act: Recalling the purpose of health insurance and reform. *Minnesota Journal of Law, Science, and Technology 16*, 63–144.

Blaser, M., Bork, P., Fraser, C., Knight, R., & Wang, J. (2013). The microbiome explored: Recent insights and future challenges. [10.1038/nrmicro2973]. *Nature Reviews Microbiology, 11*(3), 213–217.

Bleustein, C., Rothschild, D. B., Valen, A., Valatis, E., Schweitzer, L., & Jones, R. (2014). Wait times, patient satisfaction scores, and the perception of care. *American Journal of Managed Care, 20*(5), 393–400.

Bloche, M. G. (2011). *The Hippocratic Myth: Why doctors are under pressure to ration care, practice politics, and compromise their promise to heal*. Basingstoke, Hampshire: Palgrave Macmillan.

Bloche, M. G. (2012). Beyond the "r word?" Medicine's new frugality. *New England Journal of Medicine, 366*(21), 1951–1953. doi:10.1056/NEJMp1203521

Block, L., Jarlenski, M., Wu, A., & Bennett, W. (2013). Mammography use among women ages 40–49 after the 2009 U.S. Preventive Services Task Force recommendation. *Journal of General Internal Medicine*, 1–7. doi:10.1007/s11606-013-2482-5

Bloss, C. S., Schork, N. J., & Topol, E. J. (2014). Direct-to-consumer pharmacogenomic testing is associated with increased physician utilisation. *Journal of Medical Genetics, 51*(2), 83–89. doi:10.1136/jmedgenet-2013-101909

Blumenthal, D., Abrams, M., & Nuzum, R. (2015). The Affordable Care Act at 5 years. *New England Journal of Medicine, 372*(25), 2451–2458. doi:10.1056/NEJMhpr1503614

Blustein, J., & Marmor, T. R. (1992). Cutting waste by making rules: Promises, pitfalls, and realistic prospects. *University of Pennsylvania Law Review, 140*(5), 1543–1572. doi:10.2307/3312425

Bock, G. L. (2008). Medically valid religious beliefs. *Journal of Medical Ethics, 34*(6), 437–440. doi:10.1136/jme.2007.021964

Bogdan-Lovis, E., Fleck, L., & Barry, H. C. (2012). It's NOT FAIR! Or is it? The promise and the tyranny of evidence-based performance assessment. *Theor Med Bioeth, 33*(4), 293–311.

Boggs, C. (2015). The Medicalized Society. *Critical Sociology, 41*(3), 517–535.

Boorse, C. (1977). Health as a Theoretical Concept. *Philosophy of Science, 44*(4), 542–573. doi:10.2307/186939

Bopp, J., & Coleson, R. E. (1994). Child abuse by whom?—parental rights and judicial competency determinations: The Baby K and Baby Terry cases. *Ohio Northern University Law Review, 20*, 821–845.

Boss, R. D., Holmes, K. W., Althaus, J., Rushton, C. H., McNee, H., & McNee, T. (2013). Trisomy 18 and complex congenital heart disease: Seeking the threshold benefit. *Pediatrics, 132*(1), 161–165.

Bosslet, G. T., Pope, T. M., Rubenfeld, G. D., Lo, B., Truog, R. D., Rushton, C. H., et al. (2015). An Official ATS/AACN/ACCP/ESICM/SCCM Policy Statement: Responding to Requests for Potentially Inappropriate Treatments in Intensive Care Units. *American Journal of Respiratory and Critical Care Medicine, 191*(11), 1318–1330.

Bostan, S., Acuner, T., & Yilmaz, G. (2007). Patient (customer) expectations in hospitals. *Health Policy, 82*(1), 62–70. doi:S0168-8510(06)00188-6 [pii]10.1016/j.healthpol.2006.08.005

Botter, S. M., Neri, D., & Fuchs, B. (2014). Recent advances in osteosarcoma. *Current Opinion in Pharmacology, 16*, 15–23. Retrieved from http://dx.doi.org/10.1016/j.coph.2014.02.002

Bowker, G. C., & Starr, S. L. (1999). *Sorting things out*. Cambridge, MA: MIT Press.

Boyd, F. (1910). Faith and healing. *British Medical Journal, 2*(2590), 464.

Bracanovic, T. (2013). Against culturally sensitive bioethics. *Medicine and Health Care Philosophy, 16*(4), 647–652. Retrieved from http://dx.doi.org/10.1007/s11019-013-9504-2

Braithwaite, R. S., Meltzer, D. O., King, J. T., Jr., Leslie, D., & Roberts, M. S. (2008). What does the value of modern medicine say about the $50,000 per quality-adjusted life-year decision rule? *Medical Care, 46*(4), 349–356. doi:10.2307/40221668

Brandon, D. T., Isaac, L. A., & LaVeist, T. A. (2005). The legacy of Tuskegee and trust in medical care: Is Tuskegee responsible for race differences in mistrust of medical care? [Historical Article Research Support, Non-U.S. Gov't Research Support, U.S. Gov't, P.H.S.]. *Journal of the National Medical Association, 97*(7), 951–956.

Brase, G. L. (2009). Pictorial representations in statistical reasoning. *Applied Cognitive Psychology, 23*(3), 369–381.

Braun, M. M., Farag-El-Massah, S., Xu, K., & Coté, T. R. (2010). Emergence of orphan drugs in the United States: A quantitative assessment of the first 25 years. [10.1038/nrd3160]. *Nat Rev Drug Discov, 9*(7), 519–522. Retrieved from http://www.nature.com/nrd/journal/v9/n7/suppinfo/nrd3160_S1.html

Braveman, P., Egerter, S., & Williams, D. R. (2011). The social determinants of health: Coming of age. *Annual Review of Public Health, 32*(1), 381–398. doi:10.1146/annurev-publhealth-031210-101218

Braybrooke, D. (1987). *Meeting needs*. Princeton, NJ: Princeton University Press.

Brazier, J., Ratcliffe, J., Tsuchiya, A., & Salomon, J. (2007). *Measuring and valuing health benefits for economic evaluation*. Oxford, UK/New York: Oxford University Press.

Brekke, K. R., & Sørgard, L. (2007). Public versus private health care in a national health service. *Health Economics, 16*(6), 579–601.

Brennan, R., Eagle, L., & Rice, D. (2010). Medicalization and Marketing. *Journal of Macromarketing, 30*(1), 8–22. doi:10.1177/0276146709352221

Brett, A. S., & Jersild, P. (2003). "Inappropriate" treatment near the end of life: Conflict between religious convictions and clinical judgment. *Archives of Internal Medicine, 163*(14), 1645–1649. doi:10.1001/archinte.163.14.1645

Brierley, J., Linthicum, J., & Petros, A. (2013). Should religious beliefs be allowed to stonewall a secular approach to withdrawing and withholding treatment in children? *Journal of Medical Ethics, 39*(9), 573–577. doi:10.1136/medethics-2011-100104

Brill, S. (2015). *America's bitter pill: Money, politics, backroom deals, and the fight to fix our broken healthcare system.* New York: Random House.

Mason, C., Brindley, D. A., Culme-Seymour, E. J., & Davie, N. L. (2011). Cell therapy industry: billion dollar global business with unlimited potential. *Regenerative Medicine, 6*(3), 265–272.

Brock, G. (1998). Introduction. In G. GBrock (Ed.), *Necessary goods: Our responsibilities to meet other's needs* (pp. 1–18). Oxford, UK: Rowman and Littlefield.

Brody, H. (2005). The company we keep: Why physicians should refuse to see pharmaceutical representatives. *Annals of Family Medicine, 3*(1), 82–85. doi:10.1370/afm.259

Brody, H. (2007). *Hooked: Ethics, the medical profession, and the pharmaceutical industry* (Explorations in bioethics and the medical humanities). Lanham, MD: Rowman & Littlefield.

Brody, H. (2012). From an ethics of rationing to an ethics of waste avoidance. *New England Journal of Medicine, 366*(21), 1949–1951. doi:10.1056/NEJMp1203365

Brody, H., & Bonham, V. L., Jr. (1997). Gag rules and trade secrets in managed care contracts. Ethical and legal concerns. *Archives of Internal Medicine, 157*(18), 2037–2043.

Brook, R. H., Chassin, M. R., Fink, A., Solomon, D. H., Kosecoff, J., & Park, R. (1986). A method for the detailed assessment of the appropriateness of medical technologies. *Int J Technol Assess Health Care, 2*(01), 53–63.

Brooks, G. A., Li, L., Sharma, D. B., Weeks, J. C., Hassett, M. J., Yabroff, K. R., et al. (2013). Regional variation in spending and survival for older adults with advanced cancer. *Journal of the National Cancer Institute, 105*(9), 634–642. doi:10.1093/jnci/djt025

Brouwers, M. C., Haynes, R. B., Jadad, A. R., Hayward, R. S., Padunsky, J. A., & Yang, J. L. (1997). Evidence-based health care and the Cochrane Collaboration. *Clin Perform Qual Health Care, 5*(4), 195–201.

Brown, R. C. H. (2013). Moral responsibility for (un)healthy behaviour. *Journal of Medical Ethics,* doi:10.1136/medethics-2012-100774

Brownlee, S. (2008). *Overtreated: Why too much medicine is making us sicker and poorer.* New York: Bloomsbury.

Bruns, D., & Campbell, E. (2014). Twenty-two survivors over the age of 1 year with full trisomy 18: Presenting and current medical conditions. *American Journal of Medical Genetics Part A, 164*(3), 610–619. doi:10.1002/ajmg.a.36318

Buchanan, A. (2008). Enhancement and the ethics of development. *Kennedy Institute Ethics Journal, 18*(1), 1–34.

Buchanan, A., Brock, D. W., Daniels, N., & Wikler, D. (2000). *From chance to choice. Genetics and justice.* New York: Cambridge University Press.

Burnyeat, M. F. (1982). Gods and heaps. In M. C. Nussbaum, & M. Schofield (Eds.), *Language and logos: Studies in ancient Greek philosophy presented to G.E.L. Owen* (pp. 333–334). Cambridge, UK/New York: Cambridge University Press.

Buryska, J. F. (2001). Assessing the ethical weight of cultural, religious and spiritual claims in the clinical context. *Journal of Medical Ethics, 27*(2), 118–122. doi:10.1136/jme.27.2.118

Bustamante, A. V., Fang, H., Garza, J., Carter-Pokras, O., Wallace, S. P., Rizzo, J. A., et al. (2012). Variations in healthcare access and utilization among Mexican immigrants: The role of documentation status. *Journal of Immigrant and Minority Health*, *14*(1), 146–155. doi:10.1007/s10903-010-9406-9

Butterworth, J. F. (2009). Case reports: Unstylish but still useful sources of clinical information. *Regional Anesthesia and Pain Medicine*, *34*(3), 187–188. doi:10.1097/AAP.0b013e31819a277500115550-200905000-00002 [pii.

Cadieux, G., Abrahamowicz, M., Dauphinee, D., & Tamblyn, R. (2011). Are physicians with better clinical skills on licensing examinations less likely to prescribe antibiotics for viral respiratory infections in ambulatory care settings? *Medical Care*, *49*(2), 156–165. doi: 110.1097/MLR.1090b1013e3182028c3182021a

Calabresi, G., & Bobbitt, P. (1978). *Tragic choices*. New York: W. W. Norton.

Califf, R. M., McCall, J., & Harrington, R. A. (2013). Assessing research results in the medical literature: Trust but verify. *Journal of the American Medical Association Internal Medicine*, *173*(12), 1053–1055.

Callahan, D. (1987). *Setting limits: Medical goals in an aging society*. New York: Simon and Schuster.

Callahan, D. (1990). *What kind of life. The limits of medical progress*. New York: Simon and Shuster.

Callahan, D. (1991). Medical futility, medical necessity: The-problem-without-a-name. *Hastings Cent Rep*, *21*(4), 30–35. doi:10.2307/3562999

Callahan, D. (1998). *False hopes. Why America's quest for perfect health is a recipe for failure*. New York: Simon and Shuster.

Callahan, D. (2009). *Taming the beloved beast*. Princeton, NJ: Princeton University Press.

Callahan, D. (2012). Must we ration health care for the elderly? *The Journal of Law, Medicine & Ethics*, *40*(1), 10–16. doi:10.1111/j.1748-720X.2012.00640.x

Callan, M. J., Dawtry, R. J., & Olson, J. M. (2012). Justice motive effects in ageism: The effects of a victim's age on observer perceptions of injustice and punishment judgments. *Journal of Experimental Social Psychology*, *48*(6), 1343–1349. doi:10.1016/j.jesp.2012.07.003

Callison, K., & Kaestner, R. (2014). Do higher tobacco taxes reduce adult smoking? New evidence of the effect of recent cigarette tax increases on adult smoking. *Economic Inquiry*, *52*(1), 155–172, doi:10.1111/ecin.12027

Cameron, D. J. (2010). Proof that chronic Lyme disease exists. *Interdisciplinary Perspectives on Infectious Diseases 2010*, 1–4, doi:doi:10.1155/2010/876450.

Campbell, E. G., Pham-Kanter, G., Vogeli, C., & Iezzoni, L. I. (2013). Physician acquiescence to patient demands for brand-name drugs: Results of a national survey of physicians. *JAMA Internal Medicine*, *173*(3), 237–239. doi:10.1001/jamainternmed.2013.1539

Canguilhem, G. (1991). *The normal and the pathological* (Normal et le pathologique. English). New York: Zone Books.

Card, D., Dobkin, C., & Maestas, N. (2004). The impact of nearly universal insurance coverage on health care utilization and health: evidence from Medicare. Cambridge (MA): National Bureau of Economic Research.

Carman, K. L., Maurer, M., Yegian, J. M., Dardess, P., McGee, J., Evers, M., et al. (2010). Evidence that consumers are skeptical about evidence-based health care. *Health Affairs*, *29*(7), 1400–1406. doi:10.1377/hlthaff.2009.0296

Carpenter, J., Hutchings, A., Raine, R., & Sanderson, C. (2007). An experimental study of the influence of individual participant characteristics on formal consensus development. *International Journal of Technology Assessment in Health Care*, *23*(01), 108–115.

Carr-Hill, R. A. (1989). Assumptions of the QALY procedure. *Social Science & Medicine, 29*(3), 469–477. Retrieved from http://dx.doi.org/10.1016/0277-9536(89)90296-7

Cassel C., & Guest, J. A. (2012). Choosing wisely: Helping physicians and patients make smart decisions about their care. *Journal of the American Medical Association, 307*(17), 1801–1802. doi:10.1001/jama.2012.476

Cassell, E. J. (1982). The nature of suffering and the goals of medicine. *New England Journal of Medicine, 306*(11), 639–645. doi:10.1056/NEJM198203183061104

Cassell, E. J. (1983). The relief of suffering. *Archives of Internal Medicine, 143*(3), 522–523. doi:10.1001/archinte.1983.00350030136022

Cassell, E. J. (1991). Recognizing suffering. *Hastings Cent Rep, 21*(3), 24–31.

Cassell, E. J. (1999*a*). Diagnosing suffering: A perspective. *Annals of Internal Medicine, 131*(7), 531–534.

Cassell, E. J. (1999*b*). Pain, suffering, and the goals of medicine. In M. J. Hanson, & D. Callahan (Eds.), *The goals of medicine: The forgotten issue in health care reform* (pp. 101–117). Washington, DC: Georgetown University Press.

Catalano, D., Chan, F., Wilson, L., Chiu, C.-Y., & Muller, V. R. (2011). The buffering effect of resilience on depression among individuals with spinal cord injury: A structural equation model. *Rehabilitation Psychology, 56*(3), 200.

Catalona, W. J., D'Amico, A. V., Fitzgibbons, W. F., Kosoko-Lasaki, O., Leslie, S. W., Lynch, H. T., et al. (2012). What the U.S. Preventive Services Task Force missed in its prostate cancer screening recommendation. *Annals of Internal Medicine, 157*(2), 137–138. doi:10.7326/0003-4819-157-2-201207170-00463

Catlin, E. A., Cadge, W., Ecklund, E. H., Gage, E. A., & Zollfrank, A. A. (2008). The spiritual and religious identities, beliefs, and practices of academic pediatricians in the United States. *Academic Medicine, 83*(12), 1146–1152. doi:1110.1097/ACM.1140b1013e31818c31 864a31815

Ceaser, J. W. (2012). The origins and character of American exceptionalism. *Origins, 1*, 1–25.

Cerdá, M., Diez-Roux, A. V., Tchetgen, E. T., Gordon-Larsen, P., & Kiefe, C. (2010). The relationship between neighborhood poverty and alcohol use: Estimation by marginal structural models. *Epidemiology (Cambridge, Mass.), 21*(4), 482.

Chahine, T., Subramanian, S. V., & Levy, J. I. (2011). Sociodemographic and geographic variability in smoking in the U.S.: A multilevel analysis of the 2006–2007 Current Population Survey, Tobacco Use Supplement. *Social Science & Medicine, 73*(5), 752–758. Retrieved from http://dx.doi.org/10.1016/j.socscimed.2011.06.032

Chaloupka, F. J., Yurekli, A., & Fong, G. T. (2012). Tobacco taxes as a tobacco control strategy. *Tob Control, 21*(2), 172–180. doi:10.1136/tobaccocontrol-2011-050417

Chan, T., Pinto, N., & Bratton, S. (2012). Racial and Insurance Disparities in Hospital Mortality for Children Undergoing Congenital Heart Surgery. *Pediatric Cardiology, 33*(7), 1026–1039. doi:10.1007/s00246-012-0221-z

Charlifue, S., Apple, D., Burns, S. P., Chen, D., Cuthbert, J. P., Donovan, W. H., et al. (2011). Mechanical ventilation, health, and quality of life following spinal cord injury. *Archives of Physical Medicine and Rehabilitation, 92*(3), 457–463. Retrieved from http://dx.doi.org/10.1016/j.apmr.2010.07.237

Charpak, G. (2004). *Debunked!: ESP, telekinesis, and other pseudoscience* (Devenez sorciers, devenez savants. English). Baltimore, MD: Johns Hopkins University Press.

Chau, N. G., Li, Y. Y., Jo, V. Y., Rabinowits, G., Lorch, J. H., Tishler, R. B., et al. (2016). Incorporation of next-generation sequencing into routine clinical care to direct treatment of head and neck squamous cell carcinoma. *Clinical Cancer Research.* doi:10.1158/1078-0432.ccr-15-2314

Chen, D. T., Wynia, M. K., Moloney, R. M., & Alexander, G. C. (2009). U.S. physician knowledge of the FDA-approved indications and evidence base for commonly prescribed drugs: Results of a national survey. *Pharmacoepidemiology and Drug Safety, 18*(11), 1094–1100. doi:10.1002/pds.1825

Chidi, A. P., Bryce, C. L., Myaskovsky, L., Fine, M. J., Geller, D. A., Landsittel, D. P., et al. (2015). Differences in physician referral drive disparities in surgical intervention for hepatocellular carcinoma: A retrospective cohort study. *Annals of Surgery.* Advance online publication. doi:10.1097/sla.0000000000001111

Childress, J. F. (2007). Must we always respect religious belief? *Hastings Center Report, 37*(1), 3.

Churchill, L. R., & Churchill, S. C. (2013). Buying health: The costs of commercialism and an alternative philosophy. *International Journal of Health Policy and Management, 1*(2), 91.

Clark, P. A. (2009). Prejudice and the medical profession: A five-year update. [Historical Article]. *The Journal of law, medicine & ethics: A journal of the American Society of Law, Medicine & Ethics, 37*(1), 118–133. doi:10.1111/j.1748-720X.2009.00356.x

Clarke, S. (2012). When they believe in miracles. *Journal of Medical Ethics.* doi:10.1136/medethics-2012-100677

Clayton, E. W. (1995). Commentary: What is really at stake in Baby K? Response to Ellen Flannery. *Journal of Law, Medicinel & Ethics, 23*, 13–14.

Steinberg, E., Greenfield, S., Mancher, M., Wolman, D. M., & Graham, R. (2011). *Clinical practice guidelines we can trust.* Washington, DC: National Academies Press.

Coglianese, E., Samsi, M., Liebo, M., & Heroux, A. (2015). The value of psychosocial factors in patient selection and outcomes after heart transplantation. *Current Heart Failure Reports, 12*(1), 42–47. doi:10.1007/s11897-014-0233-5

Cohen, I. G., Daniels, N., & Eyal, N. M. (Eds.). (2015). *Identified versus statistical lives: An interdisciplinary perspective* (Population-level bioethics series). Oxford, UK/New York: Oxford University Press.

Cohen, J. (1996). Preferences, needs and QALYs. *Journal of Medical Ethics, 22*(5), 267–272. doi:10.1136/jme.22.5.267

Cohen, J., Wilson, A., & Faden, L. (2009). Off-label use reimbursement. *Food and Drug Law Journal, 64*(2), 391–403.

Cohen, P., Rogol, A. D., Deal, C. L., Saenger, P., Reiter, E. O., Ross, J. L., et al. (2008). Consensus statement on the diagnosis and treatment of children with idiopathic short stature: A summary of the Growth Hormone Research Society, the Lawson Wilkins Pediatric Endocrine Society, and the European Society for Paediatric Endocrinology Workshop. *The Journal of Clinical Endocrinology & Metabolism, 93*(11), 4210–4217. doi:10.1210/jc.2008-0509

Collins, F. S. (2006). *The language of God: A scientist presents evidence for belief.* New York: Free Press.

Collins, S., Rasmussen, P., & Doty, M. (2015). The rise in health care coverage and affordability since health reform took effect: Findings from the Commonwealth Fund Biennial Health Insurance Survey, 2014. *Issue brief (Commonwealth Fund), 2*, 1–16.

Colombo, C., Mosconi, P., Villani, W., & Garattini, S. (2012). Patient organizations' funding from pharmaceutical companies: Is disclosure clear, complete and accessible to the public? An Italian survey. *PLoS ONE, 7*(5), e34974.

Colver, A., Thyen, U., Arnaud, C., Beckung, E., Fauconnier, J., Marcelli, M., et al. (2012). Association between participation in life situations of children with cerebral palsy and their physical, social, and attitudinal environment: A cross-sectional multicenter European Study. *Archives of Physical Medicine and Rehabilitation, 93*(12), 2154–2164. Retrieved from http://dx.doi.org/10.1016/j.apmr.2012.07.011

Conrad, P., Mackie, T., & Mehrotra, A. (2010). Estimating the costs of medicalization. *Social Science & Medicine, 70*(12), 1943–1947.

Conroy, T., Desseigne, F., Ychou, M., Bouché, O., Guimbaud, R., Bécouarn, Y., et al. (2011). FOLFIRINOX versus Gemcitabine for metastatic pancreatic cancer. *New England Journal of Medicine, 364*(19), 1817–1825. doi:10.1056/NEJMoa1011923

Cooke, B. K., Delalot, D., & Werner, T. L. (2015). Hall v. Florida: Capital punishment, IQ, and persons with intellectual disabilities. *Journal of the American Academy of Psychiatry and the Law Online, 43*(2), 230–234.

Cookson, R., McCabe, C., & Tsuchiya, A. (2008). Public healthcare resource allocation and the Rule of Rescue. [Research Support, Non-U.S. Gov't Review]. *Journal of Medical Ethics, 34*(7), 540–544. doi:10.1136/jme.2007.021790

Cooper, R. (2006). *Classifying madness: A philosophical examination of the Diagnostic and Statistical Manual of Mental Disorders.* Dordrecht (The Netherlands): Springer Netherlands.

Cooper, R. S., Ferguson, A., Bodurtha, J. N., & Smith, T. J. (2014). AMEN in challenging conversations: Bridging the gaps between faith, hope, and medicine. *Journal of Oncology Practice.*

Courtney, A. E., & Maxwell, A. P. (2009). The challenge of doing what is right in renal transplantation: Balancing equity and utility. *Nephron Clinical Practice, 111*(1), c62–c68.

Cousin, G., Schmid Mast, M., & Jaunin-Stalder, N. (2013). When physician-expressed uncertainty leads to patient dissatisfaction: A gender study. *Medical Education, 47*(9), 923–931. doi:10.1111/medu.12237

Craig, A. (2012). Resilience in people with physical disabilities. In P. Kennedy (Ed.), *The Oxford handbook of rehabilitation psychology* (pp. 474–491). Oxford, UK: Oxford University Press.

Crisp, R. (2002). Treatment according to need: Justice and the British National Health Service. In R. Rhodes, M. P. Battin, & A. Silvers (Eds.), *Medicine and social justice* (pp. 134–155). New York: Oxford University Press.

Cruden, N., Din, J., Janssen, C., Smith, R., Carere, R., Klinke, W., et al. (2013). Prolonged clopidogrel use improves clinical outcomes following drug eluting but not bare metal stent implantation. *European Heart Journal, 34*(suppl 1), 2589.

Cruz-Oliver, D. M., Thomas, D. R., Scott, J., Malmstrom, T. K., De Jesus-Monge, W. E., & Paniagua, M. A. (2010). Age as a deciding factor in the consideration of futility for a medical intervention in patients among internal medicine physicians in two practice locations. *Journal of the American Medical Directors Association, 11*(6), 421–427. doi:10.1016/j.jamda.2010.01.011

Cunningham, P. J. (2010). The growing financial burden of health care: National and state trends, 2001–2006. *Health Affairs, 29*(5), 1037–1044. doi:10.1377/hlthaff.2009.0493

Cunningham, P. J. (2015). The share of people with high medical costs increased prior to implementation of the Affordable Care Act. *Health Affairs, 34*(1), 117–124. doi:10.1377/hlthaff.2014.0216

Cupler, E. J., Berger, K. I., Leshner, R. T., Wolfe, G. I., Han, J. J., Barohn, R. J., et al. (2012). Consensus treatment recommendations for late-onset Pompe disease. *Muscle Nerve*, *45*(3), 319–333.

Curlin, F. A., Chin, M. H., Sellergren, S. A., Roach, C. J., & Lantos, J. D. (2006). The association of physicians' religious characteristics with their attitudes and self-reported behaviors regarding religion and spirituality in the clinical encounter. *Medical Care*, *44*(5), 446–453.

Curlin, F. A., Lantos, J. D., Roach, C. J., Sellergren, S. A., & Chin, M. H. (2005). Religious Characteristics of U.S. Physicians. *Journal of General Internal Medicine*, *20*(7), 629–634. doi:10.1111/j.1525-1497.2005.0119.x

Cydulka, R. K., Tamayo-Sarver, J., Gage, A., & Bagnoli, D. (2011). Association of patient satisfaction with complaints and risk management among emergency physicians. *The Journal of emergency medicine*, *41*(4), 405–411.

Daniels, N. (1983). Justice between age groups: Am I my parents' keeper? *The Milbank Memorial Fund Quarterly. Health and Society*, *61*(3), 489–522. doi:10.2307/3349870

Daniels, N. (1991). Is the Oregon rationing plan fair? *The Journal of the American Medical Association*, *265*(17), 2232–2235. doi:10.1001/jama.1991.03460170086039

Daniels, N. (2000). Accountability for reasonableness. [Comment Editorial]. *BMJ*, *321*(7272), 1300–1301.

Daniels, N. (2008). *Just health:Meeting health needs fairly*. New York: Cambridge University Press.

Daniels, N. (2015). Why we should care about the social determinants of health. *The American Journal of Bioethics*, *15*(3), 37–38. doi:10.1080/15265161.2015.1000062

Daniels, N., & Sabin, J. (1998). The ethics of accountability in managed care reform. *Health Affairs(Millwood)*, *17*(5), 50–64.

Daniels, N., & Sabin, J. (2008). *Setting limits fairly. Learning to share resources for health* (2nd ed.). Oxford, UK: Oxford University Press.

Dart, A. B., Martens, P. J., Rigatto, C., Brownell, M. D., Dean, H. J., & Sellers, E. A. (2014). Earlier onset of complications in youth with type 2 diabetes. *Diabetes Care*, *37*(2), 436–443.

David, A., Hwa, V., Metherell, L. A., Netchine, I., Camacho-Hübner, C., Clark, A. J., et al. (2011). Evidence for a continuum of genetic, phenotypic, and biochemical abnormalities in children with growth hormone insensitivity. *Endocrine reviews*, *32*(4), 472–497.

Davis, F. (1960). Uncertainty in medical prognosis clinical and functional. *American Journal of Sociology*, *66*(1), 41–47. doi:10.2307/2773220

Davis, K., & Ballreich, J. (2014). Equitable access to care—how the United States ranks internationally. *New England Journal of Medicine*, *371*(17), 1567–1570. 10.1056/NEJMp1406707

Davis, K., Stremikis, K., Squires, D., & Schoen, C. (2014). Mirror, mirror on the wall. *The Commonwealth Fund*:www.resbr.net.br/wp-content/uploads/historico/Espelhoespelhomeu.pdf.

De Block, A., & Adriaens, P. R. (2013). Pathologizing sexual deviance: A history. *The Journal of Sex Research*, *50*(3–4), 276–298. doi:10.1080/00224499.2012.738259

de Groot, R. J., Baker, S. C., Baric, R. S., Brown, C. S., Drosten, C., Enjuanes, L., et al. (2013). Middle East Respiratory Syndrome Coronavirus (MERS-CoV): Announcement of the Coronavirus Study Group. *Journal of Virology*, *87*(14), 7790–7792. doi:10.1128/jvi.01244-13

De Nardi, M., French, E., Jones, J. B., & McCauley, J. (2015). *Medical spending of the US elderly*. No. w21270. National Bureau of Economic Research (Cambridge, MA).

Dekay, M. L., Nickerson, C. A. E., Ubel, P. A., Hershey, J. C., Spranca, M. D., & Asch, D. A. (2000). Further explorations of medical decisions for individuals and for groups. *Medical Decision Making, 20*(1), 39–44. doi:10.1177/0272989x0002000105

DeMarco, V. G., Aroor, A. R., & Sowers, J. R. (2014). The pathophysiology of hypertension in patients with obesity. [Review]. *Nature Reviews Endocrinology, 10*(6), 364–376. doi:10.1038/nrendo.2014.44

Demicheli, V., Rivetti, A., Debalini, M. G., & Di Pietrantonj, C. (2012). Vaccines for measles, mumps and rubella in children. *Cochrane Database of Systematic Reviews*(2), doi:10.1002/14651858.CD004407.pub3.

Dershowitz, A. M. (2013). *Reversal of fortune: Inside the Von Bulow case* (reissue ed.), New York: Random House LLC.

Detsky, A. S. (2012). Underestimating the value of reassurance. *Journal of the American Medical Association, 307*(10), 1035–1036. doi:10.1001/jama.2012.235

DeVita, V. T., Jr., Serpick, A. A., & Carbone, P. P. (1970). Combination chemotherapy in the treatment of advanced Hodgkin's Disease. *Annals of Internal Medicine, 73*(6), 881.

Dickenson, D. (2013). *Me medicine vs. we medicine: Reclaiming biotechnology for the common good.* New York: Columbia University Press.

Diem, S. J., Lantos, J. D., & Tulsky, J. A. (1996). Cardiopulmonary resuscitation on television. Miracles and misinformation. *New England Journal of Medicine, 334*(24), 1578–1582.

Disch, L. (1996). Publicity-Stunt Participation and Sound Bite Polemics: The Health Care Debate 1993–94. *Journal of Health Politics, Policy and Law, 21*(1), 3–33, doi:10.1215/03616878-21-1-3.

Dixon-Woods, M., Amalberti, R., Goodman, S., Bergman, B., & Glasziou, P. (2011). Problems and promises of innovation: Why healthcare needs to rethink its love/hate relationship with the new. *BMJ Quality & Safety, 20*(Suppl 1), i47–i51. doi:10.1136/bmjqs.2010.046227

Djulbecovic, B., Hozo, I., & Greenland, S. (2011). Uncertainty in clinical medicine. In F. Gifford (Ed.), *Handbook of the philosophy of science* (Vol. 16). Oxford, UK/ Burlington, MA: North Holland.

Djulbegovic, B., & Paul, A. (2011). From efficacy to effectiveness in the face of uncertainty: Indication creep and prevention creep. *Journal of the American Medical Association, 305*(19), 2005–2006. doi:10.1001/jama.2011.650

Doan, T. L., Pollastri, M., Walters, M. A., Georg, G. I., & Macor, J. (2011). The future of drug repositioning: Old drugs, new opportunities. *Annual Reports in Medicinal Chemistry, 46*, 385–401.

Dobbin, F. R. (1992). The origins of private social insurance: Public policy and fringe benefits in America, 1920–1950. *American Journal of Sociology, 97*(5), 1416–1450. doi:10.2307/2781420

Docter, S. P., Street, J., Braunack-Mayer, A. J., & van der Wilt, G. J. (2011). Public perceptions of pandemic influenza resource allocation: A deliberative forum using Grid/Group analysis. [Research Support, Non-U.S. Gov't]. *Journal of Public Health Policy, 32*(3), 350–366. doi:10.1057/jphp.2010.49

Doe *v.* Bolton (1973). *U.S.* (Vol. 410, pp. 179): U.S. Supreme Court.

Donna, T. C., Matthew, K. W., Rachael, M. M., & Alexander, G. C. (2009). U.S. physician knowledge of the FDA-approved indications and evidence base for commonly prescribed drugs: Results of a national survey. *Pharmacoepidemiology and Drug Safety, 18*(11), 1094–1100.

Donne, J. (2010). *The complete poems of John Donne: Epigrams, verse letters to friends, love-lyrics, love-elegies, satire, religion poems, wedding celebrations, verse epistles to patronesses, commemorations and anniversaries* (Longman annotated English poets). Harlow, England/New York: Longman.

Doyal, L., & Gough, I. (1991). *A theory of human need*. New York: Guilford.

Dranove, D., Garthwaite, C., & Ody, C. (2014). Health spending slowdown is mostly due to economic factors, not structural change in the health care sector. *Health Affairs, 33*(8), 1399–1406.

Drosten, C., Preiser, W., Günther, S., Schmitz, H., & Doerr, H. W. (2003). Severe acute respiratory syndrome: Identification of the etiological agent. *Trends in Molecular Medicine, 9*(8), 325–327. Retrieved from http://dx.doi.org/10.1016/S1471-4914(03)00133-3

Drummond, M., Brixner, D., Gold, M., Kind, P., McGuire, A., Nord, E., et al. (2009). Toward a Consensus on the QALY. *Value in Health, 12*, S31–S35. doi:10.1111/j.1524-4733.2009.00522.x

Duffin, J. (2007). The Doctor was surprised: Or, how to diagnose a miracle. *Bulletin of the History of Medicine, 81*(4), 699–729.

Duffy, J. P., Kao, K., Ko, C. Y., Farmer, D. G., McDiarmid, S. V., Hong, J. C., et al. (2010). Long-term patient outcome and quality of life after liver transplantation: Analysis of 20-year survivors. *Annals of surgery, 252*(4), 652–661. 610.1097/SLA.1090b1013e3181f1095f1023a

Duggan, M., Starc, A., & Vabson, B. (2014). Who Benefits when the Government Pays More? Pass-Through in the Medicare Advantage Program. Cambridge (MA): National Bureau of Economic Research.

Dutkowski, P., Oberkofler, C. E., Slankamenac, K., Puhan, M. A., Schadde, E., Müllhaupt, B., et al. (2011). Are there better guidelines for allocation in liver transplantation? A novel score targeting justice and utility in the model for end-stage liver disease era. *Annals of Surgery, 254*(5), 745–754. 710.1097/SLA.1090b1013e3182365081

Dworkin, R. (1981). What is equality? Part 2: Equality of resources. *Philosophy & Public Affairs, 10*(4), 283–345.

Dworkin, R. (2003). Equality, luck and hierarchy. *Philosophy & Public Affairs, 31*(2), 190–198. doi:10.1111/j.1088-4963.2003.00190.x

Dworkin, R. H., Turk, D. C., Peirce-Sandner, S., Burke, L. B., Farrar, J. T., Gilron, I., et al. (2012). Considerations for improving assay sensitivity in chronic pain clinical trials: IMMPACT recommendations. *Pain, 153*(6), 1148–1158. Retrieved from http://dx.doi.org/10.1016/j.pain.2012.03.003

Dwyer-Lindgren, L., Mokdad, A. H., Srebotnjak, T., Flaxman, A. D., Hansen, G. M., & Murray, C. J. (2014). Cigarette smoking prevalence in US counties: 1996–2012. *Population Health Metrics, 12*(1), 5.

Dyrbye, L. N., West, C. P., Burriss, T. C., & Shanafelt, T. D. (2012). Providing primary care in the United States: The work no one sees. *Archives of Internal Medicine, 172*(18), 1420–1421. doi:10.1001/archinternmed.2012.3166

Dzau, V. J., Ackerly, D. C., Sutton-Wallace, P., Merson, M. H., Williams, R. S., Krishnan, K. R., et al. (2010). The role of academic health science systems in the transformation of medicine. *The Lancet, 375*(9718), 949–953.

Ecklund, E. H., & Park, J. Z. (2009). Conflict between religion and science among academic scientists? *Journal for the Scientific Study of Religion, 48*(2), 276–292. doi:10.1111/j.1468-5906.2009.01447.x

Eddy, D. M. (1984). Variations in physician practice: The role of uncertainty. *Health Affairs, 3*(2), 74–89. doi:10.1377/hlthaff.3.2.74

Eddy, D. M. (1992a). Clinical decision making: From theory to practice. Applying cost-effectiveness analysis. The inside story. [Practice Guideline]. : The Journal of the American Medical Association, 268(18), 2575–2582.

Eddy, D. M. (1992b). Clinical decision making: From theory to practice. Cost-effectiveness analysis. Is it up to the task? [Research Support, Non-U.S. Gov't]. : The Journal of the American Medical Association, 267(24), 3342–3348.

Eddy, D. M. (1992c). Clinical decision making: From theory to practice. Cost-effectiveness analysis. Will it be accepted? : The Journal of the American Medical Association, 268(1), 132–136.

Eddy, D. M. (1996). Benefit language: Criteria that will improve quality while reducing costs. Journal of the American Medical Association, 275(8), 650–657. doi:10.1001/jama.1996.03530320074047

Eddy, D. M. (1997). Investigational treatments. How strict should we be? : The Journal of the American Medical Association, 278(3), 179–185.

Eddy, D. M., Adler, J., Patterson, B., Lucas, D., Smith, K. A., & Morris, M. (2011). Individualized guidelines: The potential for increasing quality and reducing costs. Annals of Internal Medicine, 154(9), 627–634. doi:10.7326/0003-4819-154-9-201105030-00008

Eichler, H.-G., Kong, S. X., Gerth, W. C., Mavros, P., & Jönsson, B. (2004). Use of cost-effectiveness analysis in health-care resource allocation decision-making: How are cost-effectiveness thresholds expected to emerge? Value in Health, 7(5), 518–528. Retrieved from http://dx.doi.org/10.1111/j.1524-4733.2004.75003.x

Eisenberg, D., Freed, G. L., Davis, M. M., Singer, D., & Prosser, L. A. (2011). Valuing health at different ages. Applied Health Economics and Health Policy, 9(3), 149–156. Retrieved from http://dx.doi.org/10.2165/11587340-000000000-00000

Ellis, L., Coleman, M. P., & Rachet, B. (2012). How many deaths would be avoidable if socioeconomic inequalities in cancer survival in England were eliminated? A national population-based study, 1996–2006. European Journal of Cancer, 48(2), 270–278.

Ellis, L. M., Bernstein, D. S., Voest, E. E., Berlin, J. D., Sargent, D., Cortazar, P., et al. (2014). American Society of Clinical Oncology perspective: Raising the bar for clinical trials by defining clinically meaningful outcomes. Journal of Clinical Oncology, 32(12), 1277–1280.

Ellis, S. D., Carpenter, W. R., Minasian, L. M., & Weiner, B. J. (2012). Effect of state-mandated insurance coverage on accrual to community cancer clinical trials. Contemp Clin Trials, 33(5), 933–941. Retrieved from http://dx.doi.org/10.1016/j.cct.2012.06.001

Emanuel, E. J. (1999). What is the great benefit of legalizing euthanasia or physican-assisted suicide? Ethics, 109(3), 629–642. doi:10.1086/233925

Emanuel, E. J. (2002). Patient v. population: Resolving the ethical dilemmas posed by treating patients as members of populations. In M. Danis, C. Calncy, & L. R. Churchill (Eds.), Ethical dimensions of health policy (pp. 227–245). New York: Oxford University Press.

Emanuel, E. J. (2012, October 27). Four myths about doctor-assisted suicide. NY Times.

Emanuel, E. J. (2014). Why I hope to die at 75. The Atlantic. http://www.garyvollbracht.com/wp-content/uploads/14.09.17-TheAtlantic-Why-I-Hope-Do-Die-at-75.pdf

Emanuel, E. J., & Fuchs, V. R. (2008). The perfect storm of overutilization. Journal of the American Medical Association, 299(23), 2789–2791. doi:10.1001/jama.299.23.2789

Emanuel, E. J., & Wertheimer, A. (2006). Public health. Who should get influenza vaccine when not all can? Science, 312(5775), 854–855.

Epstein, R. M., Alper, B. S., & Quill, T. E. (2004). Communicating evidence for participatory decision making. *Journal of the American Medical Association, 291*(19), 2359–2366. doi:10.1001/jama.291.19.2359

Epstein, R. M., & Gramling, R. E. (2013). What is shared in shared decision making? Complex decisions when the evidence is unclear. *Medical Care Research and Review, 70*(1 Suppl), 94S–112S. doi:10.1177/1077558712459216

Epstein, R. M., Korones, D. N., & Quill, T. E. (2010). Withholding information from patients—when less is more. *New England Journal of Medicine, 362*(5), 380.

Esserman, L. J., Thompson, I. M., Jr, & Reid, B. (2013). Overdiagnosis and overtreatment in cancer: An opportunity for improvement. *Journal of the American Medical Association, 310*(8), 797–798. doi:10.1001/jama.2013.108415

Estelle, et al. *v.* Gamble (1976). (Vol. 429 U.S. 97): Supreme Court of the United States.

Evans, D. A. P. (1968). Genetic variations in the acetylation of isoniazid and other drugs. *Ann N Y Acad Sci, 151*(2), 723–733. doi:10.1111/j.1749-6632.1968.tb48255.x

Evans, D. A. P., Manley, K. A., & McKusick, V. A. (1960). Genetic control of isoniazid metabolism in man. *British Medical Journal, 2*(5197), 485.

Evans, J. H., & Evans, M. S. (2008). Religion and science: Beyond the epistemological conflict narrative. *Annual Review of Sociology, 34*(1), 87–105. 10.1146/annurev.soc.34.040507.134702

Eyal, N. (2011). Why treat noncompliant patients? Beyond the decent minimum account. *Journal of Medicine and Philosophy, 36*(6), 572–588. doi:10.1093/jmp/jhr051

Fagerlin, A., Wang, C., & Ubel, P. A. (2005). Reducing the influence of anecdotal reasoning on people's health care decisions: Is a picture worth a thousand statistics? *Medical Decision Making, 25*(4), 398–405. doi:10.1177/0272989x05278931

Fairrow, A. M., McCallum, T. J., & Messinger-Rapport, B. J. (2004). Preferences of older African-Americans for long-term tube feeding at the end of life. *Aging & mental health, 8*(6), 530–534.

Fang, A., Matheny, N. L., & Wilhelm, S. (2014). Body dysmorphic disorder. *Psychiatric Clinics of North America, 37*(3), 287–300. Retrieved from http://dx.doi.org/10.1016/j.psc.2014.05.003

Feder, H. M., Johnson, B. J. B., O'Connell, S., Shapiro, E. D., Steere, A. C., & Wormser, G. P. (2007). A critical appraisal of "chronic lyme disease." *New England Journal of Medicine, 357*(14), 1422–1430. doi:10.1056/NEJMra072023

Feiring, E. (2008). Lifestyle, responsibility and justice. *Journal of Medical Ethics, 34*(1), 33–36. doi:10.1136/jme.2006.019067

Fenton, J. J., Jerant, A. F., Bertakis, K. D., & Franks, P. (2012). The cost of satisfaction: A national study of patient satisfaction, health care utilization, expenditures, and mortality. *Archives of Internal Medicine, 172*(5), 405–411. doi:10.1001/archinternmed.2011.1662

Feroze, U., Noori, N., Kovesdy, C. P., Molnar, M. Z., Martin, D. J., Reina-Patton, A., et al. (2011). Quality-of-life and mortality in hemodialysis patients: Roles of race and nutritional status. *Clinical Journal of the American Society of Nephrology 6*, 1100–1111.

Committee on Child Health Financing (2013). Essential contractual language for medical necessity in children. *Pediatrics, 132*(2), 398–401. doi:10.1542/peds.2013-1637

Finer, L. B., & Zolna, M. R. (2011). Unintended pregnancy in the United States: Incidence and disparities, 2006. *Contraception, 84*(5), 478–485.

Finkelstein, A., & McKnight, R. (2008). What did Medicare do? The initial impact of Medicare on mortality and out of pocket medical spending. *Journal of Public Economics, 92*(7), 1644–1668. Retrieved from http://dx.doi.org/10.1016/j.jpubeco.2007.10.005

Fiore, A. E., Shay, D. K., Broder, K., Iskander, J. K., Uyeki, T. M., Mootrey, G., et al. (2008). Prevention and control of influenza: Recommendations of the Advisory Committee on Immunization Practices (ACIP), 2008. *MMWR Recommendations andReports*, *57*(RR-7), 1–60.

Fitch, K., Bernstein, S. J., Aguilar, M. D., Burnand, B., & LaCalle, J. R. (2001). The RAND/ UCLA appropriateness method user's manual. No. RAND/MR-1269-DG-XII/RE, Santa Monica, CA: RAND Corporation.

Flannery, B., Clippard, J., Zimmerman, R. K., Nowalk, M. P., Jackson, M. L., Jackson, L. A., et al. (2015). Early estimates of seasonal influenza vaccine effectiveness-United States, January 2015. *Morbitity and Mortality Weekly Reprt*, *64*(1), 10–15.

Flannery, E. J. (1995). One advocate's viewpoint: Conflicts and tensions in the Baby K case. *Journal of Law, Medicine & Ethics*, *23*(1), 7–12.

Fleck, L. M. (2009). *Just caring. Health care rationing and democratic deliberation.* New York: Oxford University Press.

Fleck, L. M. (2010). Just caring: In defense of limited age-based healthcare rationing. *Cambridge Quarterly of Healthcare Ethics*, *19*(1), 27–37. http://dx.doi.org/10.1017/ S0963180109990223

Fleck, L. M. (2011). Just caring: Health care rationing, terminal illness, and the medically least well off. *The Journal of Law, Medicine & Ethics*, *39*(2), 156–171.

Flexner, A. (1910). *Medical educatuon in The United States and Canada.* Boston: D.B. Updike.

Fojo, T., Mailankody, S., & Lo, A. (2014). Unintended consequences of expensive cancer therapeutics—the pursuit of marginal indications and a me-too mentality that stifles innovation and creativity: The John Conley lecture. *JAMA Otolaryngol – Head Neck Surgery*, *140*(12), 1225–1236.

Fox, D. M., & Leichter, H. M. (1991). Rationing care in Oregon: The new accountability. [Research Support, Non-U.S. Gov't]. *Health Affairs*, *10*(2), 7–27.

Fox, N. J., & Ward, K. J. (2008). Pharma in the bedroom . . . and the kitchen. . . . The pharmaceuticalisation of daily life. *Sociology of Health & Illness*, *30*(6), 856–868. doi:10.1111/ j.1467-9566.2008.01114.x

Fox, R. C. (1957). Training for uncertainty. In R. K. Meron, G. G. Reader, & P. L. Kendall (Eds.), *The student-physician* (pp. 207–244). Cambridge, MA: Harvard University Press.

Frankfurt, H. G. (1984). Necessity and desire. *Philosophy and Phenomenological Research*, *45*(1), 1–13. doi:10.2307/2107323

Frankfurt, H. G. (2015). *On inequality.* Princeton, NJ: Princeton University Press.

Franzini, L., Mikhail, O. I., & Skinner, J. S. (2010). McAllen and El Paso revisited: Medicare variations not always reflected in the under-sixty-five population. *Health Affairs*, *29*(12), 2302–2309. doi:10.1377/hlthaff.2010.0492

Freda, P. U., Beckers, A. M., Katznelson, L., Molitch, M. E., Montori, V. M., Post, K. D., . . . & the Endocrine Society. Pituitary incidentaloma: An endocrine society clinical practice guideline (2011). *The Journal of Clinical Endocrinology & Metabolism*, *96*(4), 894–904. doi:10.1210/jc.2010-1048

Freeman, V. G., Rathore, S. S., Weinfurt, K. P., Schulman, K. A., & Sulmasy, D. P. (1999). Lying for patients: Physician deception of third-party payers. *Archives of Internal Medicine*, *159*(19), 2263–2270. doi:10.1001/archinte.159.19.2263

Freiherr, G. (1995). Product promotion strategy links drugs and devices. MDDI News Retrieved from http://www.mddionline.com/article/ product-promotion-strategy-links-drugs-and-devices

Fried, C. (1969). The value of life. *Harvard Law Review, 82*(7), 1415–1437.

Gabbay, E., Meyer, K. B., Griffith, J. L., Richardson, M. M., & Miskulin, D. C. (2010). Temporal trends in health-related quality of life among hemodialysis patients in the United States. *Clinical Journal of the American Society of Nephrology, 5*(2), 261–267. doi:10.2215/cjn.03890609

Gagliardi, A. R., Brouwers, M. C., Palda, V. A., Lemieux-Charles, L., & Grimshaw, J. M. (2011). How can we improve guideline use? A conceptual framework of implementability. *Implementation Science, 6*(1), 26.

Galesic, M., & Garcia-Retamero, R. (2010). Statistical numeracy for health: A cross-cultural comparison with probabilistic national samples. *Archives of Internal Medicine, 170*(5), 462–468. doi:10.1001/archinternmed.2009.481

Gallin, E. K., Bond, E., Califf, R. M., Crowley, W. F. J., Davis, P., Galbraith, R., et al. (2013). Forging stronger partnerships between academic health centers and patient-driven organizations. *Academic Medicine, 88*(9), 1220–1224.

Garcia-Retamero, R., & Cokely, E. T. (2013). Communicating health risks with visual aids. *Current Directions in Psychological Science, 22*(5), 392–399.

Garcia-Retamero, R., & Galesic, M. (2010). How to reduce the effect of framing on messages about health. *Journal of General Internal Medicine, 25*(12), 1323–1329. doi:10.1007/s11606-010-1484-9

Garcia-Retamero, R., & Hoffrage, U. (2013). Visual representation of statistical information improves diagnostic inferences in doctors and their patients. *Social Science & Medicine, 83*(0), 27–33. Retrieved from http://dx.doi.org/10.1016/j.socscimed.2013.01.034

Gargus, R. A., Vohr, B. R., Tyson, J. E., High, P., Higgins, R. D., Wrage, L. A., et al. (2009). Unimpaired outcomes for extremely low birth weight infants at 18 to 22 months. *Pediatrics, 124*(1), 112–121. doi:10.1542/peds.2008-2742

Gaskin, D. J., Thorpe, R. J., Jr., McGinty, E. E., Bower, K., Rohde, C., Young, J. H., et al. (2014). Disparities in diabetes: The nexus of race, poverty, and place. *American Journal of Public Health, 104* (11), 2147–2155.

Geist, P., & Hardesty, M. (2014). *Negotiating the crisis: DRGs and the transformation of hospitals.* New York: Routledge.

Geller, B. M., Bogart, A., Carney, P. A., Sickles, E. A., Smith, R., Monsees, B., et al. (2014). Educational interventions to improve screening mammography interpretation: A randomized controlled trial. *American Journal of Roentgenology, 202*(6), W586–W596.

Gerber, A. S., Patashnik, E. M., Doherty, D., & Dowling, C. (2010*a*). A national survey reveals public skepticism about research-based treatment guidelines. *Health Affairs, 29*(10), 1882–1884. doi:10.1377/hlthaff.2010.0185

Gerber, A. S., Patashnik, E. M., Doherty, D., & Dowling, C. (2010*b*). The public wants information, not board mandates, from comparative effectiveness research. *Health Affairs, 29*(10), 1872–1881. doi:10.1377/hlthaff.2010.0655

Gerber, A. S., Patashnik, E. M., Doherty, D., & Dowling, C. M. (2014). Doctor knows best: Physician endorsements, public opinion, and the politics of comparative effectiveness research. *Journal of Health, Politics, and Policy Law, 39*(1), 171–208. doi:10.1215/03616878-2395208

Gigerenzer, G. (2002). *Calculated risks: How to know when numbers deceive you.* New York: Simon & Schuster.

Gigerenzer, G. (2009). Making sense of health statistics. *Bulletin of the World Health Organization, 87*(8), 567.

Gigerenzer, G., Gaissmaier, W., Kurz-Milcke, E., Schwartz, L. M., & Woloshin, S. (2007). Helping doctors and patients make sense of health statistics. *Psychological Science in the Public Interest, 8*(2), 53–96. doi:10.2307/40062369

Gilens, M. (2012). *Affluence and influence: Economic inequality and political power in America.* Princeton, NJ/New York: Princeton University Press/Sage.

Gilmer, T., Schneiderman, L. J., Teetzel, H., Blustein, J., Briggs, K., Cohn, F., et al. (2005). The costs of nonbeneficial treatment in the intensive care setting. *Health Affairs, 24*(4), 961–971. doi:10.1377/hlthaff.24.4.961

Glassman, P. A., Jacobson, P. D., & Asch, S. (1997). Medical necessity and defined coverage benefits in the Oregon Health Plan. *Am J Public Health, 87*(6), 1053–1058.

Glod, S. A. (2014). Miracle. *Journal of the American Medical Association, 311*(15), 1499–1499.

Glover, J. (1977). *Causing death and saving lives* (Pelican books). Harmondsworth; New York: Penguin.

Golan, O. (2010). The right to treatment for self-inflicted conditions. *Journal of Medical Ethics 36*(11), 683–686. doi:10.1136/jme.2010.036525.

Goldsteen, R. L., Goldsteen, K., Swan, J. H., & Clemeña, W. (2001). Harry and Louise and health care reform: Romancing public opinion. *Journal of Health, Politics, and Policy Law, 26*(6), 1325–1352. doi:10.1215/03616878-26-6-1325

Goldstein, M. M., & Bowers, D. (2015). The patient as consumer: Empowerment or commodification? *Journal of Law, Medicine & Ethics, 43*(1), 162–165.

Goldstone, A. R., Callaghan, C. J., Mackay, J., Charman, S., & Nashef, S. A. (2004). Should surgeons take a break after an intraoperative death? Attitude survey and outcome evaluation. *BMJ, 328*(7436), 379.

Golenski, J. D., & Nelson, L. J. (1992). The Wanglie case: A demand for treatment clashes with medical integrity. *Clinical ethics report, 6*(1), 1–8.

Gonsalkorale, K., Sherman, J. W., & Klauer, K. C. (2013). Measures of implicit attitudes may conceal differences in implicit associations: The case of antiaging bias. *Social Psychological and Personality Science.* doi:10.1177/1948550613499239

Goodman, S. N. (1999). Probability at the bedside: The knowing of chances or the chances of knowing? *Annals of Internal Medicine, 130*(7), 604–606. doi:10.7326/0003-4819-130-7-199904060-00022

Goodwin, K., Viboud, C., & Simonsen, L. (2006). Antibody response to influenza vaccination in the elderly: A quantitative review. *Vaccine, 24*(8), 1159–1169. Retrieved from http://dx.doi.org/10.1016/j.vaccine.2005.08.105

Gostin, L. O. (2014). Legal and ethical responsibilities following brain death: The McMath and Muñoz cases. *Journal of the American Medical Association, 311*(9), 903–904. doi:10.1001/jama.2014.660

Gould, S. J. (1985). The median isn't the message. *Discover, 6*(6), 40–42.

Gould, S. J. (1997). Nonoverlapping magisteria. *Natural History,* 16.

Graf, M. D., Needham, D. F., Teed, N., & Brown, T. (2013). Genetic testing insurance coverage trends: A review of publicly available policies from the largest US payers. [Report]. *Personalized Medicine, 10*(3), 235–243.

Graham, R., Mancher, M., Wolman, D. M., Greenfield, S., & Steinberg, E. (2011). *Clinical practice guidelines we can trust.* Washington, DC: National Academies Press.

Gray, A. M., Clarke, P. M., Wolstenholme, J. L., & Wordsworth, S. (2011). *Applied methods of cost-effectiveness analysis in healthcare.* Oxford, UK: Oxford University Press.

Gray, B. H., Gusmano, M. K., & Collins, S. R. (2003). AHCPR and the changing politics of health services research. *Health Affairs, 22*(3; Suppl.), 283–307.

Greco, M. (2015). What is the DSM? Diagnostic manual, cultural icon, political battle-ground: An overview with suggestions for a critical research agenda. *Psychology & Sexuality, 7*(1), 1–17. doi:10.1080/19419899.2015.1024470

Green, E. P. (2014). Payment systems in the healthcare industry: An experimental study of physician incentives. *Journal of Economic Behavior & Organization, 106*(0), 367–378. Retrieved from http://dx.doi.org/10.1016/j.jebo.2014.05.009

Green, J. (2015). Living in hope and desperate for a miracle: NICU nurses perceptions of parental anguish. *Journal of Religion and Health, 54*(2), 731–744. doi:10.1007/s10943-014-9971-7

Greene, J., & Haidt, J. (2002). How (and where) does moral judgment work? *Trends Cogn Sci, 6*(12), 517–523.

Greene, J. A. (2007). *Prescribing by numbers: Drugs and the definition of disease.* Baltimore, MD: Johns Hopkins University Press.

Grey, M. R. (1989). Poverty, politics, and health: The Farm Security Administration medical care program, 1935–1945. *Journal of the History of Medicine and Allied Sciences, 44*(3), 320–350. doi:10.1093/jhmas/44.3.320

Grey, M. R. (1994). The medical care programs of the Farm Security Administration, 1932 through 1947: A rehearsal for national health insurance? *Am J Public Health, 84*(10), 1678–1687.

Griffin, M. D., & Prieto, M. (2008). Case studies in transplant ethics. *Transplant Review (Orlando), 22*(3), 178–183.

Grimes, D. A. (1993). Technology follies: The uncritical acceptance of medical innova-tion. *Journal of the American Medical Association, 269*(23), 3030–3033. doi:10.1001/jama.1993.03500230112038

Guallar, E., & Laine, C. (2014). Controversy over clinical guidelines: Listen to the evidence, not the noise. *Annals of Internal Medicine, 160*(5), 361–362.

Gupta, S. (2009). *Cheating death: The doctors and medical miracles that are saving lives against all odds.* New York: Wellness Central.

Gustavsson, E. (2013). From needs to health care needs. *Health Care Annal. 22* (1), 22–35. doi:10.1007/s10728-013-0241-8.

Guyatt, G., Akl, E. A., Hirsh, J., Kearon, C., Crowther, M., Gutterman, D., et al. (2010). The vexing problem of guidelines and conflict of interest: A potential solution. *Annals of Internal Medicine, 152*(11), 738–741.

Hacker, J. D. (2010). Decennial life tables for the white population of the United States, 1790–1900. *Historical methods, 43*(2), 45–79. doi:10.1080/01615441003720449

Hadler, N. M. (2008). *Worried sick: A prescription for health in an overtreated America* (H. Eugene and Lillian Youngs Lehman series). Chapel Hill: University of North Carolina Press.

Hadorn, D. C. (1991). Setting health care priorities in Oregon. Cost-effectiveness meets the rule of rescue. *Journal of the American Medical Association, 265*(17), 2218–2225.

Haidt, J. (2001). The emotional dog and its rational tail: A social intuitionist approach to moral judgment. *Psychology Review, 108*(4), 814–834.

Hall, D. V., Jones, S. C., & Hoek, J. (2011). Direct to consumer advertising versus disease awareness advertising: Consumer perspectives from down under. *Journal of Public Affairs, 11*(1), 60–69. doi:10.1002/pa.379

Hall, D. V., Jones, S. C., & Iverson, D. C. (2011). Consumer perceptions of sponsors of disease awareness advertising. *Health Education, 111*(1), 5–19.

Hall, M. A. (2003). State regulation of medical necessity: The case of weight-reduction surgery. *Duke Law Journal, 53* (2), 653–672.

Hall *v.* Florida. (2014). *S. Ct.* (Vol. 134, pp. 1986): U.S. Supreme Court.

Halpern, N. A., & Pastores, S. M. (2010). Critical care medicine in the United States 2000–2005: An analysis of bed numbers, occupancy rates, payer mix, and costs. *Critical Care Medicine, 38*(1), 65–71. doi: 10.1097/CCM.1090b1013e3181b1090d1090

Hamel, L., Norton, M., Politz, K., Levitt, L., Claxton, G., & Brodie, M. (2016). *The burden of medical debt: Results from the Kaiser Family Foundation/New York Times Medical Bills Survey.* Menlo Park, CA: The Henry J. Kaiser Family Foundation.

Hamilton, D. F., Lane, J. V., Gaston, P., Patton, J. T., MacDonald, D., Simpson, A. H. R. W., et al. (2013). What determines patient satisfaction with surgery? A prospective cohort study of 4709 patients following total joint replacement. *BMJ Open, 3*(4), e002525. doi:10.1136/bmjopen-2012-002525.

Han, P. K. J. (2013). Conceptual, methodological, and ethical problems in communicating uncertainty in clinical evidence. *Medical Care Research and Review, 70*(1 Suppl.), 14S–36S. doi:10.1177/1077558712459361

Han, P. K. J., Klein, W. M. P., & Arora, N. K. (2011). Varieties of uncertainty in health care: A conceptual taxonomy. *Medical Decision Making, 31*(6), 828–838. doi:10.1177/0272989x10393976

Hanchate, A., Kronman, A. C., Young-Xu, Y., Ash, A. S., & Emanuel, E. (2009). Racial and ethnic differences in end-of-life costs: Why do minorities cost more than Whites? *Archives of Internal Medicine, 169*(5), 493–501. doi:10.1001/archinternmed.2008.616

Hankey, H. J. (2007). Are n-of-1 trials of any practical value to clinicians and researchers? In P. M. Rothwell (Ed.), *Treating individuals: From randomised trials to personalised medicine* (pp. 231–243). London: Elsevier Health Sciences.

Hanson, M. J. (1999). The idea of progress and the goals of medicine. In M. J. Hanson, & D. Callahan (Eds.), *The goals of medicine: The forgotten issue in health care reform* (pp. 137–151). Washington, DC: Georgetown University Press.

Hanson, M. J., & Callahan, D. (Eds.). (1999). *The goals of medicine: The forgotten issue in health care reform* (Hastings Center studies in ethics). Washington, DC: Georgetown University Press.

Haque, O. S., & Waytz, A. (2012). Dehumanization in medicine: Causes, solutions, and functions. *Perspectives on Psychological Science, 7*(2), 176–186. doi:10.1177/1745691611429706

Harrington, K., Barney, J., Mcgiffin, D., Diaz-Guzman, E., Wille, K., & Sharma, N. (2014). Regional differences in access to lung transplantation before and after introduction of lung allocation score. *victoria, 1*(2), 3.

Harrington, R. A., & Califf, R. M. (2010). There is a role for industry-sponsored education in cardiology. *Circulation, 121*(20), 2221–2227.

Harris, J. (1985). *The value of life. An introduction to medical ethics.* London: Routledge & Kegan Paul.

Harris, J. (1987). QALYfying the value of life. *Journal of Medical Ethics, 13*(3), 117–123. doi:10.1136/jme.13.3.117

Hartman, M., Martin, A. B., Lassman, D., & Catlin, A. (2015). National health spending in 2013: growth slows, remains in step with the overall economy. *Health Affairs, 34*(1), 150–160.

Hartzband, P., & Groopman, J. (2012). The new language of medicine. *Obstetrics & Gynecology, 119*(2, Part 1), 369–370.

Hasman, A., Hope, T., & ØSterdal, L. P. (2006). Health care need: Three interpretations. *Journal of Applied Philosophy, 23*(2), 145–156. doi:10.1111/j.1468-5930.2006.00325.x

Hatchett, R. J., Mecher, C. E., & Lipsitch, M. (2007). Public health interventions and epidemic intensity during the 1918 influenza pandemic. *Proceedings of the National Academy of Sciences, 104*(18), 7582–7587. doi:10.1073/pnas.0610941104

Heard, E., & Martienssen, R. A. (2014). Transgenerational epigenetic inheritance: Myths and mechanisms. *Cell, 157*(1), 95–109.

Hemmerich, J. A., Elstein, A. S., Schwarze, M. L., Moliski, E. G., & Dale, W. (2012). Risk as feelings in the effect of patient outcomes on physicians' future treatment decisions: A randomized trial and manipulation validation. *Social Science & Medicine, 75*(2), 367–376. Retrieved from http://dx.doi.org/10.1016/j.socscimed.2012.03.020

Hemminki, E., Toiviainen, H. K., & Vuorenkoski, L. (2010). Co-operation between patient organisations and the drug industry in Finland. *Social Science & Medicine, 70*(8), 1171–1175.

Hendrick, R. E., & Helvie, M. A. (2011). United States Preventive Services Task Force screening mammography recommendations: Science ignored. *American Journal of Roentgenology, 196*(2), W112–W116. doi:10.2214/AJR.10.5609

Hennig-Schmidt, H., Selten, R., & Wiesen, D. (2011). How payment systems affect physicians' provision behaviour—An experimental investigation. *Journal of Health Economics, 30*(4), 637–646. Retrieved from http://dx.doi.org/10.1016/j.jhealeco.2011.05.001

Henry, M. S. (2006). Uncertainty, responsibility, and the evolution of the physician/patient relationship. *Journal of Medical Ethics, 32*(6), 321–323. doi:10.1136/jme.2005.013987

Herrnstein, R. J., & Murray, C. (1994). *The Bell Curve. Intelligence and class structure in American life.* New York: The Free Press.

Higgins, J. P. T., & Green, S. (Eds.). (2009). *Cochrane handbook for systematic reviews of interventions* (Version 5.0.2). London: The Cochrane Collaborative, Available from www.cochrane-handbook.org.

Higham, J. (1957). Social discrimination against Jews in America, 1830–1930. *Publications of the American Jewish Historical Society, 47*(1), 1–33.

Hill, A. B. (1952). The clinical trial. *New England Journal of Medicine, 247*(4), 113–119. doi:10.1056/NEJM195207242470401

Hill, A. B. S. (1984). *Principles of medical statistics* (11th ed.): New York: Oxford University Press.

Hilts, P. J. (1996). *Smokescreen: The truth behind the tobacco industry cover-up.* Reading, MA: Addison-Wesley.

Ho, B., & Liu, E. (2011). Does sorry work? The impact of apology laws on medical malpractice. *Journal of Risk and Uncertainty, 43*(2), 141–167. doi:10.1007/s11166-011-9126-0

Hoffman, A., & Pearson, S. D. (2009). "Marginal medicine": Targeting comparative effectiveness research to reduce waste. *Health Affairs, 28*(4), w710–w718. doi:10.1377/hlthaff.28.4.w710

Hoffman, J. R., & Cooper, R. J. (2012). Overdiagnosis of disease: A modern epidemic. *Archives of Internal Medicine, 172*(15), 1123–1124. doi:10.1001/archinternmed.2012.3319

Hoffman, L. R., & Ramsey, B. W. (2013). Cystic fibrosis therapeutics: The road ahead. *CHEST Journal, 143*(1), 207–213. doi:10.1378/chest.12-1639

Holgate, S. T., Komaroff, A. L., Mangan, D., & Wessely, S. (2011). Chronic fatigue syndro me: Understanding a complex illness. [10.1038/nrn3087]. *Nature Reviews Neuroscience, 12*(9), 539–544.

Holland, R. F. (1965). The miraculous. *American Philosophical Quarterly, 2*(1), 43–51. doi:10.2307/20009151

Holmes, M. V., Perel, P., Shah, T., Hingorani, A. D., & Casas, J. P. (2011). Cyp2c19 genotype, clopidogrel metabolism, platelet function, and cardiovascular events: A systematic review and meta-analysis. *Journal of the American Medical Association, 306*(24), 2704–2714. doi:10.1001/jama.2011.1880

Honeybul, S., Gillett, G. R., Ho, K. M., & Lind, C. R. P. (2011). Neurotrauma and the rule of rescue. *Journal of Medical Ethics, 37*(12), 707–710. doi:10.1136/medethics-2011-100081

Hope, T. (2001). Rationing and life-saving treatments: Should identifiable patients have higher priority? *Journal of Medical Ethics, 27*(3), 179–185. doi:10.1136/jme.27.3.179

Hope, T., ØSterdal, L. P., & Hasman, A. (2010). An inquiry into the principles of needs-based allocation of health care. *Bioethics, 24*(9), 470–480. doi:10.1111/j.1467-8519.2009.01734.x

Horbar, J. D., Carpenter, J. H., Badger, G. J., Kenny, M. J., Soll, R. F., Morrow, K. A., et al. (2012). Mortality and neonatal morbidity among infants 501 to 1500 grams from 2000 to 2009. *Pediatrics, 129*(6), 1019–1026. doi:10.1542/peds.2011-3028

Horton, R. (2000). Common sense and figures: The rhetoric of validity in medicine (Bradford Hill Memorial Lecture 1999). *Statistics in Medicine, 19*(23), 3149–3164. doi:10.1002/1097-0258(20001215)19:23<3149:AID-SIM617>3.0.CO;2-E

Hu, Y.-Y., Kwok, A. C., Jiang, W., Taback, N., Loggers, E. T., Ting, G. V., et al. (2012). High-cost imaging in elderly patients with stage IV cancer. *J Natl Cancer Inst, 104*(15), 1165–1173. doi:10.1093/jnci/djs286

Hume, D. (1999). *An enquiry concerning human understanding* (Oxford Philosophical Texts). Oxford, UK: Oxford University Press.

Hummert, M. L., Garstka, T. A., O'Brien, L. T., Greenwald, A. G., & Mellott, D. S. (2002). Using the implicit association test to measure age differences in implicit social cognitions. *Psychology and Aging, 17*(3), 482–495. doi:10.1037/0882-7974.17.3.482

Humphreys, G. (2009). *Direct-to-consumer advertising under fire.* World Health Organization marketing and dissemination. Geneva, Switzerland: World Health Organization.

Hurley, E. H., Krishnan, S., Parton, L. A., & Dozor, A. J. (2014). Differences in perspective on prognosis and treatment of children with trisomy 18. *American Journal of Medical Genetics Part A, 164*(10), 2551–2556. doi:10.1002/ajmg.a.36687

Hurst, S. A., & Danis, M. (2007). A framework for rationing by clinical judgment. [Research Support, N.I.H., Extramural Research Support, Non-U.S. Gov't]. *Kennedy Institute of Ethics Journal, 17*(3), 247–266.

Hurst, S. A., Slowther, A.-M., Forde, R., Pegoraro, R., Reiter-Theil, S., Perrier, A., et al. (2006). Prevalence and determinants of physician bedside rationing: Data from Europe. *Journal of General Internal Medicine, 21*(11), 1138–1143. doi:10.1111/j.1525-1497.2006.00551.x

Hutchings, A., & Raine, R. (2006). A systematic review of factors affecting the judgments produced by formal consensus development methods in health care. *Journal of Health Services Research and Policy, 11*(3), 172–179. doi:10.1258/135581906777641659

Hutchings, A., Raine, R., Sanderson, C., & Black, N. (2005). An experimental study of determinants of the extent of disagreement within clinical guideline development groups. *Quality and Safety in Health Care, 14*(4), 240–245. doi:10.1136/qshc.2004.013227

Hyde, D. (2014). Sorites Paradox. In E. N. Zalta (Ed.), *The Stanford encyclopedia of philosophy* (Winter, 2014), http://plato.stanford.edu/archives/win2014/entries/sorites-paradox/

Iglehart, J. K. (1982). New Jersey's experiment with DRG-based hospital reimbursement. *New England Journal of Medicine, 307*(26), 1655–1660. doi:10.1056/NEJM198212233072632

Illich, I. (1976). *Limits to medicine.* London: Marion Boyars.

Irving, M. J., Tong, A., Jan, S., Wong, G., Cass, A., Allen, R. D., et al. (2013). Community preferences for the allocation of deceased donor organs for transplantation: A focus group study. *Nephrology Dialysis Transplantation.* E-pub ahead of print: doi:10.1093/ndt/gft208

Israni, A. K., Salkowski, N., Gustafson, S., Snyder, J. J., Friedewald, J. J., Formica, R. N., et al. (2014). New national allocation policy for deceased donor kidneys in the United States and possible effect on patient outcomes. *Journal of the American Society of Nephrology, 25*(8), 1842–1848.

Jacobs, L. M., Burns, K., & Jacobs, B. B. (2008). Trauma death: Views of the public and trauma professionals on death and dying from injuries. *Archives of Surgery, 143*(8), 730–735. doi:10.1001/archsurg.143.8.730

Jacobson, M., O'Malley, A. J., Earle, C. C., Pakes, J., Gaccione, P., & Newhouse, J. P. (2006). Does reimbursement influence chemotherapy treatment for cancer patients? *Health Affairs(Millwood), 25*(2), 437–443.

Jacobson, P. D., & Parmet, W. E. (2007). A new era of unapproved drugs: The case of Abigail Alliance v. Von Eschenbach. *Journal of the American Medical Association, 297*(2), 205–208. doi:10.1001/jama.297.2.205

Janvier, A., Farlow, B., & Wilfond, B. S. (2012). The experience of families with children with Trisomy 13 and 18 in social networks. *Pediatrics, 130*(2), 293–298. doi:10.1542/peds.2012-0151

Jecker, N. S. (2013). The problem with rescue medicine. *Journal of Medicine & Philosophy, 38*(1), 64–81.

Jeffers, J. R., Bognanno, M. F., & Bartlett, J. C. (1971). On the demand versus need for medical services and the concept of "shortage." *Am J Public Health, 61*(1), 46–63.

Jha, A. K., Staiger, D. O., Lucas, F. L., & Chandra, A. (2007). Do race-specific models explain disparities in treatments after acute myocardial infarction? *American Heart Journal, 153*(5), 785–791.

Jha, P., & Peto, R. (2014). Global effects of smoking, of quitting, and of taxing tobacco. *New England Journal of Medicine, 370*(1), 60–68. doi:10.1056/NEJMra1308383

Johansson, L.-O. (2005). Fairness of allocations among groups of unknown others. *Social Justice Research, 18*(1), 43–61. doi:10.1007/s11211-005-3392-4

Johnson, J., & Kline, J. (2010). Intraobserver and interobserver agreement of the interpretation of pediatric chest radiographs. *Emergency Radiology, 17*(4), 285–290. doi:10.1007/s10140-009-0854-2

Johnson, K. S., Elbert-Avila, K. I., & Tulsky, J. A. (2005). The influence of spiritual beliefs and practices on the treatment preferences of African Americans: A review of the literature. *Journal of the American Geriatric Society, 53*(4), 711–719. doi:10.1111/j.1532-5415.2005.53224.x

Johnson, N. P., & Mueller, J. (2002). Updating the accounts: Global mortality of the 1918–1920 "Spanish" influenza pandemic. *Bulletin of the History of Medicine, 76*(1), 105–115.

Jones, D. E., Carson, K. A., Bleich, S. N., & Cooper, L. A. (2012). Patient trust in physicians and adoption of lifestyle behaviors to control high blood pressure. *Patient Education and Counseling, 89*(1), 57–62. Retrieved from http://dx.doi.org/10.1016/j.pec.2012.06.003

Jones, D. J., Barkun, A. N., Lu, Y., Enns, R., Sinclair, P., Martel, M., et al. (2012). Conflicts of interest ethics: Silencing expertise in the development of international clinical practice guidelines. *Annals of Internal Medicine, 156*(11), 809–816. doi:10.1059/0003-4819-156-11-201206050-00008

Jones, K. (2008). In whose interest? Relationships between health consumer groups and the pharmaceutical industry in the UK. *Sociology of Health & Illness, 30*(6), 929–943.

Jong, G., Stricker, B. H. C., & Sturkenboom, M. C. (2004). Marketing in the lay media and prescriptions of terbinafine in primary care: Dutch cohort study. *BMJ, 328*(7445), 931.

Jonsen, A. R. (1986). Bentham in a box: Technology assessment and health care allocation. *Law and Medical Health Care, 14*(3-4), 172–174.

Joshi, S., Gaynor, J. J., Bayers, S., Guerra, G., Eldefrawy, A., Chediak, Z., et al. (2013). Disparities among Blacks, Hispanics, and Whites in time from starting dialysis to kidney transplant waitlisting. *Transplantation, 95*(2), 309–318.

Juth, N. (2013). Challenges for principles of need in health care. *Health Care Analysis.* 23(1), 1–15. doi:10.1007/s10728-013-0242-7

Kahan, J. P., Bernstein, S. J., Leape, L. L., Hilborne, L. H., Park, R. E., Parker, L., et al. (1994). Measuring the necessity of medical procedures. *Medical Care, 32*(4), 357–365.

Kahn, S. E., Cooper, M. E., & Del Prato, S. Pathophysiology and treatment of type 2 diabetes: Perspectives on the past, present, and future. *The Lancet, 383*(9922), 1068–1083. Retrieved from http://dx.doi.org/10.1016/S0140-6736(13)62154-6

Kahneman, D. (2011). *Thinking, fast and slow.* New York: Farrar, Straus and Giroux.

Kaiser, J. (2012). New cystic fibrosis drug offers hope, at a price. *Science, 335*(10), 645.

Kaiser, K., Rauscher, G. H., Jacobs, E. A., Strenski, T. A., Ferrans, C. E., & Warnecke, R. B. (2011). The import of trust in regular providers to trust in cancer physicians among White, African American, and Hispanic breast cancer patients. [Comparative Study Research Support, N.I.H., Extramural]. *Journal of General Internal Medicine, 26*(1), 51–57. doi:10.1007/s11606-010-1489-4

Kantarjian, H. M., Fojo, T., Mathisen, M., & Zwelling, L. A. (2013). Cancer drugs in the United States: Justum pretium—the just price. *Journal of Clinical Oncology, 31*(28), 3600–3604. doi:10.1200/jco.2013.49.1845

Karlan, P. S. (2002). Ballots and bullets: The exceptional history of the right to vote. *University of Cincinnati Law Review, 71*, 1345.

Kassirer, J. P. (2005). *On the take: How America's complicity with big business can endanger your health.* New York: Oxford University Press.

Katz, M. B. (2013). *The undeserving poor: America's enduring confrontation with poverty* (2nd ed.). New York: Oxford University Press.

Keehan, S. P., Cuckler, G. A., Sisko, A. M., Madison, A. J., Smith, S. D., Stone, D. A., et al. (2015). National health expenditure projections, 2014–24: Spending growth faster than recent trends. *Health Affairs, 34*(8), 1407–1417. doi:10.1377/hlthaff.2015.0600

Keir, A., McPhee, A., & Wilkinson, D. (2014). Beyond the borderline: Outcomes for inborn infants born at ≤500 grams. *Journal of Paediatrics and Child Health, 50*(2), 146–152. doi:10.1111/jpc.12414

Keller, A. C., & Packel, L. (2013). Going for the Cure: Patient Interest Groups and Health Advocacy in the United States. *J Health Polit Policy Law, 39*(2), 331–367, doi:10.1215/03616878-2416238.

Kelley, A. S., Ettner, S. L., Morrison, R. S., Du, Q., Wenger, N. S., & Sarkisian, C. A. (2011). Determinants of medical expenditures in the last 6 months of life. *Annals of Internal Medicine, 154*(4), 235–242. doi:10.7326/0003-4819-154-4-201102150-00004

Kelley, M. (2005). Limits on patient responsibility. *Journal of Medicine and Philosophy, 30*(2), 189–206. doi:10.1080/03605310590926858

Kemmer, N., Zacharias, V., Kaiser, T., & Neff, G. (2009). Access to liver transplantation in the MELD era: Role of ethnicity and insurance. *Digestive Diseases and Sciences, 54*(8), 1794–1797. doi:10.1007/s10620-008-0567-5

Kenkel, D. S., & Wang, H. (2013). The Economics of Personalization in Prevention and Public Health. *Forum for Health Economics and Policy, 16*(2), S53–S71.

Kerns, R. D., Sellinger, J., & Goodin, B. R. (2011). Psychological treatment of chronic pain. *Annual Review of Clinical Psychology, 7*, 411–434.

King, C. D. (1945). The meaning of normal. *Yale Journal of Biological Medicine, 17*(3), 493.

King V. Burwell, 135 U.S. 2480, 2496 (2014)

Kingma, E. (2007). What is it to be healthy? *Analysis, 67*(2), 128–133.

Kirch, D. G., Henderson, M. K., & Dill, M. J. (2012). Physician workforce projections in an era of health care reform. *Annual Review of Medicine, 63*, 435–445.

Kircher, S. M., Benson, A. B., Farber, M., & Nimeiri, H. S. (2011). Effect of the Accountable Care Act of 2010 on Clinical Trial Insurance Coverage. *Journal of Clinical Oncology, 30*(5), 548–553, doi:10.1200/jco.2011.37.8190.

Kishnani, P. S., Steiner, R. D., Bali, D., Berger, K., Byrne, B. J., Case, L. E., et al. (2006). Pompe disease diagnosis and management guideline. *Genetics in Medicine, 8*(5), 267–288.

Kitzhaber, J. A. (1993). Prioritising health services in an era of limits: The Oregon experience. [Article]. *British Medical Journal,*

Klein, R. (1994). Can we restrict the health care menu? *Health Policy, 27*(2), 103–112. Retrieved from http://dx.doi.org/10.1016/0168-8510(94)90075-2

Klein, R. (1995). Big bang health care reform: Does it work? The case of Britain's 1991 National Health Service reforms. *Milbank Quarterly, 73*(3), 299–337. doi:10.2307/3350370

Klevit, H. D., Bates, A. C., Castanares, T., Kirk, E. P., Sipes-Metzler, P. R., & Wopat, R. (1991). Prioritization of health care services: A progress report by the Oregon Health Services Commission. *Archives of Internal Medicine, 151*(5), 912–916. doi:10.1001/archinte.1991.00400050062012

Kocher, R., & Roberts, B. (2014). The calculus of cures. *New England Journal of Medicine, 370*(16), 1473–1475. doi:10.1056/NEJMp1400868

Kocher, R., & Sahni, N. R. (2011). Rethinking health care labor. *New England Journal of Medicine, 365*(15), 1370–1372. doi:10.1056/NEJMp1109649

Kogut, T., & Ritov, I. (2005). The "identified victim" effect: An identified group, or just a single individual? *Journal of Behavioral Decision Making, 18*(3), 157–167. doi:10.1002/bdm.492

Kogut, T., & Ritov, I. (2007). "One of us": Outstanding willingness to help save a single identified compatriot. *Organizational Behavior and Human Decision Processes, 104*(2), 150–157. Retrieved from http://dx.doi.org/10.1016/j.obhdp.2007.04.006

Kohn, L. T., Corrigan, J. M., & Donaldson, M. S. (Eds.). (2000). *To err is human: Building a safer health system.* Washington, DC: National Academy Press.

Kohn, R., Rubenfeld, G. D., Levy, M. M., Ubel, P. A., & Halpern, S. D. (2011). Rule of rescue or the good of the many? An analysis of physicians' and nurses' preferences for allocating ICU beds. *Intensive Care Medicine, 37*(7), 1210–1217. doi:10.1007/s00134-011-2257-6

Kontos, E. Z., & Viswanath, K. (2011). Cancer-related direct-to-consumer advertising: A critical review. [10.1038/nrc2999]. *Nature Reviews Cancer, 11*(2), 142–150. Retrieved from http://www.nature.com/nrc/journal/v11/n2/suppinfo/nrc2999_S1.html

Kosko, J., Klassen, T. P., Bishop, T., & Hartling, L. (2006). Evidence-based medicine and the anecdote: Uneasy bedfellows or ideal couple? *Paediatrics & Child Health, 11*(10), 665–668.

Krag, E. (2013). Health as normal function: A weak link in Daniels's Theory of just health distribution. *Bioethics, 28*(8), 427–435. doi:10.1111/bioe.12007

Krahn, M., & Naglie, G. (2008). The next step in guideline development: Incorporating patient preferences. *Journal of the American Medical Association, 300*(4), 436–438. doi:10.1001/jama.300.4.436

Kravitz, R. L., Epstein, R. M., Feldman, M. D., & et al. (2005). Influence of patients' requests for direct-to-consumer advertised antidepressants: A randomized controlled trial. *Journal of the American Medical Association, 293*(16), 1995–2002. doi:10.1001/jama.293.16.1995

Kruskal, W. (1988). Miracles and statistics: The casual assumption of independence. *Journal of the American Statistical Association, 83*(404), 929–940. doi:10.2307/2290117

Kucirka, L. M., Grams, M. E., Balhara, K. S., Jaar, B. G., & Segev, D. L. (2012). Disparities in provision of transplant information affect access to kidney transplantation. *American Journal of Transplantation, 12*(2), 351–357doi:10.1111/j.1600-6143.2011.03865.x

Kung, J., Miller, R. R., & Mackowiak, P. A. (2012). Failure of clinical practice guidelines to meet institute of medicine standards: Two more decades of little, if any, progress. *Archives of Internal Medicine, 172*(21), 1628–1633. doi:10.1001/2013.jamainternmed.56

Ladin, K., & Hanto, D. W. (2011). Rational rationing or discrimination: Balancing equity and efficiency considerations in kidney allocation. *American Journal of Transplantation, 11*(11), 2317–2321. doi:10.1111/j.1600-6143.2011.03726.x

Lala, A., Berger, J., Sharma, G., Hochman, J., Scott Braithwaite, R., & Ladapo, J. (2013). Genetic testing in patients with acute coronary syndrome undergoing percutaneous coronary intervention: A cost-effectiveness analysis. *Journal of thrombosis and Haemostasis, 11*(1), 81–91.

Lane, C. (2007). *Shyness: How normal behavior became a sickness.* New Haven: Yale University Press.

Lantos, J. (2006). When parents request seemingly futile treatment for their children. *Mt Sinai J Med, 73*(3), 587–589.

Lantos, P. M., Auwaerter, P. G., & Wormser, G. P. (2013). A systematic review of Borrelia burgdorferi morphologic variants does not support a role in chronic lyme disease. *Clinical Infectious Diseases,* e-pub 12/13/2013. doi:10.1093/cid/cit810.

Lapostolle, F., Montois, S., Alhéritière, A., De Stefano, C., Le Toumelin, P., & Adnet, F. (2013). Dr House, TV, and Reality... *American Journal of Medicine, 126*(2), 171–173, http://dx.doi.org/10.1016/j.amjmed.2012.07.019.

Largent, E. A., & Pearson, S. D. (2012). Which orphans will find a home? The rule of rescue in resource allocation for rare diseases. *Hastings Center Report, 42*(1), 27–34.

Larmer, R. A. H. (1988). *Water into wine?: An investigation of the concept of miracle.* Kingston, Ont.: McGill-Queen's University Press.

Larson, B. A. (2013). Calculating disability-adjusted-life-years lost (DALYs) in discrete-time. *Cost Effectiveness and Resource Allocation, 11*(1), 1–6.

Larson, R. J., Schwartz, L. M., Woloshin, S., & Welch, H. (2005). Advertising by academic medical centers. *Archives of Internal Medicine, 165*(6), 645–651, doi:10.1001/archinte.165.6.645.

Lawson, E. H., Gibbons, M. M., Ko, C. Y., & Shekelle, P. G. (2012). The appropriateness method has acceptable reliability and validity for assessing overuse and underuse of surgical procedures. *J Clin Epidemiol, 65*(11), 1133–1143, http://dx.doi.org/10.1016/j.jclinepi.2012.07.002.

Lean, W. L., Arnup, S., Danchin, M., & Steer, A. C. (2014). Rapid Diagnostic Tests for Group A Streptococcal Pharyngitis: A Meta-analysis. *Pediatrics, 134*(4), 771–781, doi:10.1542/peds.2014-1094.

Leavitt, M. (2005). HHS Pandemic Influenza Plan. (pp. http://www.hhs.gov/pandemicflu/plan/appendixd.html). Washington, D.C.: U.S. Dept. Health and Human Services.

Lee, H., Andrew, M., Gebremariam, A., Lumeng, J. C., & Lee, J. M. (2014). Longitudinal Associations Between Poverty and Obesity From Birth Through Adolescence. *Am J Public Health*(0), e1–e7.

Lee, T. H., Rouan, G. W., Weisberg, M. C., Brand, D. A., Acampora, D., Stasiulewicz, C., et al. (1987). Clinical characteristics and natural history of patients with acute myocardial infarction sent home from the emergency room. *Am J Cardiol, 60*(4), 219–224, http://dx.doi.org/10.1016/0002-9149(87)90217-7.

Lee, Y.-T., Ottati, V., & Hussain, I. (2001). Attitudes toward "Illegal" Immigration into the United States: California Proposition 187. *Hisp. J. Behav. Sci., 23*(4), 430–443.

Leff B, F. T. E. (2008). GIzmo idolatry. *Journal of the American Medical Association, 299*(15), 1830–1832. doi:10.1001/jama.299.15.1830

Leidner, A. J., Chesson, H. W., Xu, F., Ward, J. W., Spradling, P. R., & Holmberg, S. D. (2015). Cost-effectiveness of hepatitis C treatment for patients in early stages of liver disease. *Hepatology, 61*(6), 1860–1869. doi:10.1002/hep.27736

Lenzer, J. (2013). Why we can't trust clinical guidelines. *BMJ, 346*(58), f3830.

Leonard, E. W. (2011). Can you really keep your health plan? The limits of grandfathering under the Affordable Care Act. *Journal of Corporation Law, 36*(4), 753.

Leveque, D. (2008). Off-label use of anticancer drugs. *Lancet Oncology, 9*(11), 1102–1107.

Levin, H. M., & McEwan, P. J. (2001). *Cost-effectiveness analysis: Methods and applications* (2nd ed.). Thousand Oaks: Sage.

Levine, J. A. (2011). Poverty and obesity in the U.S. *Diabetes, 60*(11), 2667–2668. doi:10.2337/db11-1118

Levinsky, N. G. (1993). The organization of medical care. Lessons from the Medicare end stage renal disease program. *New England Journal of Medicine, 329*(19), 1395–1399.

Levinson, J. D., Smith, R. J., & Young, D. M. (2014). Devaluing death: An empirical study of implicit racial bias on jury-eligible citizens in six death penalty states. *New York University Law Review, 89*, 513.

Lewis, T. (2013). *Divided highways: Building the interstate highways, transforming American life.* Ithaca, NY: Cornell University Press.

Lillie, E. O., Patay, B., Diamant, J., Issell, B., Topol, E. J., & Schork, N. J. (2011). The n-of-1 clinical trial: The ultimate strategy for individualizing medicine? *Personalized Medicine, 8*(2), 161–173.

Linas, B. P., Barter, D. M., Morgan, J. R., Pho, M. T., Leff, J. A., Schackman, B. R., et al. (2015). The cost-effectiveness of sofosbuvir-based regimens for treatment of hepatitis C virus genotype 2 or 3 infection. *Annals of Internal Medicine, 162*(9), 619–629.

Lindsay, R. A. (2009). Oregon's experience: Evaluating the record. *American Journal of Bioethics, 9*(3), 19–27.

Lipworth, L., Mumma, M. T., Cavanaugh, K. L., Edwards, T. L., Ikizler, T. A., Tarone, R. E., et al. (2012). Incidence and predictors of end stage renal disease among low-income blacks and whites. *PLoS ONE, 7*(10), e48407.

Liss, P.-E. (2003). The significance of the goal of health care for the setting of priorities. *Health Care Analysis, 11*(2), 161–169.

Liu, Q., & Gupta, S. (2011). The impact of direct-to-consumer advertising of prescription drugs on physician visits and drug requests: Empirical findings and public policy implications. *International Journal of Research in Marketing, 28*(3), 205–217.

Liu, R., Paxton, W. A., Choe, S., Ceradini, D., Martin, S. R., Horuk, R., et al. (1996). Homozygous defect in HIV-1 coreceptor accounts for resistance of some multiply-exposed individuals to HIV-1 infection. *Cell, 86*(3), 367–377.

Loewenstein, G., Volpp, K. G., & Asch, D. A. (2012). Incentives in health: Different prescriptions for physicians and patients. *Journal of the American Medical Association, 307*(13), 1375–1376. doi:10.1001/jama.2012.387

Loomes, G., & McKenzie, L. (1989). The use of QALYs in health care decision making. *Social Science & Medicine, 28*(4), 299–308. Retrieved from http://dx.doi.org/10.1016/0277-9536(89)90030-0

Lostao, L., Blane, D., Gimeno, D., Netuveli, G., & Regidor, E. (2014). Socioeconomic patterns in use of private and public health services in Spain and Britain: Implications for equity in health care. *Health & Place, 25*, 19–25. Retrieved from http://dx.doi.org/10.1016/j.healthplace.2013.09.011

Lott, D. A. (Ed.). (1992). *Designing a fair and reasonable basic benefit plan using clinical guidelines.* Sacramento, CA: California Public Employees' Retirement System (PERS).

Lubell, S., & Everett, W. (1938, December 17). Rehearsal for state medicine. *The Saturday Evening Post.*

Ludmerer, K. M. (2015). *Let me heal: The opportunity to preserve excellence in American medicine.* Oxford, UK/New York: Oxford University Press.

Luetke, A., Meyers, P. A., Lewis, I., & Juergens, H. (2014). Osteosarcoma treatment—Where do we stand? A state of the art review. *Cancer Treatment Reviews, 40*(4), 523–532. Retrieved from http://dx.doi.org/10.1016/j.ctrv.2013.11.006

Lunde, P., Frislid, K., & Hansleen, V. (1977). Disease and acetylation polymorphism. *Clin Pharmacokinet, 2*(3), 182–197. doi:10.2165/00003088-197702030-00003

Lyon, D. M. (1942). What do we mean by "normal?" *Clinical Journal of Sport Medicine, 71*, 239–243.

Ma, J., Dushoff, J., & Earn, D. J. D. (2011). Age-specific mortality risk from pandemic influenza. *Journal of Theoretical Biology, 288*(0), 29–34. Retrieved from http://dx.doi.org/10.1016/j.jtbi.2011.08.003

Macfarlane, J., Holmes, W., Macfarlane, R., & Britten, N. (1997). Influence of patients' expectations on antibiotic management of acute lower respiratory tract illness in general practice: Questionnaire study. *BMJ: British Medical Journal, 315*(7117), 1211.

Machida, M., Irwin, B., & Feltz, D. (2013). Resilience in competitive athletes with spinal cord injury: The role of sport participation. [Research Support, Non-U.S. Gov't]. *Qualitative Health Research, 23*(8), 1054–1065. doi:10.1177/1049732313493673

Mack, J. W., Wolfe, J., Cook, E. F., Grier, H. E., Cleary, P. D., & Weeks, J. C. (2007). Hope and prognostic disclosure. *Journal of Clinical Oncology, 25*(35), 5636–5642.

Mackenbach, J. P. (2006). The origins of human disease: A short story on "where diseases come from." *Journal of Epidemiology and Community Health (1979-), 60*(1), 81–86. doi:10.2307/40795079

Mackey, T., & Liang, B. (2012). Globalization, evolution and emergence of direct-to-consumer advertising: Are emerging markets the next pharmaceutical marketing frontier. *J Commer Biotechnol, 18*, 58–64.

Mackie, J. L. (1982). *The miracle of theism: Arguments for and against the existence of God.* Oxford, UK: Oxford University Press.

Magi, M., & Allander, E. (1981). Towards a theory of perceived and medically defined need. *Sociology of Health & Illness*, 3(1), 49–71. doi:10.1111/1467-9566.ep11343652

Magnus, D. C., Wilfond, B. S., & Caplan, A. L. (2014). Accepting brain death. *New England Journal of Medicine*, 370(10), 891–894. doi:10.1056/NEJMp1400930

Malin, J. L., Weeks, J. C., Potosky, A. L., Hornbrook, M. C., & Keating, N. L. (2013). Medical oncologists' perceptions of financial incentives in cancer care. *Journal of Clinical Oncology*, 31(5), 530–535. doi:10.1200/jco.2012.43.6063

Manganello, J. A., & Clayman, M. L. (2011). The association of understanding of medical statistics with health information seeking and health provider interaction in a national sample of young adults. *Journal of Health Communication*, 16(sup3), 163–176. doi:10.1080/10810730.2011.604704

Manning, S., & Schneiderman, L. (1996). Miracles or limits: What message from the medical marketplace? *HEC Forum*, 8(2), 103–108. doi:10.1007/BF00119174

Manning, W. G., Newhouse, J. P., Duan, N., Keeler, E. B., & Leibowitz, A. (1987). Health insurance and the demand for medical care: Evidence from a randomized experiment. *The American Economic Review*, 77(3), 251–277. doi:10.2307/1804094

Mansfield, C. J., Mitchell, J., & King, D. E. (2002). The doctor as God's mechanic? Beliefs in the southeastern United States. *Social Science and Medicine*, 54(3), 399–409.

Mantel, J. (2013). The myth of the independent physician: Implications for health law, policy, and ethics. *Case Western Reserve Law Review*, 64(2), 455–520.

Marchman Andersen, M., Dalton, S. O., Lynch, J., Johansen, C., & Holtug, N. (2013). Social inequality in health, responsibility and egalitarian justice. *Journal of Public Health*, 35(1), 4–8, doi:10.1093/pubmed/fdt012.

Marden, S., Thomas, P. W., Sheppard, Z. A., Knott, J., Lueddeke, J., & Kerr, D. (2012). Poor numeracy skills are associated with glycaemic control in Type 1 diabetes. *Diabetic Medicine*, 29(5), 662–669. doi:10.1111/j.1464-5491.2011.03466.x

Marewski, J. N., & Gigerenzer, G. (2012). Heuristic decision making in medicine. *Dialogues in Clinical Neuroscience*, 14(1), 77–89.

Marik, P. E. (2014). The cost of inappropriate care at the end of life: Implications for an aging population. *American Journal of Hospice and Palliative Medicine* 32(7), 703–708. doi:10.1177/1049909114537399

Markel, H., Lipman, H. B., Navarro, J., & et al. (2007). Nonpharmaceutical interventions implemented by us cities during the 1918–1919 influenza pandemic. *Journal of the American Medical Association*, 298(6), 644–654. doi:10.1001/jama.298.6.644

Marmor, T. R., & Sullivan, K. (2015). Medicare at 50: Why medicare-for-all did not take place. *Yale Journal of Health Policy, Law, & Ethics*, 15, 141.

Marrow, H. B., & Joseph, T. D. (2015). Excluded and Frozen Out: Unauthorised Immigrants' (Non)Access to Care after US Health Care Reform. *Journal of Ethnic and Migration Studies*, 41(14), 2253–2273, doi:10.1080/1369183X.2015.1051465

Martin, A. B., Hartman, M., Whittle, L., & Catlin, A. (2014). National health spending in 2012: rate of health spending growth remained low for the fourth consecutive year. *Health Affairs*, 33(1), 67–77.

Maslow, A. H. (1948). "Higher" and "lower" needs. *The Journal of Psychology*, 25(2), 433–436.

Maslow, A. H. (1948). Some theoretical consequences of basic need gratification. *Journal of Personality*, 16(4), 402–416. doi:10.1111/j.1467-6494.1948.tb02296.x

Mathisen, M. S., Kantarjian, H. M., Cortes, J., & Jabbour, E. J. (2014). Practical issues surrounding the explosion of tyrosine kinase inhibitors for the management of chronic myeloid leukemia. *Blood Reviews* 28(5), 179–187.

Mathur, A. K., Schaubel, D. E., Gong, Q., Guidinger, M. K., & Merion, R. M. (2010). Racial and ethnic disparities in access to liver transplantation. *Liver Transplantation*, *16*(9), 1033–1040. doi:10.1002/lt.22108

Mathur, A. K., Schaubel, D. E., Gong, Q., Guidinger, M. K., & Merion, R. M. (2011). Sex-based disparities in liver transplant rates in the United States. *American Journal of Transplantation*, *11*(7), 1435–1443. doi:10.1111/j.1600-6143.2011.03498.x

Mayberry, R. (2014). Racial disparities in health care access in the United States. In W. C. Cockerham, R. Dingwall, & S. R. Quah (Eds.), *The Wiley Blackwell Encyclopedia of health, illness, behavior, and society* (pp. 1–8). New York: John Wiley & Sons.

Mazur, D., & Hickam, D. (1991). Patients' interpretations of probability terms. *Journal of General Internal Medicine*, *6*(3), 237–240. doi:10.1007/BF02598968

McCall, M. G. (1966). Normality. *Journal of Chronic Diseases*, *19*(11–12), 1127–1132. http://dx.doi.org/10.1016/0021-9681(66)90013-0

McCormick, D., Hanchate, A. D., Lasser, K. E., Manze, M. G., Lin, M., Chu, C., et al. (2015). Effect of Massachusetts healthcare reform on racial and ethnic disparities in admissions to hospital for ambulatory care sensitive conditions: Retrospective analysis of hospital episode statistics. *BMJ*, *350*, h1480.

McGee, S. A., Durham, D. D., Tse, C.-K., & Millikan, R. C. (2013). Determinants of breast cancer treatment delay differ for African American and White Women. *Cancer Epidemiology Biomarkers & Prevention*, *22*(7), 1227–1238, doi:10.1158/1055-9965.epi-12-1432.

McGoldrick, T. A. (1945). Report of Special Committee of the Conference on Extension of the Emergency Maternal and Infant Care Program, postwar. *Journal of the American Medical Association*, *129*, 1185.

McGregor, J. A., Camfield, L., & Woodcock, A. (2009). Needs, wants and goals: Wellbeing, quality of life and public policy. *Applied Research in Quality of Life*, *4*(2), 135–154.

McKay, A., & Yackee, S. W. (2007). Interest group competition on federal agency rules. *American Politics Research*, *35*(3), 336–357.

McKenna, K., Leykum, L. K., & McDaniel, R. R., Jr. (2013). The role of improvising in patient care. *Health Care Management Review*, *38*(1), 1–8.

McKie, J., & Richardson, J. (2003). The rule of rescue. *Social Science & Medicine*, *56*(12), 2407–2419. doi:10.1016/s0277-9536(02)00244-7

McKneally, M. F., & Sade, R. M. (2003). The prisoner dilemma: Should convicted felons have the same access to heart transplantation as ordinary citizens? Opposing views. *Journal of Thoracic Cardiovascular Surgery*, *125*(3), 451–453.

McNeil, C. (2015). NCI-MATCH launch highlights new trial design in precision-medicine era. *Journal of the National Cancer Institute*, *107*(7), djv193.

McWilliams, J., Zaslavsky, A. M., Meara, E., & Ayanian, J. Z. (2003). Impact of Medicare coverage on basic clinical services for previously uninsured adults. *Journal of the American Medical Association*, *290*(6), 757–764. doi:10.1001/jama.290.6.757

McWilliams, J. M., Meara, E., Zaslavsky, A. M., & Ayanian, J. Z. (2007). Use of health services by previously uninsured Medicare beneficiaries. *New England Journal of Medicine*, *357*(2), 143–153. doi:10.1056/NEJMsa067712

Mechanic, D. (1992). Professional judgment and the rationing of medical care. *University of Pennsylvania Law Review*, *140*(5), 1713–1754. doi:10.2307/3312429

Mechanic, D. (1995). Dilemmas in rationing health care services: The case for implicit rationing. *BMJ*, *310*(6995), 1655–1659.

Mechanic, D. (2004). In my chosen doctor I trust. *BMJ*, *329*(7480), 1418–1419. doi:10.1136/bmj.329.7480.1418

Meekings, K. N., Williams, C. S. M., & Arrowsmith, J. E. (2012). Orphan drug development: An economically viable strategy for biopharma R&D. *Drug Discovery Today*, *17*(13–14), 660–664. Retrieved from http://dx.doi.org/10.1016/j.drudis.2012.02.005

Mehta, C., & Brady, W. (2012). Pulseless electrical activity in cardiac arrest: Electrocardiographic presentations and management considerations based on the electrocardiogram. *The American journal of emergency medicine*, *30*(1), 236–239. Retrieved from http://dx.doi.org/10.1016/j.ajem.2010.08.017

Mehta, J. L., Bursac, Z., Mehta, P., Bansal, D., Fink, L., Marsh, J., et al. (2010). Racial disparities in prescriptions for cardioprotective drugs and cardiac outcomes in Veterans Affairs hospitals. *American Journal of Cardiology*, *105*(7), 1019–1023. Retrieved from http://dx.doi.org/10.1016/j.amjcard.2009.11.031

Melichar, L. (2009). The effect of reimbursement on medical decision making: Do physicians alter treatment in response to a managed care incentive? *Journal of Health Economics*, *28*(4), 902–907. doi:10.1016/j.jhealeco.2009.03.004

Menchik, D. A., & Jin, L. (2014). When do doctors follow patients' orders? Organizational mechanisms of physician influence. *Social Science Research*, *48*, 171–184.

Mendelson, T. B., Meltzer, M., Campbell, E. G., Caplan, A. L., & Kirkpatrick, J. N. (2011). Conflicts of interest in cardiovascular clinical practice guidelines. *Archives of Internal Medicine*, *171*(6), 577–584.

Meyers, C. (2002). A new liver for a prisoner. *Hastings Center Report*, *32*(4), 12; discussion 12–13.

Meyers, D. S., Mishori, R., McCann, J., Delgado, J., O'Malley, A. S., & Fryer, E. (2006). Primary care physicians' perceptions of the effect of insurance status on clinical decision making. *Annals of Family Medicine*, *4*(5), 399–402.

Miles, S. H. (1991). Legal procedures in Wanglie: A two-step, not a sidestep. *Journal of Clinical Ethics*, *2*(4), 285–286.

Miller, A. C., Ziad-Miller, A., & Elamin, E. M. (2014). Brain death and Islam: The interface of religion, culture, history, law, and modern medicine. *Chest*, *146*(4), 1092–1101. doi:10.1378/chest.14-0130

Mohamed, M. A., Nada, A., & Aly, H. (2010). Day-by-day postnatal survival in very low birth weight infants. *Pediatrics*, *126*(2), e360–e366. doi:10.1542/peds.2009-2810

Monson, R. S., Kemerley, P., Walczak, D., Benedetti, E., Oberholzer, J., & Danielson, K. K. (2015). Disparities in completion rates of the medical prerenal transplant evaluation by race or ethnicity and gender. *Transplantation*, *99*(1), 236–242. doi:10.1097/tp.0000000000000271

Montez, J., Hummer, R., & Hayward, M. (2012). Educational attainment and adult mortality in the United States: A systematic analysis of functional form. *Demography*, *49*(1), 315–336. doi:10.1007/s13524-011-0082-8

Montgomery, K. (2006). *How doctors think*. New York: Oxford University Press.

Moraes Vinícius, Y., Lenza, M., Tamaoki Marcel, J., Faloppa, F., & Belloti João, C. (2014). Platelet-rich therapies for musculoskeletal soft tissue injuries. *Cochrane Database of Systematic Reviews* (4). Available from doi:10.1002/14651858.CD010071.pub3

Morden, N. E., Chang, C.-H., Jacobson, J. O., Berke, E. M., Bynum, J. P. W., Murray, K. M., et al. (2012). End-of-life care for Medicare beneficiaries with cancer is highly intensive overall and varies widely. *Health Affairs*, *31*(4), 786–796. doi:10.1377/hlthaff.2011.0650

Moriyama, I. M., Loy, R. M., Robb-Smith, A. H. T., Rosenberg, H. M., Hoyert, D. L., & National Center for Health Statistics. (2011). *History of the statistical classification of diseases and causes of death*. Washington, DC: US Department of Health and Human

Services, Centers for Disease Control and Prevention, National Center for Health Statistics.

Morra, D., Nicholson, S., Levinson, W., Gans, D. N., Hammons, T., & Casalino, L. P. (2011). US physician practices versus Canadians: Spending nearly four times as much money interacting with payers. *Health Affairs, 30*(8), 1443–1450.

Morreim, E. H. (2001). The futility of medical necessity. *Regulation, 24,* 22–26.

Morris, J., Swier-Vosnos, A., Dusold, J., & Woodworth, C. (2013). Comparison of able-bodied and spinal cord injured individuals' appraisals of disability. *Spinal Cord, 51*(4), 338–340. doi:10.1038/sc.2012.169

Moyer, V. A. (2012a). Screening for prostate cancer: U.S. Preventive Services Task Force recommendation statement. *Annals of Internal Medicine, 157*(2), 120–134. doi:10.7326/0003-4819-157-2-201207170-00459

Moyer, V. A. (2012b). What we don't know can hurt our patients: Physician innumeracy and overuse of screening tests. *Annals of Internal Medicine, 156*(5), 392–393.

Moylan, C. A., Brady, C. W., Johnson, J. L., Smith, A. D., Tuttle-Newhall, J. E., & Muir, A. J. (2008). Disparities in liver transplantation before and after introduction of the MELD score. *Journal of the American Medical Association, 300*(20), 2371–2378.

Moynihan, R., & Cassels, A. (2005). *Selling sickness: How the world's biggest pharmaceutical companies are turning us all into patients.* New York: Nation Books.

Moynihan, R. N., Cooke, G. P., Doust, J. A., Bero, L., Hill, S., & Glasziou, P. P. (2013). Expanding disease definitions in guidelines and expert panel ties to industry: A cross-sectional study of common conditions in the United States. *PLoS Med, 10*(8), e1001500.

Mukherjee, S. (2011). *The emperor of all maladies: A biography of cancer.* New York: Simon and Schuster.

Murphy, E. A. (1965). A scientific viewpoint on normalcy. *Perspectives in Biological Medicine, 9*(3), 333–348.

Murphy, E. A., & Abbey, H. (1967). The normal range—A common misuse. *Journal of Chronic Diseases, 20*(2), 79–88. Retrieved from http://dx.doi.org/10.1016/0021-9681(67)90099-9

Murray, C. J., Ezzati, M., Flaxman, A. D., Lim, S., Lozano, R., Michaud, C., et al. (2013). GBD 2010: Design, definitions, and metrics. *The Lancet, 380*(9859), 2063–2066.

Murray, C. J. L., & Lopez, A. D. (2013). Measuring the global burden of disease. *New England Journal of Medicine, 369*(5), 448–457. doi:10.1056/NEJMra1201534

Murray, C. J. L., Lopez, A. D., Chin, B., Feehan, D., & Hill, K. H. (2006). Estimation of potential global pandemic influenza mortality on the basis of vital registry data from the 1918–20 pandemic: A quantitative analysis. *The Lancet, 368*(9554), 2211–2218. Retrieved from http://dx.doi.org/10.1016/S0140-6736(06)69895-4

Murray, R., Godfrey, K., & Lillycrop, K. (2015). The early life origins of cardiovascular disease. *Current Cardiovascular Risk Reports, 9*(4), 1–8. doi:10.1007/s12170-015-0442-9

Nakagawa, K., & Obana, K. K. (2014). Willingness to favor aggressive care and live with disability following severe traumatic brain injury: A survey of healthy young adults in Hawai'i. *Hawai'i Journal of Medicine & Public Health, 73*(7), 212–216.

Nakhoul, G. N., & Hickner, J. (2013). Management of adults with acute streptococcal pharyngitis: Minimal value for backup strep testing and overuse of antibiotics. *Journal of General Internal Medicine, 28*(6), 830–834.

Nathan, D. M., Cleary, P. A., Backlund, J., Genuth, S., Lachin, J., Orchard, T., et al. (2005). Intensive diabetes treatment and cardiovascular disease in patients with type 1 diabetes. *New England Journal of Medicine, 353*(25), 2643–2653.

National Federation of Independent Business *v.* Sebelius. *567* U. S. ____ *(2012).*

Naughton, K., Schmid, C., Yackee, S. W., & Zhan, X. (2009). Understanding commenter influence during agency rule development. *Journal of Policy Analysis and Management, 28*(2), 258–277. doi:10.1002/pam.20426

Nelson, K. E., Hexem, K. R., & Feudtner, C. (2012). Inpatient hospital care of children with trisomy 13 and trisomy 18 in the United States. *Pediatrics, 129*(5), 869–876.

Neuberger, J. (2007). Public and professional attitudes to transplanting alcoholic patients. *Liver Transplantation, 13*(S2), S65–S68. doi:10.1002/lt.21337

Neuberger, J. (2012). Rationing life-saving resources—how should allocation policies be assessed in solid organ transplantation. *Transplant International, 25*(1), 3–6. doi:10.1111/j.1432-2277.2011.01327.x

Neuman, J. (2011). Prevalence of financial conflicts of interest among panel members producing clinical practice guidelines in Canada and United States: Cross sectional study. *British Medical Journal, 343*, d56521. doi:ARTN d7063 DOI 10.1136/bmj.d7063

Neuman, M. D., Goldstein, J. N., Cirullo, M. A., & Schwartz, J. (2014). Durability of class I American College of Cardiology/American Heart Association clinical practice guideline recommendations. *Journal of the American Medical Association, 311*(20), 2092–2100. doi:10.1001/jama.2014.4949

Neumann, P. J., Cohen, J. T., & Weinstein, M. C. (2014). Updating cost-effectiveness—The curious resilience of the $50,000-per-QALY threshold. *New England Journal of Medicine, 371*(9), 796–797. doi:10.1056/NEJMp1405158

Neumann, P. J., & Greenberg, D. (2009). Is the United States ready for QALYs? *Health Affairs, 28*(5), 1366–1371. doi:10.1377/hlthaff.28.5.1366

Neumann, P. J., Rosen, A. B., & Weinstein, M. C. (2005). Medicare and cost-effectiveness analysis. *New England Journal of Medicine, 353*(14), 1516–1522.

Neuzil, K. M. (2009). Pandemic influenza vaccine policy—Considering the early evidence. *New England Journal of Medicine, 361*(25), e59. doi:10.1056/NEJMe0908224

Nevitt, D. A. (1977). Demand and need. In H. Heisler (Ed.), *Foundations of social administration*. London: Macmillan. Pp. 113–128.

New York State Department of Health. (2008). *New York State Department of Health pandemic influenza plan*. Retrieved from https://www.health.ny.gov/diseases/communicable/influenza/pandemic/

Ngo-Metzger, Q., Sorkin, D., Billimek, J., Greenfield, S., & Kaplan, S. (2012). The effects of financial pressures on adherence and glucose control among racial/ethnically diverse patients with diabetes. *Journal of General Internal Medicine, 27*(4), 432–437. doi:10.1007/s11606-011-1910-7

Nguyen, G. C., LaVeist, T. A., Harris, M. L., Datta, L. W., Bayless, T. M., & Brant, S. R. (2009). Patient trust-in-physician and race are predictors of adherence to medical management in inflammatory bowel disease. [Research Support, N.I.H., Extramural Research Support, Non-U.S. Gov't]. *Inflammatory Bowel Diseases, 15*(8), 1233–1239. doi:10.1002/ibd.20883

Niederdeppe, J., Byrne, S., Avery, R., & Cantor, J. (2013). Direct-to-consumer television advertising exposure, diagnosis with high cholesterol, and statin use. *Journal of General Internal Medicine, 28*(7), 886–893. doi:10.1007/s11606-013-2379-3

Nikles, C. J., Clavarino, A. M., & Del Mar, C. B. (2005). Using n-of-1 trials as a clinical tool to improve prescribing. *British Journal of General Practice, 55*(512), 175–180.

Niu, X., Roche, L. M., Pawlish, K. S., & Henry, K. A. (2013). Cancer survival disparities by health insurance status. *Cancer Medicine, 2*(3), 403–411. doi:10.1002/cam4.84

Nord, E. (2005). Concerns for the worse off: Fair innings versus severity. *Social Science & Medicine, 60*(2), 257–263. doi:10.1016/j.socscimed.2004.05.003

Nord, E., & Johansen, R. (2014). Concerns for severity in priority setting in health care: A review of trade-off data in preference studies and implications for societal willingness to pay for a QALY. *Health Policy, 116*(2–3), 281–288. Retrieved from http://dx.doi.org/10.1016/j.healthpol.2014.02.009

Nordenfelt, L. (2001). On the goals of medicine, health enhancement and social welfare. *Health Care Analysis, 9*(1), 15–23. doi:10.1023/A:1011350927112

Norris, S. L., Holmer, H. K., Ogden, L. A., & Burda, B. U. (2011). Conflict of interest in clinical practice guideline development: A systematic review. [Article]. *PLoS ONE, 6*(10), 1–6. doi:10.1371/journal.pone.0025153

Nosek, B. A., Smyth, F. L., Hansen, J. J., Devos, T., Lindner, N. M., Ranganath, K. A., et al. (2007). Pervasiveness and correlates of implicit attitudes and stereotypes. *European Review of Social Psychology, 18*(1), 36–88. doi:10.1080/10463280701489053

Nunn, R. (2011). Mere anecdote: Evidence and stories in medicine. *Journal of Evaluation in Clinical Practice, 17*(5), 920–926. doi:10.1111/j.1365-2753.2011.01727.x

Nurgat, Z. A., Craig, W., Campbell, N. C., Bissett, J. D., Cassidy, J., & Nicolson, M. C. (2005). Patient motivations surrounding participation in phase I and phase II clinical trials of cancer chemotherapy. *British Journal of Cancer, 92*(6), 1001–1005.

Nussbaum, M. C. (2000). *Women and human development.* Cambridge, UK: Cambridge University Press.

Nussbaum, M. C., & Sen, A. K. (1993). Capability and well-being. In M. C. Nussbaum, & A. K. Sen (Eds.), *The quality of life* (pp. 30–53). New York/Oxford, UK: Clarenden Press.

Oberlander, J. (2007). Health reform interrupted: The unraveling of the Oregon Health Plan. [Research Support, Non-U.S. Gov't]. *Health Affairs, 26*(1), w96–w105. doi:10.1377/hlthaff.26.1.w96

Oberlander, J., Marmor, T., & Jacobs, L. (2001). Rationing medical care: Rhetoric and reality in the Oregon Health Plan. *Canadian Medical Association Journal, 164*(11), 1583–1587.

Ollendorf, D. A., Migliaccio-Walle, K., Colby, J. A., & Pearson, S. D. (2013). Management options for children with attention-deficit/hyperactivity disorder: A regional perspective on value. *Journal of Comparative Effectiveness Research, 2*(3), 261–271.

Ollendorf, D. A., & Pearson, S. D. (2010). An integrated evidence rating to frame comparative effectiveness assessments for decision makers. *Medical Care, 48*(6), S145–S152.

Ollendorf, D. A., & Pearson, S. D. (2013). Through the looking glass: Making the design and output of economic models useful for setting medical policy. *Journal of Comparative Effectiveness Research, 3*(1), 53–61. doi:10.2217/cer.13.82

Olshansky, S. J., Antonucci, T., Berkman, L., Binstock, R. H., Boersch-Supan, A., Cacioppo, J. T., et al. (2012). Differences in life expectancy due to race and educational differences are widening, and many may not catch up. *Health Affairs, 31*(8), 1803–1813. doi:10.1377/hlthaff.2011.0746

Oostvogels, A., DE WIT, G., Jahn, B., Cassini, A., Colzani, E., DE WAURE, C., et al. (2015). Use of DALYs in economic analyses on interventions for infectious diseases: A systematic review. *Epidemiology and infection, 143*(09), 1791–1802.

Oprea, T. I., Bauman, J. E., Bologa, C. G., Buranda, T., Chigaev, A., Edwards, B. S., et al. (2011). Drug repurposing from an academic perspective. *Drug Discovery Today: Therapeutic Strategies, 8*(3–4), 61–69. Retrieved from http://dx.doi.org/10.1016/j.ddstr.2011.10.002

Orr, R. D., & Genesen, L. B. (1997). Requests for "inappropriate" treatment based on religious beliefs. *Journal of Medical Ethics, 23*(3), 142–147.

Osler, W. (1910). The faith that heals. *British Medical Journal, 1*(2581), 1470–1472.

Osterholm, M. T. (2005). Preparing for the next pandemic. *Foreign Affairs, 84*(4), 24–37. doi:10.2307/20034418

O'Sullivan, B. P., Orenstein, D. M., & Milla, C. E. (2013). Pricing for orphan drugs: Will the market bear what society cannot? *Journal of the American Medical Association, 310*(13), 1343–1344. doi:10.1001/jama.2013.278129

Owens, D. K. (2011). Improving practice guidelines with patient-specific recommendations. *Annals of Internal Medicine, 154*(9), 638–639. doi:10.7326/0003-4819-154-9-201105030-00010

Ozar, D. T. (1983). What should count as basic health care? *Theoretical Medicine, 4*(2), 129–141. doi:10.1007/BF00562886

Paley, W. (2006). *Natural theology or evidence of the existence and attributes of the deity, collected from the appearances of nature.* Oxford, UK: Oxford University Press.

Park, R. E., Fink, A., Brook, R. H., Chassin, M. R., Kahn, K. L., Merrick, N. J., et al. (1986). Physician ratings of appropriate indications for six medical and surgical procedures. *American Journal of Public Health, 76*(7), 766–772.

Parry, V. (2003). The art of branding a condition. *Med Mark Media, 38*(5), 43–49.

Patel, R. M., Kandefer, S., Walsh, M. C., Bell, E. F., Carlo, W. A., Laptook, A. R., et al. (2015). Causes and timing of death in extremely premature infants from 2000 through 2011. *New England Journal of Medicine, 372*(4), 331–340. doi:10.1056/NEJMoa1403489

Pawlikowski, J. (2007). The history of thinking about miracles in the West. *Southern Medical Journal, 100*(12), 1229–1235.

Pearson, S. D., & Bach, P. B. (2010). How Medicare could use comparative effectiveness research in deciding on new coverage and reimbursement. *Health Affairs, 29*(10), 1796–1804. doi:10.1377/hlthaff.2010.0623

Peck, B. M., Ubel, P. A., Roter, D. L., Goold, S. D., Asch, D. A., Mstat, A. S. J., et al. (2004). Do unmet expectations for specific tests, referrals, and new medications reduce patients' satisfaction? *Journal of General Internal Medicine, 19*(11), 1080–1087. doi:10.1111/j.1525-1497.2004.30436.x

Peiris, J. S. M., de Jong, M. D., & Guan, Y. (2007). Avian influenza virus (H5N1): A threat to human health. *Clinical Microbiology Reviews, 20*(2), 243–267. doi:10.1128/cmr.00037-06

Pellegrino, E. D. (1999). The goals and ends of medicine: How are they to be defined? In M. J. Hanson, & D. Callahan (Eds.), *The goals of medicine: The forgotten issue in health care reform.* Washington, DC: Georgetown University Press.

Pellegrino, E. D., & Thomasma, D. C. (1981). *A philosophical basis of medical practice.* New York: Oxford University Press.

Pepin, J. (2011). *The origins of AIDS.* Cambridge: Cambridge University Press.

Perneger, T., & Agoritsas, T. (2011). Doctors and patients' susceptibility to framing bias: A randomized trial. *Journal of General Internal Medicine, 26*(12), 1411–1417. doi:10.1007/s11606-011-1810-x

Peschel, R. E., & Peschel, E. R. (1988). Medical miracles from a physician-scientist's viewpoint. *Perspectives in Biological Medicine, 31*(3), 391–404.

Phelps A. C., Maciejewski, P. K., Nilsson, M., et al. (2009). Religious coping and use of intensive life-prolonging care near death in patients with advanced cancer. *Journal of the American Medical Association, 301*(11), 1140–1147. doi:10.1001/jama.2009.341

Phillips, P. S. (2009). Balancing randomized trials with anecdote. *Annals of Internal Medicine, 150*(12), 885–886. doi:10.1059/0003-4819-150-12-200906160-00014

Pickett, J. T., Welch, K., Chiricos, T., & Gertz, M. (2014). Racial crime stereotypes and offender juvenility: Comparing public views about youth-specific and nonyouth-specific sanctions. *Race and Justice, 4*(4), 381–405. doi:10.1177/2153368714542007

Pilon, R. (1995). Liberty, responsibility, and philanthropy: Individual responsibility in a free society. *Contemporary Philosophy(Boulder), 17*, 9–24.

Pinsky, P. F., Gierada, D. S., Nath, P. H., Kazerooni, E., & Amorosa, J. (2013). National lung screening trial: Variability in nodule detection rates in chest CT studies. *Radiology, 268*(3), 865–873. doi:10.1148/radiol.13121530

Pittler, M., Mavergames, C., Ernst, E., & Antes, G. (2011). Evidence-based medicine and Web 2.0: Friend or foe? *British Journal of General Practice, 61*(585), 302–303. doi:10.3399/bjgp11X567342

Politi, M. C., Clark, M. A., Ombao, H., Dizon, D., & Elwyn, G. (2011). Communicating uncertainty can lead to less decision satisfaction: A necessary cost of involving patients in shared decision making? *Health Expectations, 14*(1), 84–91. doi:10.1111/j.1369-7625.2010.00626.x

Politi, M. C., Han, P. K. J., & Col, N. F. (2007). Communicating the uncertainty of harms and benefits of medical interventions. *Medical Decision Making, 27*(5), 681–695. doi:10.1177/0272989x07307270

Pont, S. J., Robbins, J. M., Bird, T. M., Gibson, J. B., Cleves, M. A., Tilford, J. M., et al. (2006). Congenital malformations among liveborn infants with trisomies 18 and 13. *American Journal of Medical Genetics Part A, 140A*(16), 1749–1756. doi:10.1002/ajmg.a.31382

Powers, B. J., Trinh, J. V., & Bosworth, H. B. (2010). Can this patient read and understand written health information? *Journal of the American Medical Association, 304*(1), 76–84. doi:10.1001/jama.2010.896

Powers, B. W., Navathe, A. S., Aung, K.-K., & Jaim, S. (2013). Patients as customers: Applying service industry lessons to health care. *Healthcare, 1*(3–4), 59–60.

Preda, A., & Voigt, K. (2015). The social determinants of health: Why should we care? *The American Journal of Bioethics, 15*(3), 25–36. doi:10.1080/15265161.2014.998374

Proctor, R. (2011). *Golden holocaust: Origins of the cigarette catastrophe and the case for abolition.* Berkeley: University of California Press.

Pronovost, P. J. (2013). Enhancing physicians' use of clinical guidelines. *Journal of the American Medical Association, 310*(23), 2501–2502. doi:10.1001/jama.2013.281334

Qaseem, A., Forland, F., Macbeth, F., Ollenschläger, G., Phillips, S., & van der Wees, P. (2012). Guidelines International Network: Toward international standards for clinical practice guidelines. *Annals of Internal Medicine, 156*(7), 525–531. doi:10.7326/0003-4819-156-7-201204030-00009

Quadagno, J. (2011). Interest-group influence on the patient protection and affordability act of 2010: Winners and losers in the health care reform debate. *Journal of Health, Politics, and Policy Law, 36*(3), 449–453.

Quale, A. J., & Schanke, A.-K. (2010). Resilience in the face of coping with a severe physical injury: A study of trajectories of adjustment in a rehabilitation setting. *Rehabilitation Psychology, 55*(1), 12–22. doi:10.1037/a0018415

Quigley, M., & Harris, J. (2008). Personal or public health? In M. Boylan (Ed.), *International public health policy and ethics: Vol. 42, International library of ethics, law, and the new medicine* (pp. 15–29). Dordrecht, Netherlands: Springer.

Quill, T. E. (1993). Uncertainty and control: Learning to live with medicine's limitations. *Humane medicine, 9*(2), 109–120.

Rabkin, J. (2012). American exceptionalism and the healthcare reform debate. *Harvard Journal of Law and Public Policy, 35*, 153–170.

Rahma, O. E., Duffy, A., Liewehr, D. J., Steinberg, S. M., & Greten, T. F. (2013). Second-line treatment in advanced pancreatic cancer: A comprehensive analysis of published clinical trials. *Annals of Oncology, 24*(8), 1972–1979. doi:10.1093/annonc/mdt166

Rakowski, E. (1991). *Equal justice*. Oxford/New York: Oxford University Press.

Ransohoff, D. F., Pignone, M., & Sox, H. C. (2013). How to decide whether a clinical practice guideline is trustworthy. *Journal of the American Medical Association, 309*(2), 139–140. doi:10.1001/jama.2012.156703

Rao, G., & Kanter, S. L. (2010). Physician numeracy as the basis for an evidence-based medicine curriculum. *Academic Medicine, 85*(11), 1794–1799.

Ratcliffe, J. (2000). Public preferences for the allocation of donor liver grafts for transplantation. *Health Economics, 9*(2), 137–148.

Rawlins, M. D., & Culyer, A. J. (2004). National Institute for Clinical Excellence and its value judgments. *BMJ, 329*(7459), 224.

Rawls, J. (1999). *A theory of justice* (revised ed.). Cambridge, MA: Belknap (Harvard University Press).

Rayner, J.-A., Pyett, P., & Astbury, J. (2010). The medicalisation of "tall" girls: A discourse analysis of medical literature on the use of synthetic oestrogen to reduce female height. *Social Science & Medicine, 71*(6), 1076–1083. http://dx.doi.org/10.1016/j.socscimed.2010.06.026

Reddy, S. R., Ross-Degnan, D., Zaslavsky, A. M., Soumerai, S. B., & Wharam, J. F. (2014). Impact of a high-deductible health plan on outpatient visits and associated diagnostic tests. *Medical Care, 52*(1), 86–92. doi:10.1097/mlr.0000000000000008

Redelmeier, D. A., Koehler, D. J., Liberman, V., & Tversky, A. (1995). Probability judgment in medicine: Discounting unspecified possibilities. *Medical Decision Making, 15*(3), 227–230. doi:10.1177/0272989x9501500305

Redelmeier, D. A., & Shafir, E. (1995). Medical decision making in situations that offer multiple alternatives. *Journal of the American Medical Association, 273*(4), 302–305. doi:10.1001/jama.1995.03520280048038

Redelmeier, D. A., & Tversky, A. (1990). Discrepancy between medical decisions for individual patients and for groups. *New England Journal of Medicine, 322*(16), 1162–1164 doi:10.1056/NEJM199004193221620

Redman, E. (2001). *The dance of legislation: An insider's account of the workings of the United States Senate*. Seattle, WA: University of Washington Press.

Reese, P. P., Caplan, A. L., Bloom, R. D., Abt, P. L., & Karlawish, J. H. (2010). How should we use age to ration health care? Lessons from the case of kidney transplantation. *Journal of the American Geriatric Society, 58*(10), 1980–1986. doi:10.1111/j.1532-5415.2010.03031.x

Reimers, D. M. (1998). *Unwelcome strangers: American identity and the turn against immigration*. New York: Columbia University Press.

Resnic, F. S., & Normand, S.-L. T. (2012). Postmarketing surveillance of medical devices: Filling in the gaps. *New England Journal of Medicine, 366*(10), 875–877. doi:10.1056/NEJMp1114865

Resnick, D. (2003). The Jesica Santillan tragedy: Lessons learned. *Hastings Center Report, 33*(4), 15–20. doi:10.2307/3528375

Rettig, R. A., Jacobson, P. D., Farquhar, C. M., & Aubry, W. M. (2007). *False hope. Bone marrow transplantation for breast cancer*. New York: Oxford University Press.

Reyna, V. F. (2008). A theory of medical decision making and health: Fuzzy trace theory. *Medical Decision Making*. doi:10.1177/0272989x08327066

Reynolds, P. P. (1997). Hospitals and civil rights, 1945–1963: The case of Simkins v Moses H. Cone Memorial Hospital. *Annals of Internal Medicine, 126*(11), 898–906. doi:10.7326/0003-4819-126-11-199706010-00009

Rice, C. M., & Saeed, M. (2014). Hepatitis C: Treatment triumphs. *Nature, 510*(7503), 43–44.

Riley, G. F., & Lubitz, J. D. (2010). Long-term trends in Medicare payments in the last year of life. *Health Services Research, 45*(2), 565–576. doi:10.1111/j.1475-6773.2010.01082.x

Risinger, C. F. (2003). Encouraging students to participate in the political process. *Social Education, 67*(6), 338–339.

Ritsinger, V., Malmberg, K., Mårtensson, A., Rydén, L., Wedel, H., & Norhammar, A. (2014). Intensified insulin-based glycaemic control after myocardial infarction: Mortality during 20 year follow-up of the randomised Diabetes Mellitus Insulin Glucose Infusion in Acute Myocardial Infarction (DIGAMI 1) trial. *The Lancet Diabetes & Endocrinology 2*(8), 627–633.

Rivers, T. J. (2008). Technology's role in the confusion of needs and wants. *Technology in Society, 30*(1), 104–109.

Robertson, C., Rose, S., & Kesselheim, A. S. (2012). Effect of financial relationships on the behaviors of health care professionals: A review of the evidence. *The Journal of Law, Medicine & Ethics, 40*(3), 452–466. doi:10.1111/j.1748-720X.2012.00678.x

Robinson, R. (1993). Cost-effectiveness analysis. *BMJ, 307*(6907), 793–795. doi:10.1136/bmj.307.6907.793

Roehrig, C., Turner, A., Hughes-Cromwick, P., & Miller, G. (2012). When the cost curve bent: Pre-recession moderation in health care spending. *New England Journal of Medicine, 367*(7), 590–593. doi:10.1056/NEJMp1205958

Rombach, S., Dijkgraaf, M., Linthorst, G., & Hollak, C. (2012). Cost-effectiveness of enzyme replacement therapy for Fabry disease. *Molecular Genetics and Metabolism, 105*(2), 5.

Rosoff, P. M. (2012). Unpredictable drug shortages: An ethical framework for short-term rationing in hospitals. *American Journal of Bioethics, 12*(1), 1–9.

Rosoff, P. M. (2014). *Rationing is not a four-letter word: Setting limits on healthcare.* Cambridge, MA: MIT Press.

Rosoff, P. M., & Coleman, D. L. (2011). The case for legal regulation of physicians' off-label prescribing. *Notre Dame Law Review, 86*(2), 649–691.

Rosoff, P. M., Patel, K. R., Scates, A., Rhea, G., Bush, P. W., & Govert, J. A. (2012). Coping with critical drug shortages: An ethical approach for allocating scarce resources in hospitals. *Archives of Internal Medicine, 172*(19), 1494–1499. doi:10.1001/archinternmed.2012.4367

Rothman, R. L., Housam, R., Weiss, H., Davis, D., Gregory, R., Gebretsadik, T., et al. (2006). Patient understanding of food labels: The role of literacy and numeracy. *American journal of preventive medicine, 31*(5), 391–398.

Rothwell, P. M. (2007). *Treating individuals: From randomised trials to personalised medicine.* London: Elsevier Health Sciences.

Rothwell, P. M., McDowell, Z., Wong, C. K., & Dorman, P. J. (1997). Doctors and patients don't agree: Cross sectional study of patients' and doctors' perceptions and assessments of disability in multiple sclerosis. *BMJ, 314*, 1580–1583.

Rowley, D. L., & Hogan, V. (2012). Disparities in infant mortality and effective, equitable care: Are infants suffering from benign neglect? *Annual Review of Public Health, 33*(1), 75–87. doi:10.1146/annurev-publhealth-031811-124542

Ryle, J. A. (1961). The meaning of normal. In B. Lush (Ed.), *Concepts of medicine: A collection of essays on aspects of medicine* (pp. 137–149). New York: Pergamon.

Ryu, A. J., Gibson, T. B., McKellar, M. R., & Chernew, M. E. (2013). The slowdown in health care spending in 2009–11 reflected factors other than the weak economy and thus may persist. *Health Affairs, 32*(5), 835–840. doi:10.1377/hlthaff.2012.1297

Sabbatini, A. K., Tilburt, J. C., Campbell, E. G., Sheeler, R. D., Egginton, J. S., & Goold, S. D. (2014). Controlling health costs: Physician responses to patient expectations for medical care. *Journal of General Internal Medicine, 29*(9), 1234–1241.

Sadegh-Zadeh, K. (2000). Fuzzy health, illness, and disease. *Journal of Medicine and Philosophy, 25*(5), 605–638.

Safranek, T. J., Lawrence, D. N., Kuriand, L. T., Culver, D. H., Wiederholt, W. C., Hayner, N. S., et al. (1991). Reassessment of the association between Guillain-Barré Syndrome and receipt of swine influenza vaccine in 1976–1977: Results of a two-state study. *American Journal of Epidemiology, 133*(9), 940–951.

Sandel, M. J. (2012). *What money can't buy. The moral limits of markets.* New York: Farrar, Straus and Giroux.

Sanmartin, C., Murphy, K., Choptain, N., Conner-Spady, B., McLaren, L., Bohm, E., et al. (2008). Appropriateness of healthcare interventions: Concepts and scoping of the published literature. *Int J Technol Assess Health Care, 24*(03), 342–349.

Santiago-Delpin, E. A. (2003). Ethical dilemmas: Transplantation in prisoners and the mentally disabled. *Transplant Proc, 35*(5), 2057–2059.

Saran, R., Li, Y., Robinson, B., Ayanian, J., Balkrishnan, R., Bragg-Gresham, J., et al. (2015). US Renal Data System 2014 annual data report: Epidemiology of kidney disease in the United States. *American Journal of Kidney Diseases, 65*(6 Suppl. 1), A7.

Sarkar, R. R., & Banerjee, S. (2005). Cancer self remission and tumor stability—a stochastic approach. *Mathematical Biosciences, 196*(1), 65–81. Retrieved from http://dx.doi.org/10.1016/j.mbs.2005.04.001

Sassi, F. (2006). Calculating QALYs, comparing QALY and DALY calculations. *Health policy and planning, 21*(5), 402–408.

Satz, D. (2010). *Why some things should not be for sale: The moral limits of markets.* New York: Oxford University Press.

Saul, S. (2008, August 30). Government gets hooked on tobacco tax billions. *New York Times.* Available at http://www.nytimes.com/2008/08/31/weekinreview/31saul.html?_r=0.

Savage, M. O., Burren, C. P., & Rosenfeld, R. G. (2010). The continuum of growth hormone–IGF-I axis defects causing short stature: Diagnostic and therapeutic challenges. *Clinical Endocrinology, 72*(6), 721–728.

Savulescu, J. (1998). Two worlds apart: Religion and ethics. *Journal of Medical Ethics, 24*(6), 382–384. doi:10.1136/jme.24.6.382

Savulescu, J., & Clarke, S. (2007). Waiting for a miracle . . . miracles, miraclism, and discrimination. *Southern Medical Journal, 100*(12), 1259–1262.

Schelling, T. C. (1968). The life you save may be your own. In I. Brookings, & S. B. Chase (Eds.), *Problems in public expenditure analysis: Papers presented at a conference of experts held Sept. 15–16, 1966* (pp. 127–162). Washington, DC: Brookings Institution.

Schenker, Y., Arnold, R. M., & London, A. J. (2014). The ethics of advertising for health care services. *The American Journal of Bioethics, 14*(3), 34–43. doi:10.1080/15265161.2013.879943

Schleifer, D., & Rothman, D. J. (2012). "The ultimate decision is yours": Exploring patients' attitudes about the overuse of medical interventions. *PLoS ONE, 7*(12), e52552.

Schneider, K. M., O'Donnell, B. E., & Dean, D. (2009). Prevalence of multiple chronic conditions in the United States' Medicare population. *Health Qual Life Outcomes, 7*(82), 82.

Schneiderman, L. J., & Jecker, N. S. (1996). Should a criminal receive a heart transplant? Medical justice vs. societal justice. *Theorerical Medicine, 17*(1), 33–44.

Schneiderman, L. J., & Jecker, N. S. (2011). *Wrong medicine: Doctors, patients, and futile treatment* (2nd ed.). Baltimore, MD: Johns Hopkins University Press.

Schneiderman, L. J., Jecker, N. S., & Jonsen, A. R. (1990). Medical futility: Its meaning and ethical implications. *Annals of Internal Medicine, 112*(12), 949–954. doi:10.1059/0003-4819-112-12-949

Schneiderman, L. J., Jecker, N. S., & Jonsen, A. R. (1996). Medical futility: Response to critiques. *Annals of Internal Medicine, 125*(8), 669–674. doi:10.1059/0003-4819-125-8-199610150-00007

Schoen, C., Osborn, R., Squires, D., Doty, M. M., Pierson, R., & Applebaum, S. (2010). How health insurance design affects access to care and costs, by income, in eleven countries. *Health Affairs, 29*(12), 2323–2334. doi:10.1377/hlthaff.2010.0862

Schoening, W. N., Buescher, N., Rademacher, S., Andreou, A., Kuehn, S., Neuhaus, R., et al. (2013). Twenty-year longitudinal follow-up after orthotopic liver transplantation: A single-center experience of 313 consecutive cases. *American Journal of Transplantation, 13*(9), 2384–2394. doi:10.1111/ajt.12384

Scholes, S., Bajekal, M., Love, H., Hawkins, N., Raine, R., O'Flaherty, M., et al. (2012). Persistent socioeconomic inequalities in cardiovascular risk factors in England over 1994–2008: A time-trend analysis of repeated cross-sectional data. *BMC Public Health, 12*(1), 129.

Schöne-Seifert, B. (2009). The "rule of rescue" in medical priority setting: Ethical plausibilities and implausibilities. *Rationality, Markets and Morals 0*, 421–430.

Schrag, P. (2010). *Not fit for our society: Immigration and nativism in America.* Berkeley/Los Angeles: University of California Press.

Schroeder, S. A., & Frist, W. (2013). Phasing out fee-for-service payment. *New England Journal of Medicine, 368*(21), 2029–2032. doi:10.1056/NEJMsb1302322

Schroeder-Lein, G. R. (2008). *The encyclopedia of Civil War medicine.* Armonk, NY: M. E. Sharpe.

Schultheiss, C. (2002). A note on the semantics of rationing as limitation. In F. Breyer, H. Kliemt, & F. Thiele (Eds.), *Rationing in medicine: Ethical, legal and practical aspects* (pp. 21–29). Berlin/New York: Springer.

Schwartz, L. M., Woloshin, S., Black, W. C., & Welch, H. G. (1997). The role of numeracy in understanding the benefit of screening mammography. *Annals of Internal Medicine, 127*(11), 966–972.

Schwartz, L. M., Woloshin, S., & Welch, H. (2011). Not so silver lining. *Archives of Internal Medicine, 171*(6), 489–490. doi:10.1001/archinternmed.2011.73

Scofea, L. A. (1994). The development and growth of employer-provided health insurance. *Monthly Labor Review, 117*(3), 3.

Scott, S. A., Sangkuhl, K., Stein, C. M., Hulot, J. S., Mega, J. L., Roden, D. M., et al. (2013). Clinical pharmacogenetics implementation consortium guidelines for CYP2C19 genotype and clopidogrel therapy: 2013 update. *Clinical Pharmacology and Therapeutics, 94*(3), 317–323. doi:10.1038/clpt.2013.105

Secunda, K., Gordon, E. J., Sohn, M. W., Shinkunas, L. A., Kaldjian, L. C., Voigt, M. D., et al. (2012). A national survey of provider opinions on controversial characteristics of liver transplant candidates. *Liver Transplantation.* 19 (4), 395–403. doi:10.1002/lt.23581

Seely, A. J. (2013). Embracing the certainty of uncertainty: Implications for health care and research. *Perspect Biol Med, 56*(1), 65–77.

Segall, S. (2007). In solidarity with the imprudent: a defense of luck egalitarianism. *Social Theory and Practice, 33*(2), 177–198.

Segev, D. L. (2009). Evaluating options for utility-based kidney allocation. *American Journal of Transplantation, 9*(7), 1513–1518. doi:10.1111/j.1600-6143.2009.02667.x

Sen, A. (2002). Why health equity? *Health Economics, 11*(8), 659–666. doi:10.1002/hec.762

Sen, A. (2005). Human rights and capabilities. *Journal of Human Development, 6*(2), 151–166. doi:10.1080/14649880500120491

Sen, A. (2009). *The idea of justice.* Cambridge, MA: Belknap (Harvard University Press).

Sendi, P., & Al, M. J. (2003). Revisiting the decision rule of cost–effectiveness analysis under certainty and uncertainty. *Social Science & Medicine, 57*(6), 969–974. Retrieved from http://dx.doi.org/10.1016/S0277-9536(02)00477-X

Shafrin, J. (2010). Operating on commission: Analyzing how physician financial incentives affect surgery rates (Comparative Study). *Health Economics, 19*(5), 562–580. doi:10.1002/hec.1495

Shah, K. K., Cookson, R., Culyer, A. J., & Littlejohns, P. (2013). NICE's social value judgements about equity in health and health care. *Health Economics, Policy and Law, 8*(02), 145–165.

Sharis, P. J., Cannon, C. P., & Loscalzo, J. (1998). The antiplatelet effects of Ticlopidine and Clopidogrel. *Annals of Internal Medicine, 129*(5), 394–405. doi:10.7326/0003-4819-129-5-199809010-00009

Sharpe, V. A. (1997). The politics, economics, and ethics of "appropriateness." *Kennedy Institute of Ethics Journal, 7*(4), 337–343.

Sheaff, W. (2002). *The need for health care.* London: Routledge.

Sheehan, M. (2007). Resources and the rule of rescue. *Journal of Applied Philosophy, 24*(4), 352–366. doi:10.1111/j.1468-5930.2007.00383.x

Shekelle, P. (2004). The appropriateness method. *Medical Decision Making, 24*(2), 228–231.

Shekelle, P., Woolf, S., Grimshaw, J. M., Schünemann, H. J., & Eccles, M. P. (2012). Developing clinical practice guidelines: Reviewing, reporting, and publishing guidelines; updating guidelines; and the emerging issues of enhancing guideline implementability and accounting for comorbid conditions in guideline development. *Implementation Science, 7*(1), 62.

Shekelle, P. G. (2014). Updating practice guidelines. *Journal of the American Medical Association, 311*(20), 2072–2073. doi:10.1001/jama.2014.4950

Shekelle, P. G., Kravitz, R. L., Beart, J., Marger, M., Wang, M., & Lee, M. (2000). Are nonspecific practice guidelines potentially harmful? A randomized comparison of the effect of nonspecific versus specific guidelines on physician decision making. *Health Services Research, 34*(7), 1429.

Shekelle, P. G., & Schriger, D. L. (1996). Evaluating the use of the appropriateness method in the Agency for Health Care Policy and Research Clinical Practice Guideline Development process. *Health Services Research, 31*(4), 453.

Shermer, M. (2004). Miracle on probability street. *Scientific American, 291,* 32.

Shinall, M. C., Ehrenfeld, J. M., & Guillamondegui, O. D. (2014). Religiously affiliated intensive care unit patients receive more aggressive end-of-life care. *Journal of Surgical Research, 190*(2), 623–627.

Shinall, M. C., Jr. (2014). Fighting for dear life: Christians and aggressive end-of-life care. *Perspectives in Biological Medicine, 57*(3), 329–340.

Shinall, M. C., Jr., & Guillamondegui, O. D. (2015). Effect of religion on end-of-life care among trauma patients. *Journal of Religion and Health, 54*(3), 977–983.

Shipman, S. A., & Sinsky, C. A. (2013). Expanding primary care capacity by reducing waste and improving the efficiency of care. *Health Affairs, 32*(11), 1990–1997.

Simoens, S., Picavet, E., Dooms, M., Cassiman, D., & Morel, T. (2013). Cost-effectiveness assessment of orphan drugs. *Applied Health Economics and Health Policy, 11*(1), 1–3.

Simoni, R. D., Hill, R. L., & Vaughan, M. (2002). The discovery of insulin: The work of Frederick Banting and Charles Best. *Journal of Biological Chemistry, 277*(26), e15.

Sinclair, D., Isba, R., Kredo, T., Zani, B., Smith, H., & Garner, P. (2013). World Health Organization guideline development: An evaluation. *PLoS ONE, 8*(5), e63715.

Singal, A. K., Guturu, P., Hmoud, B., Kuo, Y.-F., Salameh, H., & Wiesner, R. H. (2013). Evolving frequency and outcomes of liver transplantation based on etiology of liver disease. *Transplantation, 95*(5), 755–760.

Singer, S., & Bergthold, L. (2001). Cosmetic vs reconstructive surgery for cleft palate: A window into the medical necessity debate. *Journal of the American Medical Association, 286*(17), 2162–2162. doi:10.1001/jama.286.17.2162-JMS1107-6-1

Singh, H., Giardina, T., Meyer, A. D., Forjuoh, S. N., Reis, M. D., & Thomas, E. J. (2013). Types and origins of diagnostic errors in primary care settings. *JAMA Internal Medicine, 173*(6), 418–425. doi:10.1001/jamainternmed.2013.2777

Singh, J., Fanaroff, J., Andrews, B., Caldarelli, L., Lagatta, J., Plesha-Troyke, S., et al. (2007). Resuscitation in the "gray zone" of viability: Determining physician preferences and predicting infant outcomes. *Pediatrics, 120*(3), 519–526. doi:10.1542/peds.2006-2966

Singh, T. P., Naftel, D. C., Addonizio, L., Mahle, W., Foushee, M. T., Zangwill, S., et al. (2010). Association of race and socioeconomic position with outcomes in pediatric heart transplant recipients. *American Journal of Transplantation, 10*(9), 2116–2123. doi:10.1111/j.1600-6143.2010.03241.x

Sirovich, B., Gallagher, P. M., Wennberg, D. E., & Fisher, E. S. (2008). Discretionary decision making by primary care physicians and the cost of U.S. health care. *Health Affairs, 27*(3), 813–823, doi:10.1377/hlthaff.27.3.813.

Skirbekk, H., & Nortvedt, P. (2012). Inadequate treatment for elderly patients: Professional norms and tight budgets could cause "ageism" in hospitals. *Health Care Analysis, 22*(2), 192–201.

Skocpol, T. (2010). The political challenges that may undermine health reform. *Health Affairs, 29*(7), 1288–1292.

Skowronski, D., Chambers, C., Sabaiduc, S., De Serres, G., Dickinson, J., Winter, A., et al. (2015). Interim estimates of 2014/15 vaccine effectiveness against influenza A (H3N2) from Canada's Sentinel Physician Surveillance Network, January 2015. *Euro Surveillance, 20*(4), 21022.

Slashinski, M. J., McCurdy, S. A., Achenbaum, L. S., Whitney, S. N., & McGuire, A. L. (2012). "Snake-oil,""quack medicine," and "industrially cultured organisms": Biovalue and the commercialization of human microbiome research. *BMC Medical Ethics, 13*(1), 28.

Small, D. A., & Verrochi, N. M. (2009). The face of need: Facial emotion expression on charity advertisements. *Journal of Marketing Research, 46*(6), 777–787.

Smith, A. (1969 (1759)). *The theory of moral sentiments.* New Rochelle, NY: Arlington House.

Smith, A. (1994). *An inquiry into the nature and causes of the wealth of nations.* New York: Modern Library.

Smith, A. K., Sudore, R. L., & Pérez-Stable, E. J. (2009). Palliative care for Latino patients and their families: Whenever we prayed, she wept. *Journal of the American Medical Association, 301*(10), 1047–1057. doi:10.1001/jama.2009.308

Smith, T. J. (2013). Commentary: "The Lake Wobegon effect, a natural human tendency to overestimate one's capabilities" (Wikipedia). *Milbank Quarterly, 91*(4), 729–737. doi:10.1111/1468-0009.12031

Smith, T. J., & Hillner, B. E. (2010). Explaining marginal benefits to patients, when "marginal" means additional but not necessarily small. *Clinical Cancer Research, 16*(24), 5981–5986. doi:10.1158/1078-0432.ccr-10-1278

Soares, M. O. (2012). Is the QALY blind, deaf and dumb to equity? NICE's considerations over equity. *British medical bulletin, 101*(1), 17–31. doi:10.1093/bmb/lds003

Solanki, D. R., Koyyalagunta, D., Shah, R. V., Silverman, S., & Manchikanti, L. (2011). Monitoring opioid adherence in chronic pain patients: Assessment of risk of substance misuse. *Pain Physician, 14*(2), E119–E131.

Sondak, V. K., Swetter, S. M., & Berwick, M. A. (2012). Gender disparities in patients with melanoma: Breaking the glass ceiling. *Journal of Clinical Oncology, 30*(18), 2177–2178. doi:10.1200/jco.2011.41.3849

Song, Y., Skinner, J., Bynum, J., Sutherland, J., Wennberg, J. E., & Fisher, E. S. (2010). Regional variations in diagnostic practices. *New England Journal of Medicine, 363*(1), 45–53. doi:10.1056/NEJMsa0910881

Sorenson, C., & Drummond, M. (2014). Improving medical device regulation: The United States and Europe in perspective. *Milbank Quarterly, 92*(1), 114–150. doi:10.1111/1468-0009.12043

Sorenson, C., Gusmano, M. K., & Oliver, A. (2014). The politics of comparative effectiveness research: Lessons from recent history. *Journal of Health, Politics, and Policy Law, 39*(1), 139–170. doi:10.1215/03616878-2395199

Sotos, J. F., & Tokar, N. J. (2014). Growth hormone significantly increases the adult height of children with idiopathic short stature: Comparison of subgroups and benefit. *International Journal of Pediatric Endocrinology, 2014*(1), 15.

Special Supplement: The goals of medicine: Setting new priorities. (1996). *Hastings Center Report, 26*(6), S1–S27. doi:10.2307/3528765

Spence, M. M., Teleki, S. S., Cheetham, T. C., Schweitzer, S. O., & Millares, M. (2005). Direct-to-consumer advertising of COX-2 inhibitors: Effect on appropriateness of Prescribing. *Medical Care Research and Review, 62*(5), 544–559. doi:10.1177/1077558705279314

Spiro, T., Lee, E. O., & Emanuel, E. J. (2012). Price and utilization: Why we must target both to curb health care costs. *Annals of Internal Medicine, 157*(8), 586–590. doi:10.7326/0003-4819-157-8-201210160-00014

Sponga, S., Travaglini, C., Pisa, F., Piani, D., Guzzi, G., Nalli, C., et al. (2015). Does psychosocial compliance have an impact on long-term outcome after heart transplantation? *European Journal of Cardio-Thoracic Surgery, 49*(1), 64–72. doi:10.1093/ejcts/ezv120

Squiers, L. B., Holden, D. J., Dolina, S. E., Kim, A. E., Bann, C. M., & Renaud, J. M. (2011). The public's response to the U.S. Preventive Services Task Force's 2009 recommendations on mammography screening. *American journal of preventive medicine, 40*(5), 497–504. Retrieved from http://dx.doi.org/10.1016/j.amepre.2010.12.027.

Sreenivasan, G. (2015). HESC and equitable residues. *The American Journal of Bioethics, 15*(3), 54–55. doi:10.1080/15265161.2014.998388

Stabile, M., Thomson, S., Allin, S., Boyle, S., Busse, R., Chevreul, K., et al. (2013). Health care cost containment strategies used in four other high-income countries hold lessons for the United States. *Health Affairs, 32*(4), 643–652. doi:10.1377/hlthaff.2012.1252

Stahl, J. E., Tramontano, A. C., Swan, J. S., & Cohen, B. J. (2008). Balancing urgency, age and quality of life in organ allocation decisions—what would you do?: A survey. *Journal of Medical Ethics, 34*(2), 109–115. doi:10.1136/jme.2006.018291

Starfield, B. (2009). Primary care and equity in health: The importance to effectiveness and equity of responsiveness to peoples' needs. *Humanity & Society, 33*(1–2), 56–73.

Starr, P. (1982). *The social transformation of American medicine.* New York: Basic Books.

Starr, P. (2011). *Remedy and reaction: The peculiar American struggle over health care reform.* New Haven, CT: Yale University Press.

Statistics in medicine. (1950). *The British Medical Journal, 1*(4644), 68–69. doi:10.2307/25374724

Steiker, C. S., & Steiker, J. M. (2015). The American death penalty and the (in) visibility of race. *The University of Chicago Law Review, 82*(1), 243–294.

Steinbrook, R., & Lo, B. (2012). Medical journals and conflicts of interest. *The Journal of Law, Medicine & Ethics, 40*(3), 488–499. doi:10.1111/j.1748-720X.2012.00681.x

Steiner, J. F. (1999). Talking about treatment: The language of populations and the language of individuals. *Annals of Internal Medicine, 130*(7), 618–622. doi:10.7326/0003-4819-130-7-199904060-00029

Stempsey, W. (2015). Hope for health and health care. *Medicine, Health Care and Philosophy, 18*(1), 41–49. doi:10.1007/s11019-014-9572-y

Stempsey, W. E. (2002). Miracles and the limits of medical knowledge. *Medicine and Health Care Philosophy, 5*(1), 1–9.

Stern, R. S., & Epstein, A. M. (1985). Institutional responses to prospective payment based on diagnosis-related groups: Implications for cost, quality, and access. *New England Journal of Medicine, 312*(10), 621–627.

Steven, H. W., & Laudan, A. (Eds.). (2013). *U.S. health in international perspective: Shorter lives, poorer health.* Washington, DC: The National Academies Press.

Stevenson, B. (2014). *Just mercy: A story of justice and redemption.* New York: Spiegel & Grau.

Stolk, E. A., Brouwer, W. B. F., & Busschbach, J. J. V. (2002). Rationalising rationing: Economic and other considerations in the debate about funding of Viagra. *Health Policy, 59*(1), 53–63. Retrieved from http://dx.doi.org/10.1016/S0168-8510(01)00162-2

Stolk, E. A., Pickee, S. J., Ament, A. H. J. A., & Busschbach, J. J. V. (2005). Equity in health care prioritisation: An empirical inquiry into social value. *Health Policy, 74*(3), 343–355. Retrieved from http://dx.doi.org/10.1016/j.healthpol.2005.01.018

Stoll, B. J., Hansen, N. I., Bell, E. F., Shankaran, S., Laptook, A. R., Walsh, M. C., et al. (2010). Neonatal outcomes of extremely preterm infants from the NICHD Neonatal Research Network. *Pediatrics, 126*(3), 443–456. doi:10.1542/peds.2009-2959

Strech, D., Synofzik, M., & Marckmann, G. (2008). How physicians allocate scarce resources at the bedside: A systematic review of qualitative studies. *Journal of Medicine & Philosophy, 33*(1), 80–99.

Struijk, E. A., May, A. M., Beulens, J. W. J., de Wit, G. A., Boer, J. M. A., Onland-Moret, N. C., et al. (2013). Development of methodology for disability-adjusted life years (DALYs) calculation based on real-life data. *PLoS ONE, 8*(9), e74294. doi:10.1371/journal.pone.0074294

Stuebe, A. M. (2011). Level IV evidence: Adverse anecdote and clinical practice. *New England Journal of Medicine, 365*(1), 8–9. doi:10.1056/NEJMp1102632

Sulmasy, D. P. (2007). What is a miracle? *Southern Medical Journal, 100*(12), 1223–1228.

Sunderman, F. W. (1949). *Normal values in clinical medicine.* Philadelphia, PA: Saunders.

Sunderman, F. W. (1975). Current concepts of "normal values," "reference values," and "discrimination values" in clinical chemistry. *Clinical Chemistry, 21*(13), 1873–1877.

Szasz, T. S. (1961). *The myth of mental illness: Foundations of a theory of personal conduct.* New York: Harper & Row.

Taffé, P., Burnand, B., Wietlisbach, V., & Vader, J.-P. (2004). Influence of clinical and economical factors on the expert rating of appropriateness of preoperative use of recombinant erythropoietin in elective orthopedic surgery patients. *Medical Decision Making, 24*(2), 122–130. doi:10.1177/0272989x04263153

Taitsman, J. K. (2011). Educating physicians to prevent fraud, waste, and abuse. *New England Journal of Medicine, 364*(2), 102–103. doi:10.1056/NEJMp1012609

Tamblyn, R., Abrahamowicz, M., Dauphinee, D., Wenghofer, E., Jacques, A., Klass, D., et al. (2007). Physician scores on a national clinical skills examination as predictors of complaints to medical regulatory authorities. *Journal of the American Medical Association, 298*(9), 993–1001. doi:10.1001/jama.298.9.993

Tappero, J. W., & Tauxe, R. V. (2011). Lessons learned during public health response to cholera epidemic in Haiti and the Dominican Republic. *Emerging Infectious Diseases, 17,* 2087+.

Taubenberger, J. K., & Morens, D. M. (2006). 1918 influenza: The mother of all pandemics. *Emerging Infectious Diseases, 12*(1), 15–22.

Taubenberger, J. K., Reid, A. H., Lourens, R. M., Wang, R., Jin, G., & Fanning, T. G. (2005). Characterization of the 1918 influenza virus polymerase genes. *Nature, 437*(7060), 889–893. Retrieved from http://www.nature.com/nature/journal/v437/n7060/suppinfo/nature04230_S1.html

Tavaglione, N., & Hurst, S. A. (2012). Why physicians ought to lie for their patients. *The American Journal of Bioethics, 12*(3), 4–12. doi:10.1080/15265161.2011.652797

Tenner, E. (1996). *Why things bite back: Technology and the revenge of unintended consequences.* New York: Knopf.

Thom, D. H., & Campbell, B. (1997). Patient-physician trust: An exploratory study. [Research Support, Non-U.S. Gov't]. *Journal of Family Practice, 44*(2), 169–176.

Thomas, W. J. (1995–1996). The Clinton health care reform plan: a failed dramatic presentation. *Stanford Law and Policy Review, 7,* 83–105.

Thomasson, M. A. (2002). From Sickness to Health: The Twentieth-Century Development of U.S. Health Insurance. *Explorations in Economic History, 39*(3), 233–253, doi:http://dx.doi.org/10.1006/exeh.2002.0788.

Thomson, G. (2005). Fundamental needs. In S. Reader (Ed.), *The philosophy of needs* (pp. 175–186). Cambridge, UK: Cambridge University Press.

Thomson, G. E. (1997). Discrimination in health care. *Annals of Internal Medicine, 126*(11), 910–912. doi:10.7326/0003-4819-126-11-199706010-00011

Thorpe, K. E., & Philyaw, M. (2012). The medicalization of chronic disease and costs. *Annual Review of Public Health, 33,* 409–423.

Tibau, A., Bedard, P. L., Srikanthan, A., Ethier, J.-L., Vera-Badillo, F. E., Templeton, A. J., et al. (2015). Author financial conflicts of interest, industry funding, and clinical practice guidelines for anticancer drugs. *Journal of Clinical Oncology, 33*(1), 100–106. doi:10.1200/jco.2014.57.8898

Tilburt, J. C, & Cassel, C. K. (2013). Why the ethics of parsimonious medicine is not the ethics of rationing. *Journal of the American Medical Association, 309*(8), 773–774. doi:10.1001/jama.2013.368

Tilburt, J. C., Wynia, M. K., Sheeler, R. D., & et al. (2013). VIews of us physicians about controlling health care costs. *Journal of the American Medical Association, 310*(4), 380–388. doi:10.1001/jama.2013.8278

Tomlinson, T., & Brody, H. (1990). Futility and the ethics of resuscitation. *Journal of the American Medical Association, 264*(10), 1276–1280. doi:10.1001/jama.1990.03450100066027

Tong, A., Howard, K., Jan, S., Cass, A., Rose, J., Chadban, S., et al. (2010). Community preferences for the allocation of solid organs for transplantation: A systematic review. [Research Support, Non-U.S. Gov't Review]. *Transplantation, 89*(7), 796–805. doi:10.1097/TP.0b013e3181cf1ee1

Tong, A., Jan, S., Wong, G., Craig, J. C., Irving, M., Chadban, S., et al. (2013). Rationing scarce organs for transplantation: Healthcare provider perspectives on wait-listing and organ allocation. *Clinical transplantation, 27*(1), 60–71. doi:10.1111/ctr.12004

Torrance, G. W. (1987). Utility approach to measuring health-related quality of life. *Journal of Chronic Diseases, 40*(6), 593–600. Retrieved from http://dx.doi.org/10.1016/0021-9681(87)90019-1

Tsai, T. C., Orav, E. J., & Jha, A. K. (2015). Patient satisfaction and quality of surgical care in US hospitals. *Annals of Surgery, 261*(1), 2–8. doi:10.1097/sla.0000000000000765

Tsuchiya, A. (1999). Age-related preferences and age weighting health benefits. *Social Science & Medicine, 48*(2), 267–276. Retrieved from http://dx.doi.org/10.1016/S0277-9536(98)00343-8

Tsuchiya, A. (2000). QALYs and ageism: Philosophical theories and age weighting. *Health Economics, 9*(1), 57–68. doi:10.1002/(SICI)1099-1050(200001)9:1<57:AID-HEC484>3.0.CO;2-N

Tsuchiya, A., Dolan, P., & Shaw, R. (2003). Measuring people's preferences regarding ageism in health: Some methodological issues and some fresh evidence. *Social Science & Medicine, 57*(4), 687–696. doi:10.1016/s0277-9536(02)00418-5

Tsuchiya, A., Miguel, L. S., Edlin, R., Wailoo, A., & Dolan, P. (2005). Procedural justice in public health care resource allocation. [Research Support, Non-U.S. Gov't]. *Applied Health Economics and Health Policy, 4*(2), 119–127.

Turpcu, A., Bleichrodt, H., Le, Q. A., & Doctor, J. N. (2012). How to aggregate health? Separability and the effect of framing. *Medical Decision Making, 32*(2), 259–265. doi:10.1177/0272989x11418521

Tversky, A., & Kahneman, D. (1973). Availability: A heuristic for judging frequency and probability. *Cognitive Psychology, 5*(2), 207–232. Retrieved from http://dx.doi.org/10.1016/0010-0285(73)90033-9

Tversky, A., & Kahneman, D. (1974). Judgment under uncertainty: Heuristics and biases. *Science, 185*(4157), 1124–1131.

Tversky, A., & Kahneman, D. (1981). The framing of decisions and the psychology of choice. *Science, 211*(4481), 453–458.

Twight, C. (2002). *Dependent on D.C.: The rise of federal control over the lives of ordinary Americans.* New York: Palgrave for St. Martin's Press.

Ubel, P. A., & Arnold, R. M. (1995). The unbearable rightness of bedside rationing: Physician duties in a climate of cost containment. *Archives of Internal Medicine, 155*(17), 1837–1842.

Ubel, P. A., Arnold, R. M., & Caplan, A. L. (1993). Rationing failure: The ethical lessons of the retransplantation of scarce vital organs. *Journal of the American Medical Association, 270*(20), 2469–2474. doi:10.1001/jama.1993.03510200075035

Ubel, P. A., & Goold, S. (1997). Recognizing bedside rationing: Clear cases and tough calls. *Annals of Internal Medicine, 126*(1), 74–80.

Ubel, P. A., & Loewenstein, G. (1996a). Distributing scarce livers: The moral reasoning of the general public. *Social Science & Medicine, 42*(7), 1049–1055. Retrieved from http://dx.doi.org/10.1016/0277-9536(95)00216-2

Ubel, P. A., & Loewenstein, G. (1996b). Public perceptions of the importance of prognosis in allocating transplantable livers to children. *Medical Decision Making, 16*(3), 234–241. doi:10.1177/0272989x9601600307

Ubel, P. A., Nord, E., Marthe, G., Menzel, P., Prades, J.-L. P., & Richardson, J. (2000). Improving value measurement in cost-effectiveness analysis. *Medical Care, 38*(9), 892–901. doi:10.2307/3766898

Ulmer, C., Ball, J., McGlynn, E., & Hamdounia, S. B. (2012). *Essential health benefits: Balancing coverage and cost.* Washington, DC: National Academies Press.

Ulmer, C., McFadden, B., & Cacace, C. (2012). *Perspectives on essential health benefits* (Workshop report). Washington, DC: National Academies Press.

U.S. Preventive Services Task Force. (2009). Screening for breast cancer: U.S. Preventive Services Task Force recommendation statement (2009). *Annals of Internal Medicine, 151*(10), 716–726. doi:10.7326/0003-4819-151-10-200911170-00008

van Dijk, C. E., van den Berg, B., Verheij, R. A., Spreeuwenberg, P., Groenewegen, P. P., & de Bakker, D. H. (2013). Moral hazard and supplier-induced demand: Empirical evidence in general practice. *Health Economics, 22*(3), 340–352. doi:10.1002/hec.2801

Vandvik, P. O., Brandt, L., Alonso-Coello, P., Treweek, S., Akl, E. A., Kristiansen, A., et al. (2013). Creating clinical practice guidelines we can trust, use, and share: A new era is imminent. *CHEST Journal, 144*(2), 381–389. doi:10.1378/chest.13-0746

Vater, L. B., Donohue, J. M., Arnold, R., White, D. B., Chu, E., & Schenker, Y. (2014). What are cancer centers advertising to the public?A content analysis of cancer center advertisements. *Annals of Internal Medicine, 160*(12), 813–820. doi:10.7326/M14-0500

Verdin, E., & Ott, M. (2015). 50 years of protein acetylation: From gene regulation to epigenetics, metabolism and beyond. *Nature Reviews Molecular Cell Biology, 16*(4), 258–264. doi:10.1038/nrm3931

Vesely, M. D., Kershaw, M. H., Schreiber, R. D., & Smyth, M. J. (2011). Natural innate and adaptive immunity to cancer. *Annual Review of Immunology, 29*(1), 235–271. doi:10.1146/annurev-immunol-031210-101324

Vidal, M., Chan, D. W., Gerstein, M., Mann, M., Omenn, G. S., Tagle, D., et al. (2012). The human proteome: A scientific opportunity for transforming diagnostics, therapeutics, and healthcare. *Clinical Proteomics, 9*(1), 6.

Villanueva, M. T. (2015). Epigenetics: Chromatin marks the spot. *Nature Reviews Cancer, 15*(4), 196–197.

Vogeli, C., Shields, A. E., Lee, T. A., Gibson, T. B., Marder, W. D., Weiss, K. B., et al. (2007). Multiple chronic conditions: Prevalence, health consequences, and implications for quality, care management, and costs. *Journal of General Internal Medicine, 22*(3), 391–395.

Volk, R. J., & Wolf, A. D. (2011). Grading the new us preventive services task force prostate cancer screening recommendation. *Journal of the American Medical Association, 306*(24), 2715–2716. doi:10.1001/jama.2011.1893

Volpp, K. G., Loewenstein, G., & Asch, D. A. (2012). Choosing wisely: Low-value services, utilization, and patient cost sharing. *Journal of the American Medical Association, 308*(16), 1635–1636. doi:10.1001/jama.2012.13616

Vos, T., Barber, R. M., Bell, B., Bertozzi-Villa, A., Biryukov, S., Bolliger, I., et al. (2015). Global, regional, and national incidence, prevalence, and years lived with disability for 301 acute and chronic diseases and injuries in 188 countries, 1990–2013: A systematic analysis for the Global Burden of Disease Study 2013. *The Lancet, 386*(9995), 743–800. doi:10.1016/S0140-6736(15)60692-4

Vranic, G. M., Ma, J. Z., & Keith, D. S. (2014). The role of minority geographic distribution in waiting time for deceased donor kidney transplantation. *American Journal of Transplantation, 14*(11), 2526–2534. doi:10.1111/ajt.12860

Wailoo, A., & Anand, P. (2005). The nature of procedural preferences for health-care ration-ing decisions. *Social Science & Medicine, 60*(2), 223–236. Retrieved from http://dx.doi.org/10.1016/j.socscimed.2004.04.036

Wailoo, K., Livingston, J., & Guarnaccia, P. (Eds.). (2006). *A death retold.* Chapel Hill: University of North Carolina Press.

Ward, A. (2007). Needs, medical necessity, and the problem of helping the uninsured. *Theoria, 54*(112), 73–98.

Ward, A., & Johnson, P. (2013). Necessary health care and basic needs: Health insur-ance plans and essential benefits. *Health Care Analysis, 21*(4), 355–371. doi:10.1007/s10728-011-0197-5

Ward, B. W., & Schiller, J. S. (2013). Prevalence of multiple chronic conditions among US adults: Estimates from the National Health Interview Survey, 2010. *Preventing Chronic Disease, 10*, E65. doi:10.5888/pcd10.120203

Wastfelt, M., Fadeel, B., & Henter, J. I. (2006). A journey of hope: Lessons learned from studies on rare diseases and orphan drugs. *Journal of Internal Medicine, 260*(1), 1–10. doi:10.1111/j.1365-2796.2006.01666.x

Wegwarth, O., Gaissmaier, W., & Gigerenzer, G. (2011). Deceiving numbers: Survival rates and their impact on doctors' risk communication. *Medical Decision Making, 31*(3), 386–394, doi:10.1177/0272989x10391469.

Wegwarth, O., Schwartz, L. M., Woloshin, S., Gaissmaier, W., & Gigerenzer, G. (2012). Do physicians understand cancer screening statistics? A national survey of primary care physicians in the United States. *Annals of Internal Medicine, 156*(5), 340–349. doi:10.7326/0003-4819-156-5-201203060-00005

Weinstein, M., C. (2008). How much are americans willing to pay for a quality-adjusted life year? *Medical Care, 46*(4), 343–345. doi:10.2307/40221666

Weinstein, M. C., & Stason, W. B. (1977). Foundations of cost-effectiveness analysis for health and medical practices. *New England Journal of Medicine, 296*(13), 716–721. doi:10.1056/NEJM197703312961304

Welch, H., Sharp, S. M., Gottlieb, D. J., Skinner, J. S., & Wennberg, J. E. (2011). Geographic variation in diagnosis frequency and risk of death among medicare beneficiaries. *Journal of the American Medical Association, 305*(11), 1113–1118. doi:10.1001/jama.2011.307

Welch, H. G. (2011). *Overdiagnosed: Making people sick in the pursuit of health.* Boston, MA: Beacon Press.

Welch, H. G., & Black, W. C. (2010). Overdiagnosis in cancer. *Journal of the National Cancer Institute, 102*(9), 605–613. doi:10.1093/jnci/djq099

Wells, R. E., & Kaptchuk, T. J. (2012). To tell the truth, the whole truth, may do patients harm: The problem of the nocebo effect for informed consent. *The American Journal of Bioethics, 12*(3), 22–29. doi:10.1080/15265161.2011.652798

Wells, S. A. (2009). Health disparities in kidney transplantation: An equity analysis. *J. Health Disparitiers Research and Practice, 3*(2), 1–12.

Wennberg, J. E. (2002). Unwarranted variations in healthcare delivery: Implications for aca-demic medical centres. *British Medical Journal, 325*(7370), 961.

Werner, R. M., Alexander, G. C., Fagerlin, A., & Ubel, P. A. (2004). Lying to insurance com-panies: The desire to deceive among physicians and the public. *The American Journal of Bioethics, 4*(4), 53–59. doi:10.1080/15265160490518566

Whitehead, S. J., & Ali, S. (2010). Health outcomes in economic evaluation: The QALY and utilities. *British medical bulletin, 96*(1), 5–21. doi:10.1093/bmb/ldq033

Whitmarsh, T. (2015). *Battling the gods: Atheism in the ancient world*. New York: Alfred A. Knopf.

Whitty, J. A., & Littlejohns, P. (2014). Social values and health priority setting in Australia: An analysis applied to the context of health technology assessment. *Health Policy*. 119 (2), 127–136. Retrieved from http://dx.doi.org/10.1016/j.healthpol.2014.09.003

Widera, E. W., Rosenfeld, K. E., Fromme, E. K., Sulmasy, D. P., & Arnold, R. M. (2011). Approaching patients and family members who hope for a miracle. *J Pain Symptom Manage*, *42*(1), 119–125. Retrieved from http://dx.doi.org/10.1016/j.jpainsymman.2011.03.008

Wiechers, I. R., Perin, N. C., & Cook-Deegan, R. (2013). The emergence of commercial genomics: Analysis of the rise of a biotechnology subsector during the Human Genome Project, 1990 to 2004. *Genome Medicine*, *5*(9), 83.

Wiesner, R., Edwards, E., Freeman, R., Harper, A., Kim, R., Kamath, P., et al. (2003). Model for end-stage liver disease (MELD) and allocation of donor livers. *Gastroenterology*, *124*(1), 91–96. Retrieved from http://dx.doi.org/10.1053/gast.2003.50016

Wiggins, D. (1998). *Needs, values, truth: Essays in the philosophy of value* (3rd ed.). Oxford, UK: Clarendon Press.

Wiggins, D., & Dermen, S. (1987). Needs, need, needing. *Journal of Medical Ethics*, *13*(2), 62–68. doi:10.2307/27716574

Wille, K. M., Harrington, K. F., deAndrade, J. A., Vishin, S., Oster, R. A., & Kaslow, R. A. (2013). Disparities in lung transplantation before and after introduction of the lung allocation score. *The Journal of Heart and Lung Transplantation*, *32*(7), 684–692. Retrieved from http://dx.doi.org/10.1016/j.healun.2013.03.005

Williams, A. (1997). Intergenerational equity: An exploration of the "fair innings" argument. *Health Economics*, 6(2), 117–132. doi:10.1002/(sici)1099-1050(199703)6:2<117:Aid-hec256>3.0.co;2-b

Williams, A. W. (2015). Health policy, disparities, and the kidney. *Advances in Chronic Kidney Disease*, *22*(1), 54–59. Retrieved from http://dx.doi.org/10.1053/j.ackd.2014.06.002

Williams, W. W., Cherikh, W. S., Young, C. J., Fan, P. Y., Cheng, Y., Distant, D. A., et al. (2015). First report on the OPTN national variance: Allocation of A2/A2B deceased donor kidneys to blood group B increases minority transplantation. *American Journal of Transplantation*, *15*(12), 3134–3142. doi:10.1111/ajt.13409

Wilmot, S., & Ratcliffe, J. (2002). Principles of distributive justice used by members of the general public in the allocation of donor liver grafts for transplantation: A qualitative study. *Health Expectations*, *5*(3), 199–209. doi:10.1046/j.1369-6513.2002.00176.x

Wish, D., Johnson, D., & Wish, J. (2014). Rebasing the Medicare payment for dialysis: Rationale, challenges, and opportunities. *Clinical Journal of the American Society of Nephrology*, *9*(12), 2195–2202. doi:10.2215/cjn.03830414

Wolf, J. H., & Wolf, K. S. (2013). The Lake Wobegon effect: Are all cancer patients above average? *Milbank Quarterly*, *91*(4), 690–728. doi:10.1111/1468-0009.12030

Wolfe, B., Del Rio, E., Weiss, S., Mendelson, A., Elbaga, T., Huser, F., et al. (2001). Validation of a single-patient drug trial methodology for personalized management of gastroesophageal reflux disease. *Journal of Managed Care Pharmacy*, *8*(6), 459–468.

Woloshin, S., & Schwartz, L. M. (2006). Giving legs to restless legs: A case study of how the media helps make people sick. *PLoS Med*, *3*(4), e170.

Woloshin, S., & Schwartz, L. M. (2011). Communicating data about the benefits and harms of treatment: A randomized trial. *Annals of Internal Medicine*, *155*(2), 87–96. doi:10.7326/0003-4819-155-2-201107190-00004

Wong, D. A., Bishop, G. A., Lowes, M. A., Cooke, B., Barnetson, R. S. C., & Halliday, G. M. (2000). Cytokine profiles in spontaneously regressing basal cell carcinomas. *British Journal of Dermatology*, 143(1), 91–98. doi:10.1046/j.1365-2133.2000.03596.x

Wong, S. S., & Yuen, K. Y. (2006). Avian influenza virus infections in humans. *Chest*, 129(1), 156–168.

Woolf, S. H. (2012). The price of false beliefs: Unrealistic expectations as a contributor to the health care crisis. *The Annals of Family Medicine*, 10(6), 491–494. doi:10.1370/afm.1452

World Health Organization. (2008). *Closing the gap in a generation: Health equity through action on the social determinants of health: Commission on Social Determinants of Health final report*. Geneva: Author.

World Health Organization. (2011). *Closing the gap: Policy into practice on social determinants of health* (Discussion paper). Geneva: Author.

World Health Organization. (2012). *International classification of diseases* (ICD). Geneva: Author.

Wynia, M. K., Cummins, D. S., VanGeest, J. B., & Wilson, I. B. (2000). Physician manipulation of reimbursement rules for patients: Between a rock and a hard place. *The Journal of the American Medical Association*, 283(14), 1858–1865. doi:10.1001/jama.283.14.1858

Wynia, M. K., VanGeest, J. B., Cummins, D. S., & Wilson, I. B. (2003). Do physicians not offer useful services because of coverage restrictions? *Health Affairs*, 22(4), 190–197. doi:10.1377/hlthaff.22.4.190

Yackee, J. W., & Yackee, S. W. (2006). A bias towards business? Assessing interest group influence on the US bureaucracy. *Journal of Politics*, 68(1), 128–139.

Yackee, S. W. (2006). Sweet-talking the fourth branch: The influence of interest group comments on federal agency rulemaking. *Journal of Public Administration Research and Theory*, 16(1), 103–124.

Yackee, S. W. (2012). The politics of ex parte lobbying: Pre-proposal agenda building and blocking during agency rulemaking. *Journal of Public Administration Research and Theory*, 22(2), 373–393. doi:10.1093/jopart/mur061

Yang, Y., & Lee, L. C. (2010). Dynamics and heterogeneity in the process of human frailty and aging: Evidence from the U.S. older adult population. *The Journals of Gerontology Series B: Psychological Sciences and Social Sciences*, 65B(2), 246–255. doi:10.1093/geronb/gbp102

Yankelovich, D. (1995). The debate that wasn't: the public and the Clinton plan. *Health Affairs*, 14(1), 7–23, doi:10.1377/hlthaff.14.1.7.

Zarcadoolas, C. (2011). The simplicity complex: exploring simplified health messages in a complex world. *Health Promotion International*, 26(3), 338–350, doi:10.1093/heapro/daq075.

Zgierska, A., Rabago, D., & Miller, M. M. (2014). Impact of patient satisfaction ratings on physicians and clinical care. *Patient preference and adherence*, 8, 437.

Zhang, Y., Baicker, K., & Newhouse, J. P. (2010). Geographic variation in the quality of prescribing. *New England Journal of Medicine*, 363(21), 1985–1988.

Zier, L. S., Burack, J. H., Micco, G., Chipman, A. K., Frank, J. A., Luce, J. M., et al. (2008). Doubt and belief in physicians' ability to prognosticate during critical illness: The perspective of surrogate decision makers. *Critical Care Medicine*, 36(8), 2341–2347. doi:10.1097/CCM.0b013e318180ddf9

Zier, L. S., Burack, J. H., Micco, G., Chipman, A. K., Frank, J. A., & White, D. B. (2009). Surrogate decision makers' responses to physicians' predictions of medical futility. *Chest*, 136(1), 110–117. doi:cHest.08-2753 [pii]10.1378/chest.08-2753

Zier, L. S., Sottile, P. D., Hong, S. Y., Weissfield, L. A., & White, D. B. (2012). Surrogate decision makers' interpretation of prognostic information: A mixed-methods study. *Annals
   of Internal Medicine, 156*(5), 360–366. doi:10.7326/0003-4819-156-5-201203060-00008
Ziv, T. A., & Lo, B. (1995). Denial of care to illegal immigrants. Proposition 187 in California.
   New England Journal of Medicine, 332(16), 1095–1098.
Zoungas, S., Woodward, M., Li, Q., Cooper, M. E., Hamet, P., Harrap, S., et al. (2014). Impact
   of age, age at diagnosis and duration of diabetes on the risk of macrovascular and micro-
   vascular complications and death in type 2 diabetes. *Diabetologia, 57*(12), 2465–2474.
Zuckerman, D. M., Brown, P., & Nissen, S. E. (2011). Medical device recalls and the FDA
   approval process. *Archives of Internal Medicine, 171*(11), 1006–1011. doi:10.1001/
   archinternmed.2011.30

INDEX

Page numbers followed by f refer to figures on respective pages

interventions. *see also* demands for
   interventions; miracles; needs
   appealing to RAM panels, 223n113
   assigning monetary value to, 33
   clinical appropriateness, 82–86
   evaluating cost variations, 38
   freedom of choice, 108
   illegitimate requests, 151–152, 155
   medical necessity, 55
   public view of advances
      in, 112–113
   uncertainty of effectiveness, 107
   unproved, experimental, or
      "investigational", 86–93
investigational drugs, 77–78
investigational interventions, 86–93
investment refinement of life cycle
   principle, 12–13
IOM (Institute of Medicine), 91
IQ, cutoff point based on, 17–19,
   18f, 208n51
Isoniazid, 122
ivacaftor (Kalydeco), 123

Jacobs, L. M., 160
Jersild, Paul, 161
joint replacement surgery, 85
Jones, Booker T., 242n16
judging others for actions, 179, 186
just healthcare, 66
Juth, Niklas, 218n56

Kahan, J. P., 84
Kalydeco (ivacaftor), 123
kidney transplantation, 169
knee replacement surgery, 85

Landscape Survey, 240n82
Larmer, Robert, 155
LAS (Lung Allocation Score), 167
leukemia, 100–101, 138, 215n17, 233n99
levels of assessment of need, 75
life expectancy, cutoff points based
   on, 46–50
lifestyle choices
   considering in healthcare reform, 177–178,
   184–186

luck and, 176
   punishment for, 180
life support, 61, 76–77, 161. *see also*
   miracles
literacy skills of Americans, 228n28
little-by-little arguments, 24
liver transplants, 167, 184–185
losers, 166
luck
   background, 165–167
   brute versus option, 175–176, 177
   decision-making power, 181–184
   general discussion, 174–181
   luck egalitarianism, 176–178,
      179–180, 183
   misfortune and organ transplantation,
      167–170
   social determinants of
      disease, 170–174
Lung Allocation Score (LAS), 167
lung cancer, 46, 48, 52, 103
lung transplantation, 167–169
luxuries versus needs, 63
Lyme disease, chronic, 231n66, 232n81

Magi, M., 75
male pattern baldness, 118–120
mammogram screening, 95–96, 247n38
marginally beneficial effects, 108
market-driven healthcare products
   industry, 121
Marmor, T. R., 226n147
Maslow, Abraham H., 218n54
Massachusetts state health insurance
   plan, 242n14
mastectomy for cancer, cosmetic surgery
   after, 74
MATCH (Molecular Analysis of Therapy
   Choice) program, 233n99
McClure, Jessica, 135–136
McGregor, J. A., 217n40
McMath, Jahi, 76, 220n68
Mechanic, David, 181–182, 243n38
media, exploitation of Rule of Rescue in,
   138, 139–141
Medicaid, 4, 31, 191–192
medical condition, defined, 89